Obstetrics & Gynecology

ANNUAL REVIEW 1989

Pergamon Titles of Related Interest

Barber PERIMENOPAUSAL AND GERIATRIC GYNECOLOGY
Knapp & Berkowitz GYNECOLOGIC ONCOLOGY
Rosenwaks/Benjamin/Stone GYNECOLOGY: Principles
and Practice

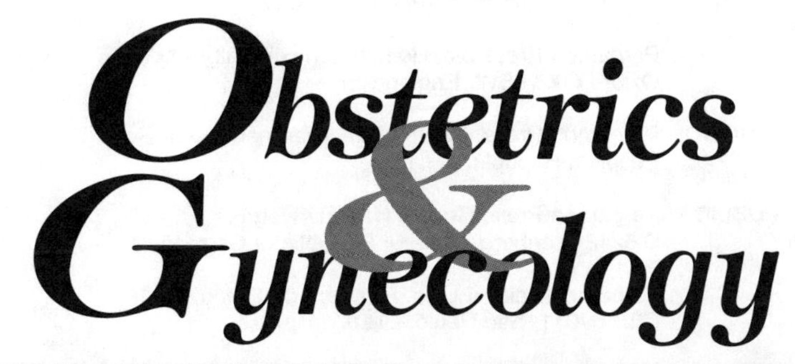

by

Harrison H. Sheld, M.D.

Chairman and Associate Professor
University of Nevada
School of Medicine
Reno, Nevada

PERGAMON PRESS
New York • Oxford • Beijing • Frankfurt • São Paulo • Sydney • Tokyo • Toronto

Pergamon Press Offices:

U.S.A.	Pergamon Press, Inc., Maxwell House, Fairview Park, Elmsford, New York 10523, U.S.A.
U.K.	Pergamon Press plc, Headington Hill Hall, Oxford OX3 0BW, England
PEOPLE'S REPUBLIC OF CHINA	Pergamon Press, Room 4037, Qianmen Hotel, Beijing, People's Republic of China
FEDERAL REPUBLIC OF GERMANY	Pergamon Press GmbH, Hammerweg 6, D-6242 Kronberg, Federal Republic of Germany
BRAZIL	Pergamon Editora Ltda, Rua Eça de Queiros, 346, CEP 04011, São Paulo, Brazil
AUSTRALIA	Pergamon Press Australia Pty Ltd., P.O. Box 544, Potts Point, NSW 2011, Australia
JAPAN	Pergamon Press, 8th Floor, Matsuoka Central Building, 1-7-1 Nishishinjuku, Shinjuku-ku, Tokyo 160, Japan
CANADA	Pergamon Press Canada Ltd., Suite 271, 253 College Street, Toronto, Ontario M5T 1R5, Canada

---

First printing 1989

Library of Congress Cataloging in Publication Data

Sheld, Harrison H.
  Obstetrics and gynecology, 1989 / by Harrison H. Sheld.
  p.   cm.
  Questions based on articles published in the American journal of obstetrics and gynecology and Obstetrics and gynecology.
  Includes bibliographies and index.
  ISBN 0-08-037906-0 (pbk.) :
  1. Gynecology--Examinations, questions, etc. 2. Obstetrics--Examinations, question, etc. I. American journal of obstetrics and gynecology. II. Obstetrics and gynecology. III. Title.
  [DNLM: 1. Gynecology--examination questions. 2. Obstetrics--examination questions.   WP 18 S544o]
RG111.S48   1989
618'.076--dc20
DNLM/DLC
for Library of Congress   89-16134
                                                                  CIP

ISSN 0957-3038

Printed in the United States of America

The paper used in this publication meets the minimum requirements of American National Standard for Information Sciences -- Permanence of Paper for Printed Library Materials, ANSI Z39.48-1984

PREFACE

This book can serve as a means for students and practitioners alike to assess their
understanding of current developments in obstetrics and gynecology. Further, as multiple
choice tests become a way of life for licensure and certification, use of this book can
sharpen examination taking skills in test preparation.

Five topics have been chosen to expedite study: Gynecology, Reproductive Endocrinology,
Gynecologic Oncology, Obstetrics and Perinatal Medicine. Some editorial liberty has been
taken in following this classification. For each topic there is a question section and answer
section.

Four basic types of questions are used: one best answer, matching, both-neither, and
multiple true-false. The authoring style of the questions conforms to that recommended by
standard testing authorities. Questions are derived from articles appearing in either *The
American Journal of Obstetrics and Gynecology* or *Obstetrics and Gynecology* and are
intended to be illustrative of basic and timely information. In the answer section, there is
an outline from the referenced article. For clarity, the outline is constructed into segments
entitled "Facts and Issues", bracketed as "F & I" and keyed into a "Facts" noted by "•",
"Detail" noted by a "°", and "Issues" noted by a "»". Facts are generally accepted
statements; issues are are suppositions or conclusions suggested by the investigators.
Some facts and issues may be at variance with standard or traditional concepts. The
abstract may contain much more material than that pertaining directly to the question. In
any case, for specific details of management refer to the original article or standard texts.

For those whose learning style peaks at the challenge of pen and pencil tests this
compendium will provide a valuable exercise which can instill an appreciation of the time,
effort and expense the scholars in our specialty have spent in pursuit of scientific
accomplishment.

With the enthusiasm and encouragement of our new publisher we hope to use this unique
format to provide an overview of obstetrical and gynecological developments as reflected in
the current medical literature.

Harrison H. Sheld, M.D.
Las Vegas, Nevada
March, 1989

TABLE OF CONTENTS

Gynecology

Directions: Each of the questions or incomplete statements below is followed by several suggested answers or completions. Select the BEST answer in each case.

1. Fecal continence is primarily dependent upon the

    A. anorectal angle
    B. external anal sphincter
    C. levator ani muscle
    D. puborectalis muscle
    E. transverse superficial perineal
       muscle

2. The mechanism by which dextran decreases post-operative intraabdominal adhesions is

    A. activation plasminogen-induced
       fibrinolysis.
    B. enhancement plasminogen activator.
    C. impairment the secretion of
       plasminogen activator.
    D. production of a polymeric coating on
       the peritoneal surface.
    E. suppression tissue bound plasminogen
       activator.

3. Which of the following treatments results in the highest pregnancy rate in the treatment of mild endometriosis (no endometriomas)?

    A. danazol alone
    B. no therapy except chromotubation
    C. operative laparoscopy (sharp excision)
       followed by danazol
    D. operative laparoscopy (sharp excision)
       alone
    E. pseudopregnancy

4. Which of the following changes can be expected in a normal patient after three month's usage of a triphasic oral contraceptive containing norethindrone?

    A. decreased plasma glucose
    B. decreased plasma insulin
    C. increased plasma glucose
    D. increased plasma insulin
    E. no change in either plasma glucose or
       insulin levels.

5. In approximately what percentage of patients with ovarian cancer has the disease spread beyond the pelvis?

    A. 20
    B. 40
    C. 60
    D. 80
    E. 92

6. The single most important prognostic factor for successful sterilization reversal

    A. absence of obesity
    B. ampullary anastomoses
    C. interval between sterilization and
       reversal
    D. tubal length
    E. use of operating microscope

7. Associated with highly aggressive and rapidly progressive type of cervical cancer, human papilloma virus type

    A. 6
    B. 11
    C. 16
    D. 18
    E. 35

8. Lumbar spine bone mineral density increases with

    A. birth control pill contraception
    B. breast feeding
    C. full term pregnancies
    D. maternal height
    E. none of the above

9. Lipoprotein levels in patients with polycystic ovarian disease are at male levels because of

    A. elevation of intermediary adrenal
       steroid levels
    B. hypothalamic driven dietary
       cravings
    C. hepatic dysfunction
    D. insulin resistance
    E. obesity

10. Normally ovulating women have a volume of peritoneal fluid at midcycle of about (ml)

     A. 5
     B. 10
     C. 15
     D. 30
     E. 50

11. Estrogen and progesterone receptor status in patients with endometrial carcinoma is most strongly associated with

     A. age
     B. depth of invasion
     C. histology
     D. menopausal status
     E. stage

12. The most common sexually transmitted pathogen in the United States is

     A. herpesvirus
     B. gonococcus
     C. crabs
     D. condylomata
     E. chlamydia

13. Intraoperative autotransfusion is advisable in which of the following situations where there is heavy blood loss?

     A. Cesarean section for cephalopelvic disproportion.
     B. Cesarean section for chorioamnionitis and failure to progress.
     C. Ovarian cystectomy for bleeding corpus luteum in a patient with chronic hepatic failure.
     D. Ovarian resection for stage III ovarian cancer.
     E. Salpingectomy for ruptured tubal ectopic pregnancy from chronic pelvic inflammatory disease.

14. Which of the following is NOT associated with accelerated oocyte depletion?

     A. autoimmune disease
     B. insensitive ovary syndrome
     C. pelvic irradiation for treatment of cervical cancer
     D. systemic chemotherapy for the treatment of ovarian cancer
     E. XO/XX mosaicism

15. The predominant aerobic isolate recovered from pelvic infected sites after hysterectomy

     A. E. coli
     B. Group B streptococcus
     C. staph. aureus
     D. staph. epidermidis
     E. strep. faecalis

16. The treatment of choice for a prolapsed submucous myoma is

     A. abdominal myomectomy
     B. antibiotics, GnRH agonist, followed by abdominal hysterectomy.
     C. immediate hysterectomy.
     D. replacement of myoma, antibiotics, and administration of GnRH agonist.
     E. vaginal myomectomy

17. Treatment of choice for stage I adenocarcinoma of the cervix in a 23 year old nulligravida is

     A. conization
     B. radiation therapy
     C. radical hysterectomy
     D. total hysterectomy followed by radiation
     E. total hysterectomy

18. Which of the following sites of endometrial implantation is most conducive to excision by the laser through the laparoscope?

     A. broad ligament
     B. fallopian tube
     C. ovary
     D. peritoneum
     E. uterus

19. The most common cause of genitourinary
fistula in the United States is

    A. abdominal hysterectomy
    B. obstetrical trauma
    C. radiation
    D. surgery for stress urinary
       incontinence
    E. vaginal hysterectomy

20. In assessing the effect of estrogen on postmenopausal urinary tract function, it may be
correctly stated that estrogen replacement
increases

    A. bladder capacity
    B. diurnal micturation frequency
    C. nocturia
    D. number of incontinence episodes
    E. proprioceptive sensory threshold

21. Approximately what percentage of patients with
urodynamically proven pure stress urinary
incontinence will develop detrussor instability
after anti-incontinence surgery?

    A. 30-35
    B. 21-29
    C. 10-20
    D. 3-5
    E. < 1

22. Associated with an increased incidence of ureteral
displacement

    A. endometriosis
    B. pelvic inflammatory disease
    C. pelvic relaxation
    D. previous appendectomy
    E. uterine size greater than 12 weeks

23. Which of the following benign conditions is the
serum CA 125 level likely to be elevated
(> 65 U/mL)?

    A. endometriosis
    B. inflammatory disease
    C. leiomyomata uteri
    D. molar disease
    E. ovarian epithelial tumors

24. What is the percentage of patients with lower
abdominal pain, abdominal tenderness, a
temperature of 38.8° C, and sedimentation rate of
40 mm/hr that will have identifiable salpingitis
on laparoscopic examination?

    A. 90
    B. 80
    C. 70
    D. 60
    E. 50

25. A patient with circulating ß-hCG is being treated
medically for a tubal ectopic pregnancy and is
noted to have a sudden significant elevation of
serum progesterone and 17-OH progesterone. It
may be correctly concluded that she has

    A. a second corpus luteum
    B. an abdominal pregnancy
    C. an adrenal tumor
    D. an ovarian neoplasm
    E. developed choriocarcinoma

26. Which of the following hemostatic factors is
decreased in women with a familial history of
thromboembolism?

    A. antithrombin III
    B. beta thromboglobulin
    C. fibrinogen
    D. fibrinopeptide A
    E. platelet factor 4

27. A patient who had a Burch procedure complains
of recurrent stress urinary incontinence.
Urodynamic testing confirms genuine stress
incontinence but a low urethral closure pressure
is noted. The operation of choice to correct the
recurrent incontinence is

    A. anterior colporrhaphy and Kelly
       plication
    B. Burch procedure
    C. Marshall-Marchetti-Krantz
       procedure
    D. Pereyra procedure
    E. sling procedure

28. Which of the following is most predictive of endometrial pathology when found on a cervical cytological smear?

    A. histiocytes
    B. nonspecific infection
    C. elevated squamous cell maturation index
    D. degree of cytological atypia of endometrial glandular cells
    E. bleeding unrelated to smear trauma

29. Which of the following progestins has the most adverse effect on lipid and lipoprotein changes?

    A. alpha-hydroxyprogesterone
    B. ethynodiol diacetate
    C. levonorgestrel
    D. norethindrone acetate
    E. norethindrone

30. The most effective diagnostic procedure for detecting asymptomatic recurrent cervical cancer is

    A. chest x-ray
    B. IVP
    C. physical examination
    D. serum alkaline phosphatase
    E. vaginal cytology

31. Endocervical curettage is indicated for the surveillance of abnormal cytology when

    A. colposcopy is adequate and directed biopsies are negative.
    B. colposcopy is adequate and directed biopsies show invasive carcinoma.
    C. colposcopy is adequate and directed biopsies show severe dysplasia.
    D. colposcopy is inadequate and directed biopsies are negative.
    E. colposcopy is performed.

32. What condition is the most likely cause of recurrent uterine bleeding in a patient in the reproductive age group, after a previous curettage was reported as secretory endometrium?

    A. endometrial atrophy
    B. endometrial polyp
    C. irregular shedding
    D. submucous myoma
    E. subseptate uterus

33. Which of the following is the most helpful historical finding in patients with masculinizing tumors?

    A. age
    B. history of menstrual function
    C. nature of onset of symptoms
    D. parity
    E. weight

34. Surgical correction of stress urinary incontinence is primarily achieved by

    A. cystocele reduction
    B. elevating the bladder neck
    C. lengthening the urethra
    D. narrowing the bladder neck
    E. narrowing the urethral lumen

35. Which of the following is most likely to be associated with a vaginal pH of 4?

    A. atrophic vaginitis
    B. Candida vaginitis
    C. cervical leukorrhea
    D. Gardnerella vaginitis
    E. Trichomonas vaginitis

36. What is the incidence of lymph node metastases (%) from breast cancer that will be present by the time detection through self-examination prompts a patient to seek medical attention for the average lesion size (2.5 cm)?

    A. 10
    B. 25
    C. 33
    D. 50
    E. 67

37. Which of the following lengthens the duration of
    therapy for patients with vaginismus?

    A. assertive husband
    B. desire for fertility
    C. male sexual dysfunction
    D. previous operative intervention
    E. use of vaginal dilators in therapy

38. All of the following are positively associated
    with the etiology of premenstrual tension
    EXCEPT

    A. age < 25 years
    B. history of premenstrual tension in
       patient's mother
    C. low level of exercise
    D. more than 3 children
    E. obesity

39. Clinically useful in diagnosing the ovarian
    remnant syndrome all of the following EXCEPT

    A. CT scan of abdomen
    B. IVP
    C. laparoscopy
    D. pelvic ultrasound
    E. serum FSH

Gynecology- References

Directions: Each of the questions or incomplete statements below is followed by several suggested answers or completions. Select the BEST answer in each case.

1. Fecal continence is primarily dependent upon the

   *A.   anorectal angle
   B.   external anal sphincter
   C.   levator ani muscle
   D.   puborectalis muscle
   E.   transverse superficial perineal muscle

p.782   Givens FT, and Browning G, "Repair of old complete perineal lacerations " Am J Obstet Gynecol 1988;159:779)

1. [F & I:•Background: Complete perinatal lacerations have been known since antiquity.

   °One was found in an ancient Egyptian mummy Henhenit of the Court of Mentuhotep dated about 2050 BC.

 •Material and Methods: A majority of cases (26) were repaired by a **layer method**.

   °There were six cases repaired by the **Warren flap** or apron method.

   °No cases were repaired by the Noble-Mengert technique of anterior wall advancement or the Bowers anoplasty procedure.

 •Results: Function was completely restored in six patients by the Warren flap method.

 •The time of repair in this series varied from 6 weeks to 29 years with the average > 4 years.

   °With healthy granulation tissue in an uninfected wound, a repair earlier than the recommended delay of three to six months is possible.

 •Repair of an old laceration is not appropriate at delivery if the bowel has not been prepared.

 •The Warren flap technique has the advantage over the layer technique of completely separating the fecal stream from the repaired sphincter.

   °A total of 45 cases of with no reported failures.

 •Pregnancy subsequent to a satisfactory repair, should be delivered by a cesarean section.

 •Adequate bowel preparation enhances the chances for successful repair.

 •Paradoxical sphincterotomy allows a temporary escape of gas and feces and prevents a build-up of pressure to the weakened repaired segment.

 •Current postoperative care calls for an elemental diet for 5-7 days and a low-residue diet for the next 5-7 days.

 •Although the external sphincter is easy to identify, it's not the prime muscle of continence.

   °It provides only intermittent continence during rectal peristalsis and at the end of defecation.

°It can be contracted for only 50 seconds at a time.

°Continence actually depends on the constriction of the rectum so that the anus is anterior to the rectum and there is an angulation of the anal canal in relation to the rectum.

°This anal rectal angle is important in preventing fecal incontinence just as urethrovesical angle is important in prevention of stress urinary incontinence.

°When the perineal body and the levator ani muscles are disrupted, this angulation is destroyed.

°This allows the rectum to bulge forward and produces a straight tube with no capacity for fecal storage.

°The sphincter is incapable of withstanding the resulting pressure and the result is incontinence.

°Reconstruction of the anorectal angle thus becomes an important principle in restoring proper function.

•The layer technique is the most used method of repair at present.

°It allows the surgeon the opportunity to repair the three very important structures necessary for maintaining continence: rectovaginal septum, perineal body, and external anal sphincter.

•The repair should be accomplished at the earliest time possible when there is no edema, induration or other signs of infection.]

---

2.   The mechanism by which dextran decreases post-operative intraabdominal adhesions is

    A.   activation plasminogen-induced fibrinolysis.
    B.   enhancement plasminogen activator.
    C.   impairment the secretion of plasminogen activator.
    *D.   production of a polymeric coating on the peritoneal surface.
    E.   suppression tissue bound plasminogen activator.

---

p.963   (Maycr M, Yedgar S, Hurwitz A, Palti Z, Finzi Z, and Milwidsky A, "Effect of viscous macromolecules on peritoneal plasminogen activator activity: A potential mechanism for their ability to reduce postoperative adhesion formation" Am J Obstet Gynecol 1988;159:957)

2. [F & I:•Background: Adhesions result from an inflammatory response caused by surgical trauma, ischemia, foreign bodies, hemorrhage, and infection.

•Insult to the serosal surface leads to the formation of a transient fibrous exudate.

°If not quickly removed by absorption or fibrinolysis, the initial fibrin deposition produces an inflammatory response, proliferation of fibroblasts, scar tissue formation, and adhesion of adjacent serosal surfaces.

•Local suppression of peritoneal fibrinolysis occurs as a result of tissue abrasion and ischemia, and a correlation was noted between suppression of fibrinolysis and formation of postoperative adhesions.

•Fibrin clot resolution is usually initiated through plasminogen activator activity.

°This enzyme converts inactive plasminogen into the potent fibrinolytic enzyme, plasmin.

•Dextran, a high-molecular weight and water-soluble polymer of glucose, facilitates fibrinolysis.

•Viscous hydrophilic macromolecules act by a hydroflotation effect, a siliconizing effect, and a charge-repulsion effect.

•Objective: to examine human peritoneal plasminogen activator activity and to establish the ability of dextran to modulate this activity.

•Results: Findings do **not** support the hypothesis that dextran activates plasminogen activator-induced fibrinolysis and do **not** support the contention that dextran minimizes adhesions formation by its ability to enhance plasminogen activator.

•Dextran physically masks peritoneal plasminogen activator and produces a polymeric coating on the peritoneal surface.

°The polymer coating may prevent shedding of plasminogen activator from the peritoneal cells into the abdominal cavity, which results in high local activity of plasminogen activator on the surface of the cells.

•Formation of a polymer coating could hinder the accessibility of fibrin clots formed within the abdominal cavity to the membranal sites.

°Such a barrier would prevent the initial adherence of clots to serosal surfaces and thereby hamper the development of a permanent scar.]

---

3. Which of the following treatments results in the highest pregnancy rate in the treatment of mild endometriosis (no endometriomas)?

 A. danazol alone
 B. no therapy except chromotubation
 C. operative laparoscopy (sharp excision) followed by danazol
 *D.   operative laparoscopy (sharp excision) alone
 E. pseudopregnancy

---

p. 931(Fayez JA, Collazo LM, and Vernon C, "Comparison of different modalities of treatment for minimal and mild endometriosis" Am J Obstet Gynecol 1988;159:927)

3. [F & I:•Background: In 1958 Kistner treated endometriosis with combinations of estrogens and synthetic progestins, inducing pseudopregnancy.

•In 1971 Greenblatt et al. treated endometriosis with danazol, inducing a pseudomenopausal condition.

•The conservative surgical reatment of endometriosis was by laparotomy preceded or followed by medical therapy.

•Objectives: to retrospectively analyze the results of different modalities of treatment used for two stages of endometriosis:

°A) to study danazol effect with regard to resolution of endometriosis and enhancement of conception rats in a homogenous population, and

°B) to compare pregnancy rates in patients receiving danazol alone or in conjunction with operative laparoscopy to pregnancy rates in patients undergoing operative laparoscopy only.

•Results: Danazol failed to bring complete resolution of early endometriosis in any of the patients studied and the pregnancy rate in these patients was 28%.

•Operative laparoscopy followed immediately by danazol therapy achieved a pregnancy rate of 55%, and with no danazol received postoperatively the rate was 72%.]

---

4. Which of the following changes can be expected in a normal patient after three month's usage of a triphasic oral contraceptive containing norethindrone?

    A. decreased plasma glucose
    B. decreased plasma insulin
    C. increased plasma glucose
    D. increased plasma insulin
    *E. no change in either plasma glucose or insulin levels.

p.879   (Spellacy WN, Ellingson AB, Kotlik A, and Tsibris JCM, "Prospective study of carbohydrate metabolism in women using a triphasic oral contraceptive containing norethindrone and ethinyl estradiol for 3 months" Am J Obstet Gynecol 1988;159:877)

4. [F & I:•Background: Alterations in carbohydrate metabolism secondary to the use of oral contraceptives include the development of insulin resistance as manifested by elevated plasma glucose and insulin levels.

•Alteration was principally related to the **progestin** component of oral contraceptives and possibly associated with a reduction in insulin receptor binding at key target tissues.

•Objective: to evaluate carbohydrate metabolism in women who used a triphasic preparation that contained norethindrone and ethinyl estradiol for 3 months.

•Results: **No** alteration in either glucose of insulin levels during a 3-hour oral glucose tolerence test was demonstrated.

•The 3-hour insulin value at 3 months was elevated, and this approaches statistical significance.

•Conclusion: First, norethindrone is a weaker progestin than norgestrel in its effect on carbohydrate metabolism.

•Second, Small amounts of estrogen improve carbohydrate metabolism by the alteration of insulin receptor binding and by the inhibition of insulin degradation.

•Third, data are reassuring in terms of a reduction in possible cardiovascular risks from oral contraceptive use.]

5. In approximately what percentage of patients with ovarian cancer has the disease spread beyond the pelvis?

    A. 20
    B. 40
    *C.   60
    D. 80
    E. 92

p.810   (Rodriguez MH, Platt LD, Medearis AL, Lacarra M, and Lobo RA, "The use of transvaginal sonography for evaluation of postmenopausal ovarian size and morphology " Am J Obstet Gynecol 1988;159:810)

5. [F & I:•Background: Because of late detection ovarian carcinoma is the leading cause of death from gynecologic malignancy in the United States.

•Objective: to assess the efficacy of transvaginal sonography in determining the size and morphologic findings of the postmenopausal ovary before elective surgery.

•Results: 18% of the ovaries were not visualized, but all these ovaries, with one exception, were much smaller than the mean volume of those visualized and all abnormal ovaries were visualized.

•Conclusion: Ultrasound evaluation with the vaginal transducer is an accurate reliable method for measuring ovarian size and observing morphology in the postmenopausal ovary.

•Further evaluation is necessary to assess the usefulness of transvaginal sonography as a routine screening tool for early ovarian carcinoma.]

6.   The single most important prognostic factor for successful sterilization reversal

     A.   absence of obesity
     B.   ampullary anastomoses
     C.   interval between sterilization and reversal
     *D.   tubal length
     E.   use of operating microscope

p.771   (Hulka JF, and Halme J, "Sterilization reversal: Results of 101 attempts " Am J Obstet Gynecol 1988;159:767)

6. [F & I:•Background:•There is a 1-2% rate of reversal request following tubal sterilization procedures.

•Objective: to evaluate the predictive value of preoperative studies and factors that can influence the success of sterilization reversal.

•Methods: The operation was performed with the usual microsurgical techniques including gentle handling, irrigation with heparinized Ringer's lactate, use of 6-0 to 9-0 sutures for the anastomoses, and prophylactic antibiotic coverage.

    °Postoperative hydrotubation was not used, and antiinflammatory regimens of cortisone and promethazine hydrochloride or both were used in about one third of the patients.

•The minimum length of the tube should be 4-6 cm.

    °This factor has been expressed indirectly in other ways that an isthmic-isthmic anastomosis has the best chance of success or that an initial sterilization technique that is the least damaging tends to be the most reversible.

•Tubal length emerged as the single most important prognostic factor in this analysis.

•The interval between sterilization and reversal was not a predictor of outcome.

•Loupes versus microscope did not make a difference.

•Presence of obesity does not appear to influence the outcome.

•Total motile sperm count per ejaculate may be useful as a prognostic factor sterilization reversal, as it has been found to be in ovulation induction.

•Ampullary anastomosis appeared to be more associated with ectopic pregnancies.

•All ectopic pregnancies were in tubes in which the distal segment stump was ampullary.

    °All ectopic pregnancies occurred in tubes less than 7 cm in length.

•Because the alternative of in vitro fertilization has improved efficacy (approaching 20% live births per ovum retrieval) and decreased cost (ultrasound versus laparoscopic retrieval), microsurgeons will need to continually review their success rates, risks, and cost-effectiveness of sterilization reversal compared with those of the emerging alternatives of new in vitro fertilization techniques.]

7. Associated with highly aggressive and rapidly progressive type of cervical cancer, human papilloma virus type

     A. 6
     B. 11
     C. 16
     *D.   18
     E. 35

p. 293   (Kurman RJ, Schiffman MH, Lancaster WD, Reid R, Jenson AB, Temple GF, Lorincz AT, "Analysis of individual human papillomavirus types in cervical neoplasia: A possible role for type 18 in rapid progression," Am J Obstet Gynec 1988; 159:293)

7. [F & I:•Background: Human papillomavirus is associated with invasive cervical cancer and its precursors.

     •Type 6 and 11 papillomavirus account for more than 90% of the human papillomavirus types found in condylomata acuminata whereas type 16 and 18 are detectable in nearly 70% of squamous carcinomas of the cervix.

     •Types 31, 33 and 35 account for another 20% of cervical cancers containing papillomavirus, nucleotides sequences.

     •Cervical intraepithelial neoplasia containing papillomavirus types 6 and 11 may have little likelihood of progressing to invasive cancer where lesions containing types 16 and 18 have a high likelihood of progressing.

     •Type 16 and 18 are not closely related at the nucleotide level and perhaps should not be combined.

     •Objective: to determine which papillomavirus types that are commonly grouped together are differentially distributed in cervical intraepithelial neoplasia and invasive squamous carcinomas.

     •Results: Heterogenous distribution of types in cervical intraepithelial neoplasia including those found in condylomas and carcinomas.

     •Cervical intraepithelial neoplasia containing papillomavirus type 6 and 11 may have little likelihood of progressing to invasive cancer whereas lesions containing type 16 and 18 may have a high likelihood of progressing.

          °Cervical intraepithelial neoplasia containing papillomavirus type 31 appears to be an intermediate category.

     •Papillomavirus type 16 accounted for 41% and type 18 for 22% of all invasive squamous carcinomas.

          °Type 16 was found in 37% of all grades of cervical intraepithelial neoplasia whereas type 18 was present on only 3%.

          °Thus in this data set, type 16 was no more similar to type 18 in its distribution than it was to type 6 and 11.

     •The different patterns of distribution of papillomavirus type 16 and 18 have important implications relating to screening and management of cervical neoplasia.

•Traditionally, the histogenesis of invasive squamous carcinoma of the cervix is that it develops from precursor intraepithelial lesions that progress from cervical intraepithelial neoplasia 1, 2, 3 to invasive cancer.

°The transition time from cervical intraepithelial neoplasia stage III to invasive cancer is about 10 years.

°The indolent course is the basis for mass screening; diagnosis and treatment of cervical cancer precursors can prevent the development of invasive cancer.

•Despite the use of mass screening programs, however, there are still 15,000 new cases of cervical cancer a year with 7,000 deaths in the United States.

°Some deaths may be due to a highly virulent type of cancer that evolves rapidly from cervical intraepithelial neoplasia, thereby eluding periodic cytologic screening.

°Women with this rapid course tended to be young, with a mean age of 32 years, and presented with advanced stage disease despite having had normal Papanicolaou smears within 1 year of their diagnosis.

•There is a significant underrepresentation of papillomavirus type 18 in cervical intraepithelial neoplasia compared with invasive cancer.

°This dearth of type 18 in cervical intraepithelial neoplasia could represent a rapid transit time of type 18 lesions through the intraepithelial stage.

°Papillomavirus type 18 was more frequently associated with poorly differenitated carcinomas and with a greater likelihood of lymph node metastasis than tumors containing papillomavirus type 16.

•Conclusion: Women in whom papillomavirus type 18 is detected on cervical screening, even with a normal Papnicolaou smear may require closer surveillance than do women with type 16 or other types of papillomavirus infection.]

---

8.   Lumbar spine bone mineral density increases with

     A.   birth control pill contraception
     *B.   breast feeding
     C.   full term pregnancies
     D.   maternal height
     E.   none of the above

---

p.321   (Hreshchyshyn MM, Hopkins A, Zylstra S, Anbar M, "Associations of parity, breast-feeding, and birth control pills with lumbar spine and femoral neck bone densities," Am J Obstet Gynec   1988; 159:318)

8. [F & I:•Background: Osteoporosis is characteristic of aging in women.

°Manifestations include spinal compression fractures and fractures of the femoral neck.

•Parity and breast feeding may be related to post menopausal osteoporosis.

°Specifically, increased live births and periods of lactation enhance the development of **osteopenia**, presumably due to calcium loss.

°Conversely the increased estrogen levels associated with pregnancy might inhibit or even reverse bone loss.

•The clinical manifestations of osteoporosis are associated with excessive of loss of bone mineral; the bone density at younger age combined with the rate of bone loss may predict the occurrence of symptoms in old age.

•Objective: to evaluate defects of parity, lactation and birth control pills on bone mineral density of the lumbar spine and femoral neck.

•Methods: Dual-photon absorptiometry measurements of the bone mineral density of the lumbar spine and femoral neck were conducted in 588 ambulatory white women, 21 - 95 years old.

•Results: Lumbar spine bone mineral density showed no correlation with **parity**.

•Femoral neck bone mineral density was negatively correlated with **parity**.

•When only parous women were included in the analysis, lumbar spine bone mineral density data showed a positive correlation with **lactation**.

•Femoral neck bone mineral density was **not** significantly correlated with breast feeding.

•During lactation, calcium uptake from the gut is **stimulated**.

°Lumbar spine and femoral neck changes may reflect the increase metabolically active state of **trabecular versus cortical bone**, which would be manifested by the preferential increase of lumbar spine bone mineral density because of its higher trabecular content.

•No significant relationships between **birth control pill use** and bone mineral density was found.]

---

9. Lipoprotein levels in patients with polycystic ovarian disease are at male levels because of

    A. elevation of intermediary adrenal steroid levels
    B. hypothalamic driven dietary cravings
    C. hepatic dysfunction
    *D.   insulin resistance
    E. obesity

---

p.427   (Wild RA, Bartholomew MJ, "The influence of body weight on lipoprotein lipids in patients with polycystic ovary syndrome," Am J Obstet Gynec   1988; 159:423)

9. [F & I:•Background: Women with polycystic ovary syndrome have higher triglyceride levels, lower levels of high-density lipoprotein (HDL) cholesterol, and consequently higher cholesterol/HDL and low-density lipoprotein (LDL)/(HDL) ratios than a group of regularly menstruating women with no evidence of an androgen excess.

•Differences in body weight alone do not explain the male pattern of lipoprotein lipid concentrations in women with PCOS.

•Objective: to investigate the association of hyperandrogenism in lipoprotein lipid profiles in women with PCOS.

•Material and Methods: Criteria for PCOS patients included irregularity or absence of menses, a history of oligomenorrhea or amenorrhea beginning at or near the onset of menstrual function, and acne or hirsutism.

°No patient had virilization.

°All PCOS patients had above-normal levels of serum free testosterone or dehydroepiandrosterone sulfate (DHEAS)

°Because many PCOS patients are obese and obesity is known to influence lipoprotein lipids, differences in their lipoprotein lipid profiles could be explained by the associated excess body weight.

•Results: Excess **weight** alone does **not** readily explain the differences in lipoprotein lipid levels observed.

•**Age** increases cholesterol and triglyceride levels in both men and women, and higher triglyceride levels, VLDL levels, and cholesterol/HDL ratios were seen in the younger PCOS patients.

•Older patients with PCOS had better **diets** than younger PCOS patients.

°The poorer lipoprotein lipid profiles in older PCOS patients could not be explained by alterations in the diet alone.

•The difference in frequency of atherosclerotic vascular disease between premenopausal women and men have been attributed to differences in serum lipoprotein lipid profiles.

°The basis for the metabolic variation between the sexes may be related to differences in the sex steroids.

°**Testosterone** may be a key factor regulating HDL levels and composition in men.

•Patients with PCOS display **insulin resistance**, whether or not they are obese.

°Insulin resistance associated with PCOS may lead to increased insulin concentrations that lead to increased concentrations of triglycerides and decreased HDL concentrations.

°The increased insulin production also can lead to increased ovarian androgen production.

°Hyperinsulinemia occurs in association with insulin resistance, and there are significant relationships between hyperinsulinemia and both increased plasma triglyceride and reduced plasma HDL cholesterol concentrations.

•Hyperinsulinism is known to be a risk factor for development of coronary artery disease.

°Because women with PCOS are heavier, are more sedentary, have higher blood pressure, and in some instances consume diets containing high saturated fat and low fiber, common sense regarding counseling to reduce potential risks of developing heart disease should be encouraged.]

---

10. Normally ovulating women have a volume of peritoneal fluid at midcycle of about (ml)

    A. 5
    B. 10
    *C.   15
    D. 30
    E. 50

---

p.453   (Haney AF, Weinberg JB, "Reduction of the intraperitoneal inflammation associated with endometriosis by treatment with medroxyprogesterone acetate," Am J Obstet Gynec 1988; 159:450)

10. [F & I:•Background: Infertile women have an intraperitoneal inflammatory process in the absence of mechanical compromise of the pelvic viscera, particularly when endometriosis is present.

°This is manifested by increases in the peritoneal fluid volume, leukocyte number (primarily macrophages), and concentrations proteolytic enzymes.

•For infertile women with endometriosis the inflammatory exudate may have an adverse influence on reproduction either by **sperm phagocytosis** by peritoneal macrophages or by the effects of cell-free peritoneal fluid on gametes or embryos.

•An analogous localized sterile inflammatory process within the uterus is the mechanism responsible for the contraceptive effect of intrauterine contraceptive devices.

•Objective: to investigate the relationship between ovulatory menstrual cycles and intraperitoneal inflammation with peritoneal fluid volume and leukocyte number used as markers of a peritoneal fluid exudate.

•A causal relationship between an inflammatory exudate and infertility is postulated because:

°1. The parameters used to measure the degree of peritoneal inflammation are lower in fertile women.

°2. Peritoneal fluid macrophages from women with endometriosis can act as effector cells phagocytizing increased numbers of sperm in vitro.

°3. Cell-free peritoneal fluid from women with endometriosis alters sperm motility, fimbrial ovum capture, sperm-oocyte interaction, and early embryonic growth in vitro.

•**In normal ovulatory function there is a maximum of 13 to 18 ml of peritoneal fluid at midcycle and women who are not undergoing cyclic ovulations (e.g., using oral contraceptives and after menopause) have <5 ml.**

•Some degree of retrograde menstruation is present in most regularly cycling women as evidenced by bloody peritoneal dialysates and bloody peritoneal fluid at the time of menses.

•The peritoneal fluid leukocyte number is increased during menses, and the most consistent evidence of intraperitoneal in flammation is observed in the clinical situation in which regurgitation of endometrial cells into the peritoneal cavity has been sufficient to develop endometriosis.

•These data form the basis for the hypothesis that refluxed menstrual debris represents a significant stimulus for the elicitation of an intraperitoneal inflammatory exudate.

•Results: The markers of intraperitoneal inflamamation decreased after medroxyprogesterone acetate therapy induced anovulation.

•The direct inflammatory effect of medroxyprogesterone acetate cannot be ruled out, is unlikely without clinically apparent systemic immunosuppression.

•The mean American Fertility Society score did not change as impressively as the peritoneal fluid parameters with medroxyprogesterone acetate treatment.

•When ovulatory menses are pharmacologically suppressed, retrograde menstruation ceases and the signs of intraperitoneal inflammation abate.]

11. Estrogen and progesterone receptor status in patients with endometrial carcinoma is most strongly associated with

    A. age
    B. depth of invasion
    *C. histology
    D. menopausal status
    E. stage

p.392   (Palmer DC, Miur IM, Alexander AI, Cauchi M, Bennett RC and Quinn MA, "The prognostic importance of steroid receptors in endometrial carcinoma " Obstet Gynecol 1988;71:388)

11. [F & I: Objectives: to investigate the prognostic importance of estrogen receptor and progesterone receptor content,

    °to identify the levels of estrogen receptor and progesterone receptor relating best to prognosis, and

    °to compare the prognostic importance of estrogen and progesterone receptors with other clinicopathologic features.

•Receptor status (of both estrogen and progesterone) related most strongly to histologic grade of tumor, with well-differentiated tumors more likely to be receptor-positive and to have a higher absolute receptor content.

    °A less invasive tumor was more likely to have a higher estrogen receptor and progesterone content.

    °There was a weak negative relationship with age and none with menopausal status.

    °The relationship between low receptor content and advanced stage was significant for estrogen receptor, but less so for progesterone receptor.

•There is a benefit for measuring both receptors as the composite receptor variable that will best identify the poorer prognostic group.

•If only one receptor assay can be obtained, **progesterone** receptor provides the most helpful information for the greatest number of patients.

•Patients with receptor-positive tumors have a better prognosis and have a greater likelihood of responding to hormonal manipulation.]

12. The most common sexually transmitted pathogen in the United States is

    A. herpesvirus
    B. gonococcus
    C. crabs
    D. condylomata
    *E. chlamydia

p.240   (Dattel B, Landers D, Coulter K, Hinton J, Sweet R, and Schachter J. "Isolation of Chlamydia trachomatis from sexually abused female adolescents" Obstet Gynecol 1988;72:240)

12. [F & I:•Background: ***Chlamydia trachomatis* is the most common sexually transmitted pathogen in the United States.**

°It causes endocervicitis, endometritis, pelvic inflammatory disease, infertility, ectopic pregnancy, and perinatal infection.

•Sexually active adolescents have the highest rate of sexually transmitted diseases and often have no routine medical care.

•Objective: to determine the prevalence of *C trachomatis* in adolescent females presenting for medical evaluation of sexual abuse.

•The prevalence of *C trachomatis* found in sexually abused adolescent females is similar to the expected prevalence of these pathogens in the sexually active population of this age group.

•The vast majority (89%) of positive cultures for *C trachomatis* and all of the cultures positive for *N gonorrhoeae were* from sexually active adolescents and not the recent sexual assault.

°These pathogens most likely derive from the consensual sexual activity of these adolescents and not the recent sexual assault.

°The incubation period to establish symptomatic *C trachomatis* infection is at least one to two weeks.

•Conclusion: The high rate of positive cultures in adolescents is more likely due to consensual sexual activity than recent sexual assault.

•The standard antibiotic prophylaxis for all victims of sexual assault provides coverage against *N gonorrhoeae*.

•However, the higher prevalence of *C trachomatis* in the general population, as well as in the sexually abused adolescent, suggests that if antibiotic prophylaxis is to be initiated, it be directed against both *N gonorrhoeae* and *C trachomatis*.]

---

13. Intraoperative autotransfusion is advisable in which of the following situations where there is heavy blood loss?

    A. Cesarean section for cephalopelvic disproportion.
    B. Cesarean section for chorioamnionitis and failure to progress.
    C. Ovarian cystectomy for bleeding corpus luteum in a patient with chronic hepatic failure.
    D. Ovarian resection for stage III ovarian cancer.
    *E. Salpingectomy for ruptured tubal ectopic pregnancy from chronic pelvic inflammatory disease.

---

p.949   Grimes DA, "A simplified device for intraoperative autotransfusion," Obstet Gynec   1988; 72:947)

13. [Facts and Issues:•Background: Intraoperative transfusion is used in trauma, orthopedic , and cardiovascular surgery.

•Underuse of autotransfusion in obstetrics and gynecology is probably due to lack of familiarity with the technique, complex instrumentation and expense.

•The incidence of post-transfusion, non-A, non-B hepatitis and recipients of blood from volunteer donors in the United States is ranges from 4-12% with an average of 7%.

°The hepatitis incidence increases as a function of the number of units transfused up to about 10-12 units after which it reaches a plateau.

•Testing of donated blood for elevated levels of **alanine aminotransferase** could prevent 29% of post-transfusion hepatitis, at the loss of only 1.6% of donor units.

•Approximately 2% of adult cases and 12% of pediatric cases of AIDS in the United States have been related to transfusions.

•Autotransfusion has several limitations.

°It should **not** be used in the presence of heavy bacterial contamination eg. in cases involving colon perforation.

•Autotransfusion has been used in cases of **ruptured ectopic pregnancy** complicated by chronic pelvic inflammatory disease without an increase in morbidity.

•Autotransfusion should **not** be used in the presence of **cancer** because of fear of potential blood-borne metastases.

•Autotransfusion during **cesarean delivery should be avoided** because transfusion of amniotic fluid and fetal debris may cause amniotic fluid embolism despite filtration.

•Hemolysis remains a problem.

°Autotransfusion units that wash cells before reinfusion reduce the amount of free hemoglobin and cell fragments in the final product.

•Theoretically, rapid infusion of citrated blood can cause cardiac depression which is reversible by administration of calcium.

•To avoid possible myocardial depression, blood should be infused by gravity only and calcium chloride should be administered through another intravenous line.]

---

14. Which of the following is NOT associated with accelerated oocyte depletion?

      A. autoimmune disease
      *B.   insensitive ovary syndrome
      C. pelvic irradiation for treatment of cervical cancer
      D. systemic chemotherapy for the treatment of ovarian cancer
      E. XO/XX mosaicism

---

p. 926   (Kreiner D, Droesch K, Navot D, Scott R and Rosenwaks Z, "Spontaneous and pharmacologically induced remissions in patients with premature ovarian failure," Obstet Gynec 1988; 72:926)

14. [Facts and Issues:•Background: Premature or secondary ovarian failure is defined as hypergonadotropic hypogonadism and amenorrhea occuring before age 40.

•After a thorough diagnostic work-up including a karyotype, specific antibody studies or an ovarian biopsy, the diagnosis may remain elusive..

•Ovarian failure may be caused by an acceleration of the naturally occurring process of atresia of the oocytes.

°Accelerated oocyte depletion may be associated with sex chromosomal abnormalities, exposure to radiation, chemotherapy or an autoimmune process.

°Another form of ovarian failure is the **insensitive ovary syndrome** which may be diagnosed when primordial follicles are present in women who demonstrate a hypergonadtropic hypoestrogenic state with resistance to endogenous or exogenous gonadotropins.

•Malignancy, infection or severe endometriosis or other etilogy factors that can cause secondary factors that can cause secondary ovarian failure.

°Approximately 1% of women over age 30 have secondary ovarian failure.

•Objective: to determine the fertility potential of patients with apparent ovarian failure.

•Estrogens appear to sensitize the follicles by synergizing with FSH to increase the number of FSH receptors.

°Estrogen therapy could sensitize the granulosa cells to respond to FSH.

°This etiology may be the most likely to remit spontaneously without estradiol replacement.

•The prognosis for patients with autoimmune ovarian failure may not be quite as poor as that of patients whose problem is more continuous and permanent, ie, those with idiopathic, chromosomal, or radiation etiologies.

•Ovarian biopsy was **not** predictive of future fertility as one patient with idiopathic ovarian failure who had an ovarian biopsy without follicles successfully delivered a healthy infant.

•Daily measurements of serum estradiol and FSH obtained during hormone replacement cannot identify those patients who are likely to resume normal reproductive functions.

•Patients with secondary ovarian failure should be treated with a trial of estrogen replacement and have close monitoring for ovulation before resorting to oocyte donation.]

---

15. The predominant aerobic isolate recovered from pelvic infected sites after hysterectomy

    A.   E. coli
    B.   Group B streptococcus
    C.   staph. aureus
    D.   staph. epidermidis
    *E.   strep. faecalis

---

p.877   (Hemsell DL, Heard MC, Hemsell PG, Nobles BJ, and Bawdon RE, "Alterations in lower reproductive tract flora after single-dose piperacillin and triple-dose cefoxitin at vaginal and abdominal hysterectomy," Obstet Gynec 1988; 72:875)

15. [Facts and Issues:•Background: *Streptococcus faecalis* **was the predominant aerobic isolate recovered from pelvic infection sites after hysterectomy.**

°It is suseptible to newer penicillins but resistant to most cephalosporins.

•Objective: to compare the alterations of lower reproductive tract flora and susceptibility profiles of piperacillin compared to cefoxitin.

•Preoperative hot conization almost completely eradicates pelvic infection after vaginal hysterectomy which implies that the endocervix serves as an inoculation source.

•Hysterectomy without antibiotics does alter lower reproductive tract flora as does antimicrobial administration.

°This alteration involves and increase in bacteroids sp, enterococcus, and Enterobacteriaceae, and a decrease in other gram positive cocci.

•*Streptococcus faecalis* and *Streptococcus epidermidis* were the predominant gram-positve aerobic organisms isolated from the endocervix before hysterectomy from the cardinal ligament intraoperatively from the vagina of unifected women postoperatively and from pelvic infection sites from women undergoing hysterectomy at Parkland Memorail Hospital.

•After single-dose cefoxitin, a significant increase in resistance in all bacteria but not in anerobic bacteria was seen.

•More enterococci were recovered postoperatively after both prophylactic regimens evaluated in this trial.

°This was observed even though all enterococci were sensitive to pipericllin and 97% were resistant to cefoxitin both pre and postoperatively.

•Pipercillin did prevent the significant postoperative increase in enterococcus observed with triple dose of cefoxitin and single dose cefoxitin.

•Enteroccus continued to be the gram-positive aerobic bacterium most frequently isolated from postoperative infection sites regardless of prophylactic regimen.

°The most frequently isolated anerobic species preoperative was *Bacteroides*.]

---

16. The treatment of choice for a prolapsed submucous myoma is

    A. abdominal myomectomy
    B. antibiotics, GnRH agonist, followed by abdominal hysterectomy.
    C. immediate hysterectomy.
    D. replacement of myoma, antibiotics, and administration of GnRH agonist.
    *E.   vaginal myomectomy

---

p.860   (Ben-Baruch G, Schiff E, Menashe Y, and Menczer J, "Immediate and late outcome of vaginal myomectomy for prolapsed pedunculated submucous myoma," Obstet Gynec 1988; 72:858)

16. [Facts and Issues:•Background: Submucous myomas constitute about 5% of all uterine myomas, and are likely to cause profuse bleeding and anemia.

•Some submucous tumors are pedunculated and may dilate the cervix and prolapse through it, even when they are large.

•Objective: to evaluate the immediate and long-term results of vaginal myomectomy.

•In most of the patients the uterus was not markedly enlarged and there was no correlation between the size of the myoma and the size of the uterus.

•The most common symptom was an acute episode of severe vaginal bleeding.

•A pedunculated myoma may become necrotic because of twisting the myoma around its pedicle and impairment of its blood supply.

°Necrotic myoma may become infected.

°If the myoma becomes infected, administration of broad spectrum antibiotics to prevent endometritis is indicated, particularly if abdominal myomectomy is intended.

•Vaginal myomectomy is the treatment of choice for prolapsed submucous myoma unless there are other indications necessitating total hysterectomy.

•Electrocervical resection under hysteroscopic controls, successfully used for excision of submucous myomas, may also be used for the removal of prolapsed submucous myomas.]

---

17. Treatment of choice for stage I adenocarcinoma of the cervix in a 23 year old nulligravida is

    A. conization
    B. radiation therapy
    *C.   radical hysterectomy
    D. total hysterectomy followed by radiation
    E. total hysterectomy

---

p.919   (Hopkins MP, Schmidt RW, Roberts JA, and Morely GW, "The prognosis and treatment of stage I adenocarcinoma of the cervix," Obstet Gynec   1988; 72:915)

17. [Facts and Issues:•Objectives: to analyze those patients with stage I disease,

°to determine whether differences exist among the various subtypes of adenocarcinoma and whether the grade, lymph node status, size, depth of tumor penetration, angiolymphatic invasion, age of the patient, and method of therapy influence survival.

•Results: Patients with moderately or poorly differentiated lesions had a significantly worse prognosis than those with those with differentiated lesions.

•Among patients undergoing radical hysterectomy, the **depth of cervical penetration** by the adenocarcinoma influenced survival as an individual factor in all patients who were analyzed.

°There was a better survival when the invasion was limited to the inner half of the cervix.

°The presence of of capillary/lymphatic space involvement did not significantly influence survival.

•The survival with positive lymph nodes in stage I was close to 15%.

•No patient with with the endocervical subtype and a positive lymph node has survived for 5 years.

•The method of therapy used for stage I disease did not alter the prognosis in those patients with a pretherapy diagnosis.

°Patients treated by radiation therapy alone had the lowest survival although there was no significant difference when radical hysterectomy was compared with radiation therapy or with radiation therapy and adjuvant hysterectomy.

•An adenocarcinoma of the cervix that is removed by standard hysterectomy represents a postoperative challenge.

°These patients appear to have a very high likelihood of recurrence despite adjuvant therapy.

°The addition of radiation therapy after a standard hysterectomy in squamous cell carcinoma of the cervix appears to provide a satisfactory outcome.

°Adjuvant radiation therapy after a standard hysterectomy for adenocarcimona of the cervix did not produce results similar to those reported for squamous cell carcinoma of the cervix.

°Survival was not dependent on hysterectomy margins, and patients with negative margins had an outcome similar to those with involved margins.

•Ovarian conservation at the time of radical hysterectomy is an option that can be safely considered in the young patient.]

---

18. Which of the following sites of endometrial implantation is most conducive to excision by the laser through the laparoscope?

    A. broad ligament
    B. fallopian tube
    C. ovary
    *D.   peritoneum
    E. uterus

p.819   (Davis GD, and Brooks RA, "Excision of pelvic endometriosis with the carbon dioxide laser laparoscope" Obstet Gynecol 1988;72:816)

18. [F & I:•Background: Vaporization of endometrial implants is associated with carbon deposition in the dessicated tissues.

•Carbon causes a foreign body reaction.

•Small implants can be cleanly vaporized; larger lesions leave carbon deposits.

•Ablation of a biopsy site causes bleeding which increases carbonization.

•Carbon deposits obscure visualization of incompletely removed endometriotic implants.

•Vaporization of endometriosis over the ureter or large vessels could result in undertreatment in an effort to protect these structures.

•Traction on the peritoneum can isolate endometrioic foci from large vessels and the ureters.

•Material and Methods: The most dependent pelvic structures were treated first.

•Endometriotic foci in the cul-de-sac were grasped, the peritoneum tented, and the lesion circumscribed.

•Endometriosis of the broad ligament and parietal peritoneum was removed by grasping the peritoneum, tenting it medially, and sharply incising the peritoneum superior to the endometriotic implant; this allowed access to the retroperitoneal areolar space.

•With continued traction on the peritoneum, the endometriotic implant was circumferentially excised and subsequently undercut and removed.

•Mobilization of the peritoneum of the broad ligament and pelvic wall allowed inspection of both sides of the endometriotic nodule.

•Direct visualization of the retroperitoneal space and medial traction of the peritoneal surface avoided significant vessels, nerves, and the ureter.

•Excision of the endometriosis involving the uterosacral ligaments and cul-de-sac peritoneum done similarly.

•Fibromuscular endometriosis of the uterosacral ligaments could be distinguished from the normal uterosacral ligamentous tissue during excision.

•Implants less than 5mm in diameter were vaporized.

•Ovarian endometriomas were incised and drained, and the cyst capsule was stripped and excised by laser.

•Superficial ovarian endometriosis and superficial uterine implants were vaporized.

•Removal of endometriosis can be performed at the time of diagnosis or after a course of hormonal therapy.

•Vaporization and excision of endometriosis is performed as an outpatient procedure.

•The morbidity of removal of endometriosis by laparoscopy is less than that with laparotomy.

•Second-look observations showed that **excisional** techniques do not leave large amounts of carbon, and minimize the possibility of obscuring residual endometriosis.

•**Tenting the peritoneum** and developing a peritoneal flap in the retroperitoneal areolar space decreased the amount of total vaporization.

•Evaluation of patients post-operatively disclosed that dyspareunia was relieved.

•Implants on the surface of the **ovary and uterus** were difficult to excise and were usually vaporized.

•The excision technique was not applicable to areas close to the uterus such as the broad ligament continguous with the uterine vasculature.

•Small peritoneal implants can be removed thoroughly by vaporization.]

---

19. The most common cause of genitourinary fistula in the United States is

    *A.   abdominal hysterectomy
    B.   obstetrical trauma
    C.   radiation
    D.   surgery for stress urinary incontinence
    E.   vaginal hysterectomy

p.317   (Lee RA, Symmonds RE and Williams TJ, "Current status of genitourinary fistula " Obstet Gynecol 1988;71:313)

19. [F & I:•Background: •The distribution of fistulas: 85% after operation, 10% after irradiation, and 5% from obstetric injury.

•Objective: to identify the which entities result in fistula formation.

•Material and Methods: Three hundred and three women with genitoruinary fistulas between 1970-1985 were evaluated.

•In 225 patients (74%), the fistula resulted from treatment for a **benign** condition.

•**Malignant** conditions were responsible in 42 patients (14%), with 26 originating from the cervix, 14 from the endometrium, and two from the ovary.

•Operations were responsible for 249 (82%) of the fistulas, 24 (8%) followed obstetric procedures, 17 (6%) followed various forms irradiation, and 13 (4%) followed trauma or fulguration.

•Fifty-three patients were seen for a **urethrovaginal fistula**; ten of these also had a separate vesicovaginal fistula.

   °Treatment for diverticulum of the urethra, which was the most common condition (13 patients), led to formation of a urethral fistula.

°Vaginal surgery for stress incontinence (11) and cystocele (8) were the next most common conditions.

•Of the 190 patients with **vesicovaginal fistulas**, cause could be identified in 177 patients.

•Treatment of a benign condition was responsible for 27 of the 31 **ureterovaginal fistulas.**

°Operative procedures account for 29 of the 31 fistulas.

•The onset of vaginal leakage of watery fluid, the first evidence of urinary fistula, was related to the site of the fistula.

•Another factor that influenced the time of recognition was the cause:

°1) unrecognized gross injury to the urinary tract (onset is usually immediate);

°2) unrecognized suture through the wall of the urethra, bladder, or ureter;

°3) necrosis of the urinary tract wall with associated hematoma or infection; or

°4) any combination of these.

•Patients with urethrovaginal fistulas after forceps delivery or trauma had leakage immediately or within the first 24 hours.

•**Gynecologic surgery (mainly total abdominal hysterectomy) is by far the most common cause of genitourinary fistula.**

•When the fistula first becomes symptomatic is determined by its cause, site or origin, and method of catheter drainage.

°Immediate leakage after operation probably represents unrecognized perforation or laceration of the urinary tract.

°Most patients noted leakage of urine between the second and tenth days postoperatively; this is the result of varying degrees of trauma and precarious placement of clamps or suture followed by devascularization, necrosis, and variably delayed development of a fistula.

•A **ureteral fistula** may take several days or even weeks to progress through a period of necrosis, urinoma formation, and eventual dissection through a previously "closed" vaginal suture line.

•Very early operative intervention at 10 to 15 days is a contributing factor for unsuccessful fistula operative repairs.

°With or without preoperative steroid preparation, the presence of resolving suture material, edema, and inflammation with micro- and macroabscess formation should have an adverse effect on the overall success rate of primary repair.

°Preliminary catheter drainage of the urethra or bladder (or "splinting" of a ureter) for 15-30 days may provide spontaneous healing in a significant number of patients with fistulas, thus avoiding the need for early operation that some advocate.

•In the nonirradiated patient with a postoperative urethral or vesicovaginal fistula, at about **eight to 12 weeks** after the formation of a fistula (or after a failed repair), the tissues will have a good blood supply, minimal edema and infection, little evidence of previous suture material, and readily identifiable cleavage planes in the dissection.

°This will permit wide mobilization and adequate dissection to allow accurate approximation of the tissues without tension on the suture lines.

•The general physical condition of the patient should be the prime consideration before a decision for early intervention.

•Fistulas may be repaired by vaginal, abdominal, or transvesical approach.

•The **vaginal** approach is easier, safer, and the most comfortable.

°The usual fistula resulting from an operation is located **low in the bladder, just above the interureteric ridge, in the trigone, or involving the bladder neck.**

°Repair of such fistulas through an abdominal incision would be ill-advised because it would require an incision in the bladder to expose the fistula in a deep pelvic site when it is so easily (and relatively superficially) accessible in the anterior vaginal wall.

°In the obese patient, the vaginal approach may be even more advantageous.

•A fistula **high in a fixed vaginal wall** will make dissection difficult because of limited visibility.

°The decision to make an abdominal approach is influenced by the proximity of a large vesicovaginal fistula to the ureter and the difficulty of adequate exposure with the vaginal approach, even with the use of a Schuchardt incision.

°Because of the proximity to the ureter or adherent segment of bowel the **transperitoneal approach** is preferred and permits mobilization of the bladder and ureter (usually with an indwelling ureteral catheter) allowing an accurate and safe repair under good visibility.

•With **ureterovaginal fistulas,** the patient's general condition and the degree of obstruction of the ureter will influence the timing of the operation and the method of repair.

°Preservation of kidney function must be ensured by adequate decompression of the upper renal system.

°When the overall condition of the tissues is considered optimal, an **abdominal** approach to the ureterovaginal fistula may be used.

•Choice of operative repair will be determined by the **location of the injury to the ureter** and its relationship to the bladder.

°Ureterovaginal fistulas that occur after gynecologic procedures usually result from injury close to the bladder, for these, a ureteroneocystostomy is preferred.

•When the ureter has been divided high above the point where a ureteroneocystostomy can safely be accomplished, ureteroureterostomy becomes the procedure of choice.

°Drainage of the anastomotic site is essential.

•Conclusion: A successful fistula repair (urethra, bladder, or ureter) requires sound surgical judgment during the postoperative period.

°Any tension or manipulation of the suture line must be avoided; competent bladder drainage with a large-caliber catheter, urethrally, suprapubically, or both, is mandatory.

°Overdistention of the bladder because of obstructing blood or mucus can be prevented by hourly charting of the urinary output and appropriate use of irrigation.

•Catheter drainage is provided for at least seven days and, in some patients, several weeks.

•A most difficult type of fistula involves the linear loss of a major segment of the proximal urethra and bladder neck.]

---

20. In assessing the effect of estrogen on post-menopausal urinary tract function, it may be correctly stated that estrogen replacement increases

A. bladder capacity
B. diurnal micturation frequency
C. nocturia
D. number of incontinence episodes
*E.   proprioceptive sensory threshold

---

p.827   (Fantl JA, Wyman JF, Anderson RL, Matt DW and Bump RC, "Postmenopausal urinary incontinence: Comparison between non estrogen-supplemented and estrogen-supplemented women" Obstet Gynecol 1988;71:823)

20. [F & I:•Background: Estrogenic hormones affect the urinary tract but their specific role in the etiology and pathogenesis of lower urinary tract dysfunction in older women is not clear.

•Objective: to compare two groups of women, with and without estrogen supplementation, with respect to the characteristics of their incontinence, associated lower urinary tract symptoms, and physical and urodynamic findings.

•Material and Methods: 72 women entering a clinical trial on behavioral management of urinary incontinence.

•Assessment of the filling phase of lower urinary tract function consisted of the following:

°fluid loss quantitation,

°subtracted provocative cystometry,

°passive and dynamic urethral profilometry,

°direct visualization of urine loss, and

°determination of urethral axial mobility.

•The genital and lower urinary tract in women have a common embryologic origin and similar hormonal sensitivities.

•Results: Very few objective or subjective differences in lower urinary tract function were seen between these two groups.

•None of the urethral sphincteric mechanism variables were independently affected by the estrogen supplementation status of the patient.

•The difference between the bladder volume at maximal cystometric capacity and the first sensation to void was larger in the estrogen-supplemented group in subjects with detrusor instability.

•The magnitude of the volume difference between the supplemented and nonsupplemented groups was about 75 mL.

•The increased maximal cystometric capacity/first sensation to void volume difference represents a temporally lengthened, impending-incontinence episode "warning time" for the subject with an unstable detrusor.

°This may represent a beneficial effect of estrogen on the **proprioceptive sensory** threshold of the lower urinary tract.

•Other evidence that would support a sensory-modulating effect of estrogen supplementation includes

°a significantly **lower** frequency of **nocturia,**

°a significantly **higher** prevalence of a **positive bulbocavernosus reflex**, and

°a **lower** prevalence of the symptoms of **urge incontinence** in the estrogen-supplemented subjects.

•Conclusion: Hypoestrogenism affects the sensory threshold of the urinary tract and this reduces the volume and time needed to change the first sensation to void into the feeling of imminent micturition, and involuntary detrusor contractions in some subjects.]

---

21. Approximately what percentage of patients with urodynamically proven pure stress urinary incontinence will develop detrussor instability after anti-incontinence surgery?

    A. 30-35
    B. 21-29
    *C.   10-20
    D. 3-5
    E. < 1

---

p.822   (Sand PK, Bowen, LW Ostergard DR, Brubaker L, and Panganiban R, "The effect of retropubic urethropexy on detrusor stability" Obstet Gynecol 1988;71:818)

21. [F & I:•Background: **Detrusor instability** has been found in 8-53% of incontinent women and may increase the risk of operative failure.

•Detrusor instability can be treated by medication, electrical stimulation, or behavior modification, with the latter being most successful.

°Bladder drill may be successful in 82-87% of cases.

•The effect of anti-incontinence operations on the detrusor is the new onset of detrusor instability may be caused by operative procedures.

°The incidence of operatively induced detrusor instability ranges from 2.0-20.5%.

•Objective: to evaluate the effect of retropubic urethropexy on the detrusor.

•Material and Methods: 86 consecutive women who had genuine stress incontinence and who were evaluated with preoperative and postoperative multichannel urodynamic evaluations.

•Patients were diagnosed as having unstable detrusors if an **involuntary true detrusor pressure contraction was associated with leakage or was 15 cm of water or more during urethrocystometry.**

°All patients in the study were neurologically normal and had no detrusor hyperreflexia.

•After preoperative urodynamics, all 86 women underwent modified **Burch** retropubic urethropexies.

•All patients then underwent postoperative urodynamics 12-16 weeks after retropubic urethropexy.

•The patients were considered **objectively cured** if there was **no** evidence of genuine stress incontinence and/or detrusor instability on this testing.

•Results: **There was a 23% incidence of detrusor instability in women who also had genuine stress incontinence.**

°The total incidence of detrusor instability in the incontinent population was 37%.

°Women with mixed urinary incontinence were distinguished from their stable-detrusor counterparts only by an increased incidence of urinary urgency.

•55% of the women with preoperative detrusor instability had stable bladders after retropubic urethropexy.

°These women could not be distinguished preoperatively from those women whose bladders remained unstable after operative repair.

•Retropubic urethropexy was able to cure 55% of the unstable bladders, and only cured genuine stress incontinence in 70% of these women.

•Overall, 30 patients had persistent genuine stress incontinence demonstrated objectively after operation.

°Twenty-eight of these 30 women (93%) had adequate support of the urethrovesical junction on Q-tip testing.

°None of these patients had rigid drainpipe urethras, but 22 of the 30 persistent genuine stress incontinence patients (73%) had **low-pressure urethras, which have been shown to be associated with a 54% failure rate after the modified Burch procedure.**

•The patient should be aware of the substantial risk of developing a new cause of urinary incontinence (detrusor instability) even if their anti-incontinence operation cures their genuine stress incontinence.]

---

22. Associated with an increased incidence of ureteral displacement

    A. endometriosis
    B. pelvic inflammatory disease
    C. pelvic relaxation
    D. previous appendectomy
    *E.   uterine size greater than 12 weeks

---

p.84   (Mann WJ, Arato M, Patsner B, and Stone ML,"Ureteral injuries in an Obstetric and Gynecologic Training Program: Etiology and Management" Obstet Gynecol 1988;71:82)

22. [F & I:•Background: Surgical injury is more common than obstetric trauma as a cause of iatrogenic ureteral injury.

°It is estimated to occur in 0.5-1% of all pelvic operations.

°55-75% of operative ureteral injuries are sustained during gynecologic (rather than general surgical or urologic) procedures.

•Objective: to review experience with ureteral injuries over a 7 year period.

•Material and Methods: 17 patients were studied between the ages of 46-81.

  °All injuries were unilateral.

    °°6 were explored for a benign mass (either leiomyoma or ovarian cyst).

    °°5 underwent primary exploration for a malignancy.

    °°4 underwent cancer reexploration.

    °°One patient required laparotomy for failed vaginal hysterectomy and one patient required a retropubic urethropexy for stress urinary incontinence after vaginal hysterectomy.

•Results: 14 patients had ureteral injury within 4 cm of the ureterovesical junction.

  °All of these injuries were repaired by ureteroneocystostomy over a silastic ureteral stent.

  °A **psoas hitch** was performed on the injured side to reduce tension.

  °All were drained with a soft, pliable, closed system drain, and all patients' bladders were drained with a suprapubic Foley catheter.

  °Of these 14 patients, 12 had normal-appearing kidneys and ureters before discharge from the hospital.

•One patient suffered a small distal ureterotomy.

  °This was repaired by stenting and and oversewing the injury.

•One patient suffered ureteral injury at the pelvic brim.

  °Her right ureter was transected along with the right infundibulopelvic ligament.

•All patients received cephalosporin antibiotics until stents and drains were removed.

•All 6 patients with benign pelvic masses had ureteral injury at the infundibulopelvic ligament.

•3 injuries occurred during primary cancer surgery.

•A single injury at the time of retropubic urethropexy was in retrospect due to marked displacement of the ureter at the time of a previous vaginal hysterectomy complicated by bladder injury at that time.

•Suggestions to help avoid ureteral injury.

  °The only factors associated with an increased incidence of preoperative aberrations were a uterine size of 12 weeks or greater or an ovarian cyst of 4 cm or larger.

  °**Endometriosis, pelvic inflammatory disease, pelvic relaxation, and previous intra-abdominal surgery were not associated with ureteral abnormalities.**

•On the gynecologic oncology service, all patients with cervical cancer have a preoperative IVP as part of staging, whereas patients with other malignancies are studied only if they are considered to be at risk for ureteral involvement with tumor.

•Conclusion: **Radiologic evaluation of the urinary tract in all patients with masses over 10 cm, particularly if they are obese, is recommended.**

•Ureteral injuries noted at laparotomy should be repaired primarily.

•The management of ureteral injuries postoperatively is controversial.

•Although residents actively participated in these operations, the infrequency of the procedures makes it unreasonable to assume that residents will become skillful enough to perform them.

°Rather, the **residents must learn sufficient surgical skills to avoid ureteral trauma, adequate anatomy to identify and avoid the ureter, and proper judgement to recognize when ureteral injury is a real concern or has happened.**]

---

23. Which of the following benign conditions is the serum CA 125 level likely to be elevated (> 65 U/mL)?

    *A.   endometriosis
    B. inflammatory disease
    C. leiomyomata uteri
    D. molar disease
    E. ovarian epithelial tumors

---

p.25   (Di-Xia C, Schwartz PE, Xinguo L, and Zahn Y,"Evaluation of CA 125 levels in differentiating malignant from benign tumors in patients with pelvic masses" Obstet Gynecol 1988;71:23)

23. [F & I:•Background: CA 125 greater than 65 U/mL serves as a positive criterion for the presence of a nonmucinous epithelial ovarian cancer.

°The sensitivity of CA 125 in detecting patients with epithelial ovarian cancer is 73-92.9%.

°There are two problems to be considered:

°°The false-positive rate of CA 125 and

°°the value of CA 125 assays in the detection of nonepithelial ovarian cancer.

•Objective: to study CA 125 results from 211 patients with pelvic masses.

•False-positive rates for serum CA 125 in patients with various benign pelvic masses may be high.

°These were 10% in patients with benign epithelial ovarian tumors.

°4.4% for uterine leiomyomas.

°9.5% for pelvic inflammatory masses.

°37.5% for ovarian endometriomas.

•Conclusion: Defining a serum CA 125 value > 65 U/mL as positive has a high false-positive rate in patients with benign pelvic masses.

•Based on the serum CA 125 results of the 153 patients with benign pelvic masses, a CA 125 level > 194 U/mL was defined as the positive criterion.

•According to this new criterion, the sensitivity of the CA 125 assay for epithelial ovarian cancer decreased from 93.3 to 80%, but the specificity for benign pelvic masses increased from 79.7 to 94.8%.

°False-positive serum CA 125 values were found only in patients with mucinous ovarian cystadenomas, endometriomas, hydatidiform moles, and pelvic tuberculosis.

°None of the serum CA 125 values were greater than 194 U/mL in patients with the most common pelvic masses, ie, uterine leiomyomas, benign cystic teratomas, and nonspecific inflammatory masses.

•Conclusion: A CA 125 level > 65 U/mL is a useful positivity criterion for screening ovarian cancer and monitoring ovarian cancer patients after surgery.

•CA 125 > 194 U/mL is a positivity criterion for differentiating malignant tumors from benign ones in patients with pelvic masses.

•Any patients with CA 125 results > 65 U/mL should be evaluated for ovarian cancer.]

---

24. What is the percentage of patients with lower abdominal pain, abdominal tenderness, a temperature of 38.8° C, and sedimentation rate of 40 mm/hr that will have identifiable salpingitis on laparoscopic examination?

    *A.   90
    B. 80
    C. 70
    D. 60
    E. 50

---

p.11   (Soper DE and Despres B,"A comparison of two antibiotic regimens for treatment of pelvic inflammatory disease" Obstet Gynecol 1988;71:7)

24. [F & I:•Objective: to compare the effectiveness of the combination of cefoxitin and doxycycline with the combination of clindamycin and amikacin in the treatment of acute pelvic inflammatory disease.

•Material and Methods: Pelvic inflammatory disease was diagnosed by the following criteria.

°All patients had lower abdominal pain and bilateral adnexal tenderness on bimanual pelvic examination, and microscopy of a wet mount of the vaginal contents revealing a marked increase in the number of leukocytes (ie, the leukocytes outnumbered all other cellular elements in the smear).

°These patients also had at least two of the following additional critera:

    °°temperature over 38C,

    °°leukocytosis (greater than 11,000/μL),

    °°purulent material from the peritoneal cavity by culdocentesis,

    °°inflammatory complex on bimanual examination or sonography, and/or

    °°an erythrocyte sedimentation rate over 20 mm/hour.

•Patients were considered ready for discharge when they met the following criteria.

°1. Total lysis of fever (temperature less than 37.5C for over 24 hours).

°2. Total disappearance of rebound tenderness.

°3. Normalization of the white blood cell count (less than 11,000/μL).

°4. Marked amelioration of pelvic organ tenderness (decrease in the tenderness score of 66%).

°Patients with persistent adnexal masses were discharged only if they had met the other discharge criteria.

°Intravenous antibiotic therapy was continued until the therapeutic response was obtained, at which time the patient's IV therapy was discontinued and she was discharged from the hospital on an oral antibiotic regimen.

•Results: Four of the 62 study patients (3 in the clindamycin/amikacin group and 1 in the cefoxitin/doxycycline group) were treatment failures.

•Response rates and duration of hospitalization were not statistically different between the two antibiotic regimens.

•**Laparoscopy confirms the presence of acute salpingitis in only 65% of patients with the clinical diagnosis of pelvic inflammatory disease based on minimal diagnostic criteria.]**

---

25. A patient with circulating ß-hCG is being treated medically for a tubal ectopic pregnancy and is noted to have a sudden significant elevation of serum progesterone and 17-OH progesterone. It may be correctly concluded that she has

  *A.   a second corpus luteum
  B.   an abdominal pregnancy
  C.   an adrenal tumor
  D.   an ovarian neoplasm
  E.   developed choriocarcinoma

---

p.669   (Sauer MV, Gorrill MJ, Rodi IA Yeko TR and Buster JE, "Corpus luteum activity in tubal pregnancy " Obstet Gynecol 1988;71:667)

25. [F & I:•Background: The corpus luteum is essential for maintaining normal pregnancy during the first six weeks of gestation.

•About the **40**th day of pregnancy, the placenta becomes sufficiently autonomous in producing progesterone, and the corpus luteum is no longer required for pregnancy support.

•Objectives: to determine the level of corpus luteum activity at the diagnosis of ectopic pregnancy.

°to define the relationship between corpus luteum activity and data human chorionic gonadotropin (ß-hCG).

°to determine if corpus luteum activity is a predictive response to nonsurgical therapy.

°to determine if spontaneous ovulation occurs before the diappearance of serum ß-hCG.

•Material and Methods: Serum progesterone, 17-hydroxyprogesterone, and immunoreactive ß-hCG were measured in 20 women receiving nonsurgical treatment for unruptured ectopic pregnancy.

•The 20 ectopic gestations appeared similar: they were unruptured, approximately 3 cm in size, and ampullary in location.

°The clinical course was highly variable.

°Some ectopics consist of a viable, growing trophoblastic mass, producing ß-hCG that is both bioreactive and immunoreactive.

°These presentations are associated with an active, steroid-producing corpus luteum.

°In others the trophoblast is probably severely compromised or dead at the time of diagnosis, as evidenced by declining ß-hCG levels and the lack of ovarian steroids production.

•In all cases the corpus luteum secretes abnormally **low** levels of progesterone and 17-hydroxyprogesterone.

°**A deficient corpus luteum could be the etiologic factor of tubal abortion,** and subsequent spontaneous resolution of the abnormal gestation.

•The functional integrity of the corpus luteum in ectopic pregnancy appears related to immunoreactive ß-hCG, but **not dependent** upon it.

°Although the treatment with methotexate stopped ovarian steroid production, this was not preceded by a decreased immunoreactive ß-hCG signal.

°Methotrexate may be toxic to the corpus luteum, negatively affecting ovarian steroidogenesis.

•Measurement of corpus luteum activity predicts the response to nonsurgical therapy.

•**Progesterone and 17-hydroxyprogesterone fall days to weeks in advance of ß-hCG.**

°Once progesterone and 17-hydroxyprogesterone reach their nadir, ß-hCG falls predictably without further intervention.

•**Ovulation occurs despite circulating ß-hCG in ectopic gestations.**

•If progesterone and 17-hydroxyprogesterone are used to follow subjects treated nonsurgically, **a sudden or persistent elevation in these levels may represent the emergence of a second corpus luteum.**

•Women with small unruptured ectopic pregnancies without a functionally active corpus luteum had spontaneous resolution of their abnormal gestations.

°Those with functional activity responded favorably to methotrexate but required a longer time for resolution.

°In all cases, progesterone and 17-hydroxyprogesterone declined before resolution of ß-hCG.

•Conclusion: Progesterone and 17-hydroxyprogesterone may be valuable markers for following those patients treated nonsurgically.

•**Spontaneous ovulation and development of a second corpus luteum may occur up to two weeks before the disappearance of ß-hCG.]**

---

26. Which of the following hemostatic factors is **decreased** in women with a familial history of thromboembolism?

    *A.   antithrombin III
    B.   beta thromboglobulin
    C.   fibrinogen
    D.   fibrinopeptide A
    E.   platelet factor 4

p.586   (Farag AM, Bottoms SF, Mammen EF, Hosni MA, Ali AA, Moghissi KS, "Oral contraceptives and the hemostatic system " Obstet Gynecol 1988;71:584)

---

26. [F & I: Background: Women taking oral contraceptives have an increased risk of developing thromboembolic disease.

°Additional risks: cigarette smoking, obesity, older age and higher estrogen doses.

•Correlations between risk factors for thromboembolism in oral contraceptive users and hemostatic parameters have been limited to smoking and to higher estrogen dosages.

•Objective: to investigate the relationship between several clinical factors and hemostasis among pill users.

•Materials and Methods: 161 women.

°Excluded: patients with diabetes mellitus, varicose veins and hepatic, cardiac or renal disease and those who had recently taken medications which interfere with hemostasis.

•Measured: plasma levels of markers of in vitro activation of the hemostatic system:

°fibrinopeptide A which reflects thrombin generation (clotting);

°platelet factor 4 and beta thromboglobulin, two markers of platelet activation and release; and

°fibronectin, a possible indicator of **vascular endothelial injury**.

•Also assayed were several other proteins that may be related to the risk of thromboembolism;

°fibrinogen, antithrombin, prekallikrein, protein C, plasminogen, and alpha-2 antiplasmin.

•Results: Use of birth control pills was **not** associated with the change in the markers of hemostasis activation.

°Prekallikrein, plasminogen and protein C, three hemostatic parameters that may offer prophylaxis against clotting, were significantly higher in pill users.

°The other hemostatic proteins were not different.

°**Antithrombin** levels were significantly **lower** among pill users with a family history of thromboembolism.

•Obese pill users had **higher** fibrinogen and fibronectin levels.

•Conclusion 1: The absence of differences in the levels of fibrinopeptide A, platelet factor 4, and beta thromboglobulin between oral contraceptive users and controls suggests that **birth control pills do not accelerate thrombin formation or platelet activation in vivo.**

°In addition to the **higher** plasminogen and protein C levels; prekallikrein was higher among oral contraceptive users.

•Other hemostatic proteins were not different from the control group.

•The finding of decreased antithrombin among oral contraceptive users with a family history of thromboembolism, is of concern because of the high frequency of thrombosis among families with heterozygous antithrombin deficiencies.

•Conclusion 2: It does not appear that oral contraceptive use is associated with hypercoagulability.

•Conclusion 3: a family history of thromboembolism and the questions routinely asked before starting oral contraceptives and obtaining antithrombin levels in selected cases seems to be indicated.]

27. A patient who had a Burch procedure complains of recurrent stress urinary incontinence. Urodynamic testing confirms genuine stress incontinence but a low urethral closure pressure is noted. The operation of choice to correct the recurrent incontinence is

    A. anterior colporrhaphy and Kelly plication
    B. Burch procedure
    C. Marshall-Marchetti-Krantz procedure
    D. Pereyra procedure
    *E.   sling procedure

p.651   (Horback NS, Blanco JS, Ostergard DR, Bent AE, and Cornella JL, "A suburethral sling procedure with polytetrafluoroethylene or the treatment of genuine stress incontinence in patients with low urethral closure pressure " Obstet Gynecol 1988;71:648)

27. [F & I:•Background: Pubourethral sling procedures for the treatment of stress urinary incontinence were introduced by von Giordano in 1907 using a gracilis muscle sling.

    •Complications of the procedure: urinary retention requiring sling revision, urethral irritation, urethral necrosis from excessive sling tension, and graft infection or rejection with synthetic materials.

    •Pubourethral sling procedures have been suggested primarily to treat recurrent genuine stress incontinence.

    •Patients with **low** urethral closure pressures preoperatively are at risk for a failure of standard anti-incontinence procedures.

    •Objective: to describe the use of a suburethral sling procedure in the treatment of patients with genuine stress incontinence and low urethral pressures.

    •Materials and Methods: Seventeen patients with genuine stress incontinence and low urethral closure pressures documented by urodynamic testing underwent a Gore-tex suburethral sling procedure.

        °Gore-tex Soft Tissue Patch is a sheet of nonabsorbable, expanded polytetrafluoroethylene designed for use as a prosthetic material.

    •During the procedure cystoscopy was performed to rule out bladder injury.

    •Tension on the polytetrafluoroethylene graft was adjusted to create a $-5°$ Q-tip angle with the horizontal.

    •Partial closure of the urethrovesical junction with elevation of the graft was documented by urethroscopy.

    •A suprapubic catheter was inserted, and a vaginal pack was placed for 24 hours.

    •Intravenous antibiotics (cephalosporin) were administered for 24-48 hours, and oral antibiotic suppression continued until the suprapubic catheter was removed.

    •**Bladder training** began on post-operative day 3.

    •The suprapubic catheter was removed once post-void residuals remained below 100 mL and did not exceed one-fourth of the volume spontaneously voided for 48 hours.

    •Results: 17 patients underwent the surgery and 13 patients completed postoperative urodynamic evaluation.

•The average hospital stay was 6.2 days.

•The estimated blood loss was 153 mL, and no patient required a blood transfusion.

•Hospital courses were complicated by a urinary tract infection in two women and a wound seroma in one.

•The suprapubic catheter was removed after an average of 29.2 days (range 10 to 61 days).

•Three patients have shown evidence of urinary retention, with intermittent post-void residuals over 100 mL.

°Two of these patients have required intermittent self-catheterization.

•There were no cases involving erosion of the graft into the bladder.

•Previous sling procedures have used autologous fascia or synthetic materials such as silastic, Marlex, mersilene, or Lyodura.

•Harvesting fascia lata requires an additional operative site, and rectus fascia may be difficult to use because of poor tissue quality or insufficient fascial length.

•The disadvantage of most synthetic materials is that they must be removed in the presence of an acute infection.

°The porous structure of polytetrafluoroethylene allows one to treat an infection in situ with antibiotics.

•This procedure includes blunt perforation into the retropubic space from the vagina, allowing dissection of the bladder from the pubic ramus and preventing bladder perforation.

°Although this is similar to Pereyra's approach, the use of polytetrafluoroethylene to encircle the urethra (rather than perivaginal sutures) provides excellent closure and obstruction of the proximal urethra, as seen on urethroscopy.

°This is essential in patients with low urethral pressures whose intrinsic urethral sphincter tone is inadequate to achieve continence.

•Ideally, repeat objective urodynamic testing should be performed at two-and five-year intervals.]

---

28. Which of the following is most predictive of endometrial pathology when found on a cervical cytological smear?

    A. histiocytes
    B. nonspecific infection
    C. elevated squamous cell maturation index
    *D.   degree of cytological atypia of endometrial glandular cells
    E. bleeding unrelated to smear trauma

---

p.243   (Cherkis RC, Patten SF, Andrews TJ, Dickinson JC, Patten FW, "Significance of normal endometrial cells detected by cervical cytology " Obstet Gynecol 1988;71: 242)

28. [F & I: Background: Normal endometrial cells and in vaginal or cervicovaginal smears in the second half of the menstrual cycle or in the postmenopausal period is often associated with coexistent endometrial pathology.

°These findings were associated with endometrial disease in women over 40 years of age in from 20-60%, and with adenocarcinoma of the endometrium from 1-13%.

•Objectives:

°to evaluate the histologic changes that accompany the finding of abnormally shed endometrial cells detected on routine cervical cytology;

°to define the predictive value with regard to endometrial disease.

•The following cervical cytologic parameters in menopausal women have been examined: histiocytes, nonspecific infection, bleeding unrelated to smear trauma, elevated squamous maturation index, and **degree of cytologic atypicality of endometrial glandular cells.**

°Only the last parameter was reported as predictive of endometrial pathology.

•Results: 11.2% of women with abnormally shed endometrial cells had adenocarcinoma, and this association was age-dependent.

•Of the 20 women with proved adenocarcinoma, five had no symptoms.

°The cytologic presence of **normal** endometrial cells triggered the initial endometrial sampling that identified the occult malignancy.

•There appears to be a continuum of risk for endometrial adenocarcinoma based on the cytologic atypicality of the endometrial cells.

•Type II atypia was defined by moderate nuclear enlargement (40-60 μm^2), nuclear hyperchromasia, and focal alteration distribution

•Type III atypia was associated with further increased nuclear size (60-80 μm^2), irregular distribution of chromatin particles, and the presence of nucleoli.

•The greatest chance of harboring cancer occurs among older patients for all endometrial cell types.

°The highest risk can be assigned to those with type III cells, which is a 19-fold increase over the younger age with normal-appearing endometrial cells.

•Conclusion: The cytologic finding of endometrial cells in the second half of the menstrual cycle or in the menopausal period is associated in an age-dependent manner with endometrial disease and adenocarcinoma.]

---

29. Which of the following progestins has the most adverse effect on lipid and lipoprotein changes?

    A.   alpha-hydroxyprogesterone
    B.   ethynodiol diacetate
  *C.   levonorgestrel
    D.   norethindrone acetate
    E.   norethindrone

---

p.37   (Burkman RT, Robinson JC, Kruszon-Moran D, Kimball AW, Kwiterovich P, and Burford RG.Lipid and lipoprotein changes associated with oral contraceptive use: A randomized clinical trial: Obstet Gynecol 71:33,1988)

29. [F & I: •Background: Increased plasma levels of total cholesterol and its major lipoprotein carrier, low density (beta) lipoproteins, are associated with increased risk of coronary heart disease.

°Conversely, a low level of high-density (alpha) lipoprotein cholesterol is an independent predictor of coronary heart disease.

°The major apolipoprotein of low-density lipoprotein, apolipoprotein B, and of high-density lipoprotein, apolipoprotein A1, provide additional discriminatory power to detect coronary heart disease.

°Thus, an **elevated** apolipoprotein B, or **depressed** level of apolipoprotein A-1 (or a high ratio of apolipoprotein B/apolipoprotein A-1) are associated with coronary artery disease.

•Objective: to examine by means of a randomized trial, lipids, apolipoprotein B and A-1, and lipoproteins in young women before oral contraceptive use and after three and six months of use.

•Results: Within the four oral contraceptive groups, several trends occurred over the six-month interval:

°an **increase** in plasma total **cholesterol** and **triglycerides**;

°parallel **increases** in **low-density lipoprotein-apolipoprotein B**: and

°an apolipoprotein A-1 **increase** not in proportion to high-density lipoprotein cholesterol, which either did not change or decreased in value.

•The increased plasma triglyceride may reflect an increased synthesis of very low-density lipoprotein by the liver or the decreased lipolysis of very low-density lipoprotein in blood by lipoprotein lipase.

•Steroid hormones affect the activity of hepatic triglyceride lipase.

°Estrogen **increases** high-density lipoprotein, but **lowers** low-density lipoprotein and hepatic triglyceride lipase in postmenopausal women, whereas hormones with an androgenic effect have the opposite action.

•The ratio of low-density lipoprotein-apolipoprotein B/apolipoprotein A-1 tended to increase for three of the four preparations.

°Inexplicably, the higher-dosage norethindrone preparation showed no change, whereas the lower-dosage norethindrone preparation showed approximately a 10% increase in the ratio over six months.

°Based on our current understanding of risk for coronary artery disease, an increase in this ratio represents an adverse trend.

•Elevation of low-density lipoprotein cholesterol and lowering of high-density lipoprotein cholesterol with oral contraceptive use–an adverse change–are believed to be an effect of the progestin component.

°**Levonorgestrel** produces greater adverse changes than do either ethynodiol diacetate or norethindrone, which appear to be equipotent.

°These changes are related to the dosage as well as to the type of progestin.

•The risk of myocardial infarction is increased among current users, and the risk diminishes substantially after use is discontinued.

•The Walnut Creek Oral Contraceptive Study reported that standardized rates of acute myocardial infarction for past users of oral contraceptives were less than the rates for those who never used oral contraceptives.

°These finding suggest that a thrombotic mechanism, as opposed to an atherogenic mechanism alone, may be etiologically important.

•Information on myocardial infarction in relation and oral contraceptive use involves preparations containing dosages of estrogen and progestin often three to four times higher than those in current use.

•Data from the Bogalusa Heart Study supports the concept that changes in lipid and lipoprotein levels in young individuals correlate with the potential for atherosclerotic change in blood vessels.

•Conclusion: Despite a paucity of clinical information involving current oral contraceptive preparations, the use of preparations that minimize adverse effects on lipids and lipoproteins is supported].

---

30. The most effective diagnostic procedure for detecting asymptomatic recurrent cervical cancer is

    A. chest x-ray
    B. IVP
    *C.   physical examination
    D. serum alkaline phosphatase
    E. vaginal cytology

---

p.9   (Larson DM, Copeland LJ, Malone Jr JM, Stringer CA, Gershenson DM, and Edwards CL.Diagnosis of recurrent cervical carcinoma after radical hysterectomy: Obstet Gynecol 71:6,1988)

30. [F & I:•Background: Recurrent carcinoma occurs in 10-20% of patients with stage IB cervical carcinoma treated with radical hysterectomy and pelvic lymphadenectomy.

•Objective: to evaluate the effectiveness of surveillance procedures in identifying patients with recurrent cervical carcinoma.

•Approximately 90% of patients who develop recurrent carcinoma after radical hysterectomy will do so within two years of surgery.

•Results: Recurrence developed in only 4% of patients with stage IB cervical carcinoma who were treated with radical hysterectomy and pelvic lymphadenectomy and who were asymptomatic at follow-up.

•Examinations at 3-4 month intervals are adequate to diagnose the small number of patients who will be asymptomatic and yet develop recurrent carcinoma.

•Any symptoms, especially those involving pain are significant.

•Clinical history suggests recurrence in 63% of patients and in 75% of patients from other studies.

•**Results: Physical examination was the most effective diagnostic procedure.**

°Examination should be performed on each visit and should include palpation of the supraclavicular lymph node region, auscultation of the lungs, palpation of the abdomen, and pelvic examination.

°Physical examination identified 81% of patients with recurrent carcinoma.

°The combination of clinical history and examination alone identified 89% of patients with recurrent carcinoma.

•Vaginal cytology was of **limited** diagnostic value.

°Vaginal cytology may identify the rare asymptomatic patient with a subclinical vaginal recurrence who can be treated successfully with radiotherapy.

°Because vaginally cytology is a simple, painless and inexpensive addition to the routine pelvic examination, a vaginal cytologic examination at each visit is recommended.

•Routine chest radiography detected pulmonary metastases in only 1% of asymptomatic patients.

•Routine evaluation of the urinary tract for diagnosing early ureteral obstruction due to subclinical pelvic sidewall recurrent carcinoma was without benefit.

•Every patient identified with ureteral obstruction had either symptoms of pelvic sidewall recurrence or a palpable pelvic mass.

•Yearly IVPs did not add to overall diagnostic accuracy in other studies].

---

31. Endocervical curettage is indicated for the surveillance of abnormal cytology when

    A. colposcopy is adequate and directed biopsies are negative.
    B. colposcopy is adequate and directed biopsies show invasive carcinoma.
    C. colposcopy is adequate and directed biopsies show severe dysplasia.
    D. colposcopy is inadequate and directed biopsies are negative.
    *E.   colposcopy is performed.

---

p.110   (Soisson AP, Molina CY, and Benson WL, "Endocervical curettage in the evaluation of cervical disease in patients with adequate colposcopy" Obstet Gynecol 71:109,1988)
31. [F & I: •Background: The outpatient evaluation of abnormal cervical cytology has two primary goals:

°to detect all cases of cervical pathology and

°to reduce the incidence of conization and its associated morbidity.

•**Diagnostic** measures used to evaluate these patients include

°colposcopic inspection of the cervix,

°directed biopsies of the cervix, and

°curettage of the endocervical canal.

•There may be a 2-17% risk of invasive cancer when the endocervical curettings are positive for dysplasia, indicating that endocervical curettage should be performed.

•Objective: to compare the experience in a colposcopy clinic and to evaluate the prognostic implications of endocervical curettage positive for dysplasia.

•In nonpregnant patients, the protocol which calls for conization

°1) in all cases in which colposcopic examination is inadequate

°2) in all cases with adequate colposcopic examination and with an endocervical curettage that shows any form of dysplastic epithelium.

•Results: 122 of 1450 patients (8%) had dysplastic curettings despite an adequate colposcopic examination.

•In a subgroup of patients with an adequate colposcopic examination, positive endocervical curettage, and directed biopsy showing less than invasive cancer, the risk of finding microinvasion or invasive cancer appears to be **less than the 2-17% risk in the total endocervical curettage-positive group.**

°11 patients with abnormal cytology, had adequate colposcopic examination, and negative directed biopsy, but positive endocervical curettage.

°°Nine of the 11 had cervical intraepithelial neoplasia identified in the cone specimen, and two had no disease.

°In another 11 patients with adequate colposcopic examination, no ectocervical lesion was identified and ectocervical biopsy was not done; endocervical curettage revealed dysplastic epithelium and conization confirmed **cervical intraepithelial neoplasia in ten patients**.

°Thus, **endocervical curettage** is important in patients with adequate colposcopic examination when no ectocervical lesion is diagnosed.

•Conclusion: The value of endocervical curettage depends largely on the adequacy of colposcopic examination and the presence or absence of an ectocervical intraepithelial lesion.

°When examination is adequate, and colposcopy reveals findings of invasive cancer, endocervical curettage should be done to rule out an intraepithelial or invasive lesion.

°When colposcopic examination is adequate, directed biopsy specimens reveal a cervical intraepithelial neoplasia lesion, and endocervical curettings are positive, the risk of invasion appears to be **lower** than previously reported.

•When colposcopy is adequate, endocervical curettage is positive, and no cervical intraepithelial neoplasia lesion is detected on the ectocervix, however, conization should be done to find cervical intraepithelial neoplasia or invasive lesion within the canal.]

---

32. What condition is the most likely cause of recurrent uterine bleeding in a patient in the reproductive age group, after a previous curettage was reported as secretory endometrium?

    A. endometrial atrophy
    B. endometrial polyp
    C. irregular shedding
    *D.   submucous myoma
    E. subseptate uterus

---

p.1355 (Brooks PG and Serden SP, "Hysteroscopic findings after unsuccessful dilatation and curettage for abnormal uterine bleeding.," Am J Obstet Gynecol 1987;158:1354)

32. [F & I:•Background: The diagnostic dilatation and curettage is a frequently performed surgical procedure in the United States.

•After introduction in 1843 by Recamier, its popularity wavered opposing opinions expressed by influential physicians and teachers until the past 50 years, its use has increased.

°Dilatation and curettage may increase the risk of uterine adhesions, tubal damage, and infertility.

•There is a complication rate of 2% and the lack of a pathologic diagnosis for as msuch as 60% of the tissue obtained.

•Objective: to report the hysteroscopic findings in women with persistent abnormal uterine bleeding after having undergone dilatation and curettage for that problem.

•Material and Methods: 29 patients with a history of persistent abnormal uterine bleeding for whom a dilatation and curettage procedure had been performed by a previous physician within the previous year, was evaluated by hysteroscopy.

•The hysteroscopy was performed with carbon dioxide as the distension medium with the Storz 2.7 mm diagnostic hysterscope.

•Results: 19 of 29 patients (66%) had totally unsuspected **myomata.**

•Reacting to Pantaleoni's 1869 use of a lead pipe and a candle to perform the first hysteroscopy, Munde described his feelings: "Compared with the information imparted to the real eye of the gynecologist, the tip of the index finger, this brief glimpse of the endometrium possesses little value."]

---

33. Which of the following is the most helpful historical finding in patients with masculinizing tumors?

     A. age
     B. history of menstrual function
     *C.   nature of onset of symptoms
     D. parity
     E. weight

---

p.1318   (Surrey ES, deZiegler D, Gambone JC, and Judd HL, "Preoperative localization of androgen-secreting tumors: Clinical, endocrinologic, and radiologic evaluation of ten patients," Am J Obstet Gynecol 1988;158:1313)

33. [F & I:•Background: Important diagnostic steps during the evaluation of androgenization in women include:

°determining the presence of an androgen-secreting tumor and

°if present, accurately locating it preoperatively.

•Criteria that strongly suggest the presence of an androgen-secreting tumor:

°history of rapid onset of symptoms,

°presence of virilizing signs, and

°measurement of serum testosterone in excess of 2 ng/ml and/or dehydroepiandrosterone sulfate levels in excess of 7000 ng/ml.

•Objective: to report experience with the identification and preoperative localization of 10 androgen-secreting tumors.

•Results: Although the onset of symptoms was abrupt in each patient, medical attention was not sought for on average 7.4 years after onset.

°In only 2 patients did masculinizing symptoms begin during puberty.

•6 women complained primarily and 2 secondarily of masculinizing symptoms (hirsutism, baldness, voice change).

°The other primary complaints were secondary amenorrhea, infertility, and postmenopausal vaginal bleeding.

•Seven patients were postmenopausal, including one who experienced premature hypergonadotropic ovarian failure at age 17 years, but at age 41 years began bleeding intermittently 2 years before the onset of virilization.

•**Clitoromegaly**, defined as a basal transverse clitoral diameter > 1 cm, was observed in eight patients.

•Pelvic examination revealed an abnormal **adnexal mass** in only one woman.

•**Serum testosterone** concentrations were clearly abnormal in all 10 patients in comparison with values observed in normal pre- and postmenopausal women.

°In only 5 patients was a screening testosterone level in excess of 2 ng/ml.

°The percentage of **free testosterone** was elevated above the range observed in normal premenopausal women in the 8 patients with tumor in whom the value was measured.

•The levels of **androstenedione** were elevated in seven patients with tumor compared with the range of values obtained in normal premenopausal and postmenopausal women.

°In premenopausal women with functional androgen excess, however, androstenedione levels may be as high as 5.8 ng/ml.

•Serum estrogen levels were assessed in eight patients with tumor.

°In one premenopausal woman the estrone level of 310 pg/ml was clearly higher than normal.

°In the postmenopausal women the levels of estrone and estradiol were outside the normal range in 2 and 4 patients, respectively

•The primary hormone secreted by 8 of the ovarian tumors was assessed by calculating steroid hormone gradients from the effluent vein of the tumor-bearing organ to a peripheral vein.

°Two of the tumors primarily secreted testosterone, 4 primarily secreted androstenedione, 1 primarily secreted **cortisol** and 1 primarily secreted **dehydroepiandrosterone.**

•Pelvic **ultrasonography** was performed in the last five patients; it correctly identified the location of a tumor to a specific ovary in 2, **incorrectly** localized a neoplasm to a specific ovary in 2 others it was **not helpful** in the remaining patient.

•**CT scans** of the adrenal glands showed normal glandular images in 4 patients with ovarian tumors, the only patients with an adrenal tumor was evaluated prior to the availability of this imaging technique.

•**All of the tumors were benign.**

°9 were ovarian, and included five **hilus cell,** one **Sertoli-Leydig cell,** and three **lipoid cell** tumors; the tenth tumor was an **adrenal adenoma.**

•6 of the ovarian neoplasms were **2 cm or smaller.**

•The **most helpful historical finding** was the **abrupt onset of symptoms** in women who had experienced several to many years of normal menstruation without signs of androgenization.

•7 women were postmenopausal with **elevated** gonadotropin levels.

»**This observation raises the possibility that the high gonadotropin levels present in these women with various types of ovarian failure may have stimulated the neoplastic transformation of their tumors.**

•2 patients initially had symptoms of **estrogen** excess, that is, **postmenopausal bleeding,** and not complaints of virilism.

°These women had tumors that primarily secreted androstenedione, and through extraglandular aromatization their peripheral levels of estrone and estradiol were elevated, leading to the initial complaints.

°The presence of virilizing signs (90% of patients), in particular **clitoromegaly**, was very helpful in the preoperative evaluation.

°°Although clitoromegaly is occasionally seen in patients with **functionally** androgen excess, it presence should alert the physician to the necessity of carefully eliminating the possibility of a tumor.

•The recommended laboratory assessment of a virilized patient has focused on the measurement of **testosterone** and **dehydroepiandrosterone** sulfate in the peripheral circulation.

•All androgen levels are lower in older women because of menopause and adrenopause.

°**Values of testosterone, androstenedione, and dehydroepiandrosterone sulfate > 1, 2, and 4000 ng/ml, respectively, in older women should be viewed with concern.**

•Functional ovarian and adrenal tumors may predominantly secrete ovarian hormones other than testosterone and dehydroepiandrosterone sulfate.

»The secretory product of a tumor may **not** reflect the usually hormonal steroidogenesis of the gland in which it arose.

•**Adrenal tumors can secrete principally testosterone, and ovarian tumors can secrete mainly dehydroepiandrosterone or cortisol .]**

---

34. Surgical correction of stress urinary incontinence is primarily achieved by

    A. cystocele reduction
    *B.   elevating the bladder neck
    C. lengthening the urethra
    D. narrowing the bladder neck
    E. narrowing the urethral lumen

---

p.137   (van Geelen JM, Theeuwes AGM, Eskes TKAB, and Martin CB. "The clinical and urodynamic effects of anterior vaginal repair and Burch colposuspension," Am J Obstet Gynec 1988; 159:137)

34. [F & I:•Background: Urinary continence is maintained by the properties of the urethral sphincter mechanism and by adequate transmission of intraabdominal pressure to the bladder and proximal urethra.

•**Stress incontinence** is defined as involuntary loss of urine when the intravesical pressure exceeds the maximum urethral pressure in the absence of detrusor activity.

•Objective: to evaluate the clinical and urodynamic effects of anterior vaginal repair and Burch colposuspension for the correction of genuine stress incontinence.

•Material and Methods: 90 women with symptoms of stress urinary incontinence.

•In all women the diagnosis of genuine stress incontinence was confirmed by a codified history, physical examination, observation of urine loss during straining with a bladder volume of 300 ml, and urodynamic assessment.

•None of the 90 women had previous surgery for urinary incontinence or genital prolapse.

•Anterior vaginal repair with bladder neck plication and tightening of the pubovesicocervical fascia with interrupted 2-0 chromic catgut sutures was performed in 56 women.

°In eighteen women anterior vaginal repair was combined with vaginal hysterectomy.

•34 women underwent Burch colposuspension.

°The colposuspension was performed by placing two absorbable sutures (Vicryl 1) on each side of the proximal urethra and bladder neck.

°In 9 of these 34 women Burch colposuspension was combined with abdominal hysterectomy.

•Regardless of the surgical procedure, postoperative bladder drainage by an indwelling Foley catheter for 5 to 7 days was used.

•The choice of surgical procedure was based on the degree of genital prolapse and the mobility of the anterior vaginal wall.

•Preoperative assessment included simultaneous urethrocystometry by means of a soft dual-channel microtransducer catheter.

•The degree of genital prolapse was estimated during straining with the patient in supine position and was assigned a vaginal relaxation grade as follows:

°0, Normal;

°1, descent to halfway to hymen;

°2, progression to hymen; or

°3, progression halfway through the hymen.

•The severity of stress incontinence was classified into three degrees as follows:

°I, Incontinence with severe stress such as coughing, sneezing, or jumping:

°II, incontinence already at rapid movements, walking stairs, or changing from a sitting to a standing position; or

°III, incontinence in standing position without strain.

•The cure rate was assessed 1 to 2 years postoperatively; cure was defined both subjectively (patient's history) and objectively (no urine loss during staining with bladder volume of 300 ml in any position).

°The term "improved" was used for those patients who subjectively experienced improvement of their symptoms.

•Because the choice of operation was determined mainly by the degree of genital prolapse, the women treated by vaginal repair generally had a higher degree of anterior vaginal wall descent than the women treated by Burch colposuspension.

•Results: Surgical outcome was not affected by the clinical variables of age, height, weight, parity and menopausal status nor by the degree of genital prolapse.

•A higher cure rate was generally associated with a milder degree of incontinence.

•Urodynamic investigation 1 to 2 years postoperatively and clinical assessment at the 5-year follow-up did not show significant differences between those women treated by anterior vaginal repair with and without hysterectomy.

•Burch colposuspension was much more effective in restoring urinary continence than anterior vaginal repair.

•The most constant finding in women with stress incontinence is defective transmission of increased intraabdominal pressure to the urethra, resulting a decrease in urethral closure pressure.

•The static urethral pressure profile variables after surgical correction of stress urinary incontinence in any of the three positions was not changed.

•Postural changes characteristic of stress urinary incontinence were still present even after restoration of continence.

•Pressure transmission in the proximal urethra and in the midurethra was significantly increased in all recording positions in all women who were successfully treated by Burch colposuspension.

°Coloposuspension restored continence by improved passive transmission of intraabdominal pressure increases rather than by activation of urethral sphincter mechanisms.

•The overall objective cure rate for the colposuspension procedure after 1 to 2 years was 85%. Five years postoperatively, 75.8% of the women reported to be free of symptoms; another 13.2% believed their symptoms to be alleviated.

•After successful correction of incontinence by anterior vaginal repair, the increase in pressure transmission was less obvious.

•An objective cure rate for the anterior vaginal repair was 45% after 1 to 2 years; another 36% of the women felt improved.

•Five years postoperatively, 31% of the women reported to be free of symptoms; another 31% felt alleviated.

•Conclusion: Surgical correction of stress urinary incontinence is achieved primarily by repositioning and elevating the bladder neck and limiting urethral mobility during stress.]

---

35. Which of the following is most likely to be associated with a vaginal pH of 4?

    A. atrophic vaginitis
    *B.   Candida vaginitis
    C. cervical leukorrhea
    D. Gardnerella vaginitis
    E. Trichomonas vaginitis

---

p.986   (Kaufman RH, "Establishing a correct diagnosis of vulvovaginal infection" Am J Obstet Gynecol 1987;158:986)

35. [F & I:•Background: Approximately 25% of women with symptoms of vulvovaginal candidiasis do not respond to initial therapy.

•*Candida albicans* accounts for most candidal infections, symptoms can be induced by other species of *Candida*, such as *C. tropicalis* or *C. glabrata*.

°Correct diagnosis can be made clinically, but should be supported by confirmatory testing.

•**Vulvar candidiasis:**

°Mild erythema of the inner labia minor, satellite pustules, and a slight creamy vaginal discharge.

•The **saline wet mount** and **potassium hydroxide** (KOH) preparations are the simplest, most useful, and fastest office procedures for identifying the causative organism in vulvovaginal infection.

°The three most common causative organisms-

°°*Candida* species, identified by visualization of spores and filaments

°°°A **Nickerson medium**, the most common culture technique, has a sensitivity of about 90% but a false positive rate of about 30%.

°°°The most **reliable** means of indentifying *Candida* is provided by the use of **Sabouraud medium.**

°°°A **cervical smear** can detect fungal infections in 80% of patients with positive cultures.

°°*Trichomonas vaginalis,* identified by visualization of motile trichomonads

°°*Gardnerella vaginalis*- identified by visualization of "clue" cells

°A wet mount with 20% potassium hydroxide is also an accurate means of diagnosing candidiasis.

•A pH within the normal range (3.8 to 4.2) essentially **eliminates** the possibility of trichomoniasis or *G. vaginalis* vaginitis (bacterial vaginosis).

•*Candida* is can be present at all pH ranges, but most *Candida* infections occur in the normal pH range of 3.5 to 4.0 or 4.5.]

---

36. What is the incidence of lymph node metastases (%) from breast cancer that will be present by the time detection through self-examination prompts a patient to seek medical attention for the average lesion size (2.5 cm)?

    A. 10
    B. 25
    C. 33
    *D.   50
    E. 67

p.147   (Knaus JV, Dolan JR, and Isaacs JH,, "Detection of localized breast cancer by prospective mammographic screening criteria" Am J Obstet Gynecol 1988;158: 147)

36. [F & I:•One in 10 American women will develop carcinoma of the breast.

•In 1987 an estimated 130,000 new cases and 40,000 deaths will occur in the United States from breast cancer.

•By the time detection through breast self-examination compels patients to seek medical attention, the average lesion size (2.5 cm) has already resulted in a 50 % incidence of lymph node metastasis.

•Despite aggressive treatment approaches, overall survival for patients with breast cancer has remained unchanged for decades.

•Objective: to determine the diagnostic accuracy of mammography when indicated by specific prospective criteria and confirmed by needle-localized excisional breast biopsy.

•Material and Methods: Any patient with a palpable breast mass was excluded from the study.

•Patients with a dominant mass, spiculated or nodular lesion, or clustered microcalcifications identified on mammogram as suspicious for malignancy had an initial excisional breast biopsy performed under general anesthesia.

•Patients with biopsy specimens demonstrating carcinoma underwent subsequent outpatient preoperative work-up, including bone scan an serum liver enzyme determinations.

°The treatment alternatives of ipsilateral axillary lymph node sampling and radiation or modified radical mastectomy were explained, and each patient participated in the selection of therapy.

•In patients choosing axillary lymph node sampling, simultaneous reexcision of the original biopsy site was performed when microscopic examination showed that the breast cancer was <1 cm from the biopsy border.

°The same axillary lymph node sampling group subsequently received whole-breast irradiation, plus a tumor-site boost with external beam electrons or an afterloading iridium 192 needle implant.

°In addition, combination chemotherapy (cyclophosphamide, methotrexate, or doxorubicin and fluorouracil) was given selectively to any patients with positive lymph nodes.

•Results: Twenty-one non palpable limited breast cancers were found out of 1110 mammograms.

°Positive first-degree family history and age over 35 years equaled age over 50 years alone in enabling the detection of these nonpalpable breast cancers.

°These two groups comprised two thirds of the patients (12/18) found to have breast cancer.

°The age factor was significant in this study (mean, 55 years) because of the gynecology only nature of the practice from which the study population as derived.

°In the remaining one third of the group diagnosed with breast cancer (6/18), four patients had persistent subjective symptoms only, and two patients had vague objective findings (one questionable skin dimpling and the other questionable nipple retraction).]

---

37. Which of the following lengthens the duration of therapy for patients with vaginismus?

    A. assertive husband
    B. desire for fertility
    C. male sexual dysfunction
    *D.   previous operative intervention
    E. use of vaginal dilators in therapy

---

p.234   (Scholl GM. "Prognostic variables in treating vaginismus" Obstet Gynecol 1988;72:231)

37. [F & I:•Background: Vaginismus has been defined as a spastic involuntary reflex contraction of the muscles around the vagina that is brought about by real, imagined, or anticipated attempts at vaginal penetration.

•The diagnosis of classical vaginismus has centered on a history of an unconsummated marriage in which there is neither erectile difficulty nor any anatomic pathology.

°During pelvic examination there is contractions of perivaginal muscles, with adduction of the thighs and extension of the back.

•Traditional insight-oriented psychotherapy has never proved particularly effective in treating this disorder.

•Remarkable success has been reported with short-term treatment schedules using systematic desensitization.

°This technique uses fantasized images of a feared situation while the patient is relaxed.

•Traditional psychoanalysis portrays this as an hysterical or conversion symptom of a specific unconscious intrapsychic conflict.

°As a revenge for having been castrated, the woman castrates her husband and destroys his potency.

•Vaginismus has also been seen as a learned conditioned response to a real or imagined painful experience.

•Objective: to determine the prognostic variables for a patient with vaginismus and to review the experience in a sexual dysfunction program.

•Patients who persist in their belief that their vaginismus is caused by an anatomic problem, and that the medical profession does not believe them, will go fro doctor to doctor until someone agrees to operate.

•**Operative intervention will be detrimental to achieving success.**

°The surgeon will have joined the patient in her fantasy of the etiology, and when she still cannot have coitus after operation, she feels frustrated, angry, and betrayed.

•The longer the duration of vaginismus, the more difficult it is to cure.

•Masters and Johnson believe that vaginismus results after a childhood characterized by excessively severe control from religious orthodoxy, a history of sexual trauma, or after attempted heterosexual activity by a woman with previous homosexual identification.

°The few patients with these histories were no different in their resistance to treatment.

•Fifteen of the 23 patients in this study demonstrated a definite lack of sexual sophistication, and took longer to treat.

°The ignorance may be a symptom rather than a cause of the difficulty, with refusal to accept or seek information about sex being a part of the personality problem.

•Five of 20 couples who completed therapy has a male sexual dysfunction, but there was no difference in this groups difficulty in being treated.

•Patients whose husbands were more assertive, and the driving force behind seeking therapy, had a shorter treatment course.

•The longer duration of therapy needed for couples with a longer history of an unconsummated marriage was not an unexpected finding.

•Cases involving previous anatomic abnormalities that had been remedied but had resulted in a conditioned response of vaginismus wee particularly difficult to treat.

•Negative feelings about genitalia antedated the onset of the problem.

•The patients use of dilator prevents the situation form becoming one in which she passively acquiesces.

°The dilators help her to gain confidence and to extinguish the conditioned response.

•When resistances to emerge, relaxation and systematic desensitization with images of the feared situation are usually successful in overcoming the obstacle.

•Women whose primary reason for seeking help was fertility-related had a significantly shorter course of therapy.]

---

38. All of the following are positively associated with the etiology of premenstrual tension EXCEPT

      A. age < 25 years
      B. history of premenstrual tension in patient's mother
      C. low level of exercise
      D. more than 3 children
      *E.   obesity

---

p.238   (Freeman E, Sondheimer SJ, and Rickels K. "Effects of medical history factors on symptom severity in women meeting criteria for premenstrual syndrome" Obstet Gynecol 1988;72:236)

38. [F & I:•Background: The severity of premenstrual syndrome ranges widely, even among the small minority of women who seek medical treatment, and is one of the major problems in diagnosing this disorder.

•There is a strong relationship between severe symptoms and psychiatric illness, particularly **depression**.

•Little is known about whether other medical history factors, such as background characteristics, cycle characteristics, health status, and family history of emotional disorders, relate to the severity of PMS.

•Social and psychological variables, rather than any menstrual cycle parameters, such as dysmenorrhea, were associated with variations in premenstrual symptoms.

•**Depression** often accounts for much of the variation in symptom severity between patients, demonstrating a strong relationship between symptom severity ad psychiatric illness.

•Less education and lower occupational status associated with more severe symptoms.

•The effect of age in PMS has not been delineated, although treatment samples consistently show a mean age of approximately 34 years.

•Objective. to examine medical history variables and to identify their effects on the severity of PMS in women seeking medical treatment.

•Material and Methods: Sixty women with regular menstrual cycles were enrolled in a PMS program.

•All patients were medication-free (including hormonal contraceptives), had general good health, and had signed informed consent for medical treatment.

•Patient maintained daily symptom reports for one cycle before enrollment, one untreated cycle, and two placebo-treated cycles for evaluation of their symptom patterns.

•The daily symptom report listed 17 symptoms compiled from those most frequently reported by the first 300 patients in the program, using a Menstrual Symptom Questionnaire and patient report.

°The symptoms included nervous tension, mood wings, irritability, swelling, breast tenderness, headache, food cravings, fatigue, depression, insomnia, confusion, aches, cramps, crying, loss of control, avoidance of social activity, and poor coordination.

•The measure of PMS severity, the dependent variable in this report, was calculated by summing the total daily scores for the seven worst days between days 20-28 in the cycle preceding the first visit.

•The Hamilton Depression Ratings, which screen for the present level of depression, were obtained at the first visit (cycle days 6-12 when PMS should be absent) by a social worker or psychologist with training and extensive experience in the use of the Hamilton Rating Scales.

•History of the psychiatric illness was obtained from the Schedule for Affective Disorders and Schizophrenia-Life Time interview.

•This sample represents 50% of the women in a series who sought treatment for PMS; the remaining half did not meet the diagnostic criteria stated above.

°The severity of symptoms was significantly associated with four of the medical history items: "mother had PMS," age, low level of exercise, and more children, which together explained 34% of the variance and suggest a role of familial and stress factors in PMS.

•The inverse association of PMS symptoms with age contradicts popular belief and is surprising, because PMS sufferers overall are in the upper half of the reproductive-age group.

•There was no significant association between depression, assessed in the follicular phase, and severity of PMS.

•**Depression item in premenstrual symptom ratings was the strongest discriminatory between psychiatric and nonpsychiatric status.**]

---

39. Clinically useful in diagnosing the ovarian remnant syndrome all of the following EXCEPT

    A. CT scan of abdomen
    B. IVP
    *C.   laparoscopy
    D. pelvic ultrasound
    E. serum FSH

---

p.580   (Pettit PD, and Lee RA, "Ovarian remnant syndrome: Diagnostic dilemma and surgical challenge" Obstet Gynecol 1988;71:580)

39. [F & I: Background: The **ovarian remnant syndrome** is an unusual complication of bilateral oophorectomy, usually when combined with hysterectomy; the patient presents with pain with or without a definable pelvic mass.

°Pathologic study of the excised mass reveals ovarian tissue frequently associated with functional pathologic cystic disease.

•This syndrome is to be contrasted with those patients who have signs or symptoms of a pelvic mass and in whom there was a purposeful ovarian conservation after hysterectomy--the **residual ovarian syndrome**.

•Materials and Methods: 31 patients with a diagnosis of ovarian remnant syndrome.

•The criteria for inclusion is as follows:

°1) documentation of previous bilateral oophorectomy (usually by written operative and pathology reports) and

°2) histologic documentation of ovarian tissue obtained at operation.

•Patients who have pain after undergoing bilateral oophorectomy, may harbor remnants of ovarian tissue.

•Knowledge of the clinical history of this entity is critical in making the diagnosis.

•Most patients present with pelvic pain of highly variable quality--chronic or cyclic, with periodic sharp, stabbing exacerbations.

•A palpable mass or thickening is identifiable in most patients.

•Preoperative pyelography may also define status of the **ureter**, demonstrating effects from previous operations or current ovarian problem that may foretell surgical obstacles.

•**Laparoscopic examination added little to the preoperative evaluation.**

°Either the mass was missed and the examination was reported as normal, or adhesions prevented accurate assessment.

•The FSH value lends support to the diagnosis.

°The presence of premenopausal levels of FSH in the absence of exogenous hormone confirms that residual ovarian tissue is present.

°The remaining ovarian tissue may not be not active enough to suppress hormonal levels.

•Radiotherapy may be successful in some patients given castrating levels of radiation.

•**Operative excision** with identification of the ureter in an extraperitoneal position, beginning above the level of the previous operation is favored.

°After the pararectal spaces are developed, the anterior division of the interior iliac vessels is usually ligated in preparation for further ureteral dissection.

°Staying close to the ureter, tension is applied to the mass to provide necessary countertraction for sharp dissection.

°Rather than concentrating excision on the mass, attention is directed to complete the sections of the ureter throughout its pelvic course.

°After this is accomplished, the ovarian remnant is excised with its contiguous peritoneum and surrounding tissues.

°Preoperative placement of a ureteral stent to safeguard against ureteral injury has been recommended but it may add to the risk of injury.

°If there is significant ureteral trauma or if a ureteral stent would help in delineating the ureter, an extraperitoneal or retropubic cystotomy can be performed.

°Subsequently, a catheter is placed is retrograde fashion and is left in place for an appropriate time to insure an adequate healing.

°Hemovac catheter drainage is carried out in an extraperitoneal fashion to prevent hematoma or lymphocyst formation.]

Reproductive Endocrinology

Directions: Each of the questions or incomplete statements below is followed by several suggested answers or completions. Select the BEST answer in each case.

1. Thalassemic patients develop amenorrhea secondary to

    A. diabetes mellitus
    B. endometriosis
    C. hyperprolactinemia
    D. hypothyroidism
    E. iron overload

2. Using a 6.5 MHz vaginal probe, a normal intrauterine gestational sac can be identified at 4.5 weeks menstrual age. At this time, a serum ß-hCG should not be less than

    A. 500 mIU/ml
    B. 750 mIU/ml
    C. 1000 mIU/ml
    D. 2000 mIU/ml
    E. 6500 mIU/ml

3. Which of the following can be used to monitor patients who are being superovulated and will undergo intrauterine insemination, so that multiple gestation can be avoided?

    A. amount of hMG
    B. duration of hMG administration
    C. number of preovulatory sized follicles
    D. serum estradiol concentration on day of hCG
    E. none of the above

4. Viability of a pregnancy is quite likely if fetal heart activity is identified and the gestational sac is at least (cm)

    A. 1
    B. 1.5
    C. 2
    D. 2.5
    E. 3

5. The risk of abortion in cases of IUD failure when the IUD is left in place is about (%)

    A. 85
    B. 75
    C. 67
    D. 50
    E. 33

6. A 19 year old patient with primary amenorrhea, sexual infantilism (46 XX) and a normal pelvic examination, developed hirsutism and clitoromegaly over a one year period. The next best step in management is

    A. dexamethasone suppression test
    B. exploratory laparotomy
    C. pelvic ultrasound
    D. serum CA 125 determination
    E. serum FSH and LH determination

7. Which of the following is increased in patients using a 50 µg/day transdermal estradiol patch after 4 weeks of use:

    A. Plasma renin substrate
    B. serum aldosterone
    C serum HDL cholesterol
    D. superficial cells in maturation index
    E. systolic blood pressure

8. What percent of couples with recurrent fetal wastage have major chromosomal abnormalities?

    A. 5
    B. 20
    C. 22
    D. 50
    E. 67

9. The pathogenesis of retroperitoneal endometriosis involves

    A. coelomic metaplasia
    B. endorphin deficiency
    C. hematogenous spread
    D. lymphatics
    E. tubal regurgitation

10. A change in electrical resistance of saliva consistently occurs how many days before ovulation?

    A. 3
    B. 5
    C. 7
    D. 9
    E. none of the above

11. HLA B locus homozygosity in a mating couple is a cause of infertility because of maternal

    A. cumulus resistance to hydrolytic enzymes of sperm
    B. failure to recognize trophoblastic antigens
    C. IgG antibodies to sperm antigens
    D. IgM antibodies to sperm antigens
    E. antibodies which interfere with capacitation

12. A patient had undergone tubal plastic surgery by means of microsurgical technique through a Pfannenstiel incision. A 32% solution of dextran 70 was placed and the peritoneum was not closed. Corticosteroids, antibiotics, and antihistamines were not used. What would be most likely involved in abdominal wall adhesions at subsequent laparoscopy?

    A. adnexa
    B. large intestine
    C. omentum
    D. small intestine
    E. uterus

13. Which mechanism is likely operative in explaining the effectiveness of progesterone in the treatment of the premenstrual syndrome?

    A. enhancer of adrenocorticotropic hormones
    B. suppressor of central nervous system activity
    C. suppressor of hepatic production of sex hormone binding globulin
    D. suppressor of ovarian steroid hormones
    E. suppressor of prolactin

14. Which of the following conditions is the basis for infertility associated with the inadequate corpus luteum?

    A. congenital absence of the uteroovarian ligament
    B. cystic fibrosis
    C. deficiency of immunosuppressive factors
    D. deficient cervical mucus
    E. XXX/XX karyotype

15. Pregnancy wastage is LEAST likely with

    A. uterus bicornis
    B. uterus bicomplete
    C. uterus didelphys
    D. uterus septus
    E. uterus subseptus

Directions: Each group of numbered words or phrases is preceded by a list of lettered statements. MATCH the lettered item most closely associated with the numbered word or phrase. Each item may be used once, more than once, or not at all.

A.   intrauterine synechiae
B.   polycystic ovarian disease
C.   hyperthyroidism
D.   prolactinoma
E.   hypothalamic hypogonadism

16. hirsutism and insulin resistance

17. anosmia

18. galactorrhea

Directions: Each set of lettered headings below is followed by a list of numbered words or phrases. For each numbered word or phrase select:

A.   if item is associated with (A) only
B.   if item is associated with (B) only
C.   if item is associated with both (A) and (B)
D.   if item is associated with neither (A) nor (B)

A.   ampullary tubal ectopic pregnancy
B.   isthmic tubal ectopic pregnancy
C.   both
D.   neither

19. salpingitis principal etiology

20. implantation more often intraluminal

21. absence of decidual reaction

A.   foremilk
B.   hindmilk
C.   both
D.   neither

22. primarily for hydration

23. primarily for energy

24. prolactin content significantly affects newborn
     fluid and electrolyte exchange

Reproductive Endocrinology- References

Directions: Each of the questions or incomplete statements below is followed by several suggested answers or completions. Select the BEST answer in each case.

---

1. Thalassemic patients develop amenorrhea secondary to

    A. diabetes mellitus
    B. endometriosis
    C. hyperprolactinemia
    D. hypothyroidism
    *E.   iron overload

---

p.643 (De Sanctis V, Vullo C, Katz M, Wonke B, Hoffbrand AV, and Bagni B, "Hypothalamic-pituitary-gonadal axis in thalassemic patients with secondary amenorrhea " Obstet Gynecol 1988;72:643)

1. [F & I:•Background: Secondary amenorrhea is common in patients with thalassemic major and is as frequent as primary hypogonadism.

•Objective: to investigate the etiology of secondary amenorrhea in thalassemic women who developed amneorrhea 2-15 years after menarche.

•Material and Methods: Eight women, 24-35 years of age with secondary amenorrhea were studied.

•Pituitary-gonadal function the the basal state and after an intravenous pulse of 100 µg gonadotropin-releasing hormone were evaluated.

•The pituitary-thyroid axis was evaluated by measuring basal levels of triiodothyronine (T3), thryoxine (T4), and TSH, and TSH was assayed after an intravenous bolus of 200 µg throtropin-releasing hormone.

•Serum prolactin (PRL) and growth hormone (GH) levels were measured in the basal state and after thyrotropin-releasing hormone injection.

•Serum concentrations of LH and FSH were determined.

•Delayed or absent puberty is the most common endocrine disorder in patients with thalassemia major.

•Results: Impaired pituitary and gonadal function in nearly all patients with secondary amenorrhea was found.

°The patients usually showed low basal plasma levels of E2 with a poor or absent response to human menopausal gonadotropin, and low basal serum levels of LH and FSH with poor response to a gonadotropin-releasing hormone test.

•Histologic examination of the endocrine glands in patients with thalassemia major has shown mild to moderate siderosis and a reduced number of cells in the pituitary gland.

•The abnormalities in endocrine function are probably caused by chronic iron overload due to transfusion therapy, with consequent hemosiderosis.

•Associated factors such as chronic liver disease and diabetes mellitus, may contribute to secondary amenorrhea.

•The high prevelance of ovarian failure in patients with secondary amenorrhea may be age-dependent.

•Desferrioxamine mesylate was administered by subcutaneous injection in 5 patients for about 3 ± 1.5 years before the appearance of secondary amenorrhea, and all eight patients studied still showed excessively high serum ferritin levels at the time that secondary amenorrhea occurred.

•Uterine width may be a more sensitive indicator of estrogen stimulation than uterine length or ovarian volume.

•Transvesical ultrasound is less sensitive than transvaginal ultrasound.

•Low basal and/or stimulated PRL levels were found in some patients.

°Impaired PRL release might be a consequence of several factors, such as iron infiltration in the pituitary, E_2 deficiency, low LH levels, and alteration in dopamine tone.

•Aberrant GH response to thyrotropin-releasing hormone occurs in patients with liver cirrhosis.

•Chronic active hepatits or cirrhosis was documented histologically in four patients, and this association might explain the GH release observed.

•Conclusion: Iron overload may play a part in the endocrine dysfunction in such patients.]

---

2.   Using a 6.5 MHz vaginal probe, a normal intrauterine gestational sac can be identified at 4.5 weeks menstrual age. At this time, a serum ß-hCG should not be less than

     *A.   500 mIU/ml
     B.   750 mIU/ml
     C.   1000 mIU/ml
     D.   2000 mIU/ml
     E.   6500 mIU/ml

---

p.680   (Timor-Tritsch IE, Farine D, and Rosen MG, "A close look at early embryonic development with the high-frequency transvaginal transducer " Am J Obstet Gynecol 1988;159:676)

2. [F & I:•Objective: to evaluate a first-trimester gestation with the use of high frequency transvaginal sonography.

•Patients and Methods: Singleton and uncomplicated pregnancies of 38 healthy patients were scanned by a 6.5 MHz transvaginal mechanical sector scanner.

•Results: The earliest gestational sac was seen at 4 weeks and 1 day; it measured 2 by 3 mm.

°The mean gestational age at which the first detection of a gestational sac was made was 4 weeks and 3 days.

°The mean level of the ß-subunit of human chorionic gonadotropin at the mean time of the detection of the sac was found to be 500 to 550 mIU/ml.

•The fetal pole became evident toward the end of the fifth week.

°At this time the fetal heartbeat became visible.

°By six weeks and 1 to 3 days, the heartbeat was seen in all twelve patients.

•The effective focal range of the probe used for this study was from 2 to 7 or 8 cm.

°The limitations of this relatively narrow range can be overcome by different maneuvers, such as angling, pushing, pulling and rotating the probe and by changing the position of the uterus through the use of a second hand placed on the abdomen.

•The study of embryonic anatomy was time-consuming.

°The scanning time invested at 6 weeks was 5 to 10 minutes, but as the gestational age increased so did the time required.

•Conclusions:

°1) A normal intrauterine gestational sac or a singleton pregnancy should be visible with this technique, with a 6.5 MHz probe, by $4\frac{1}{2}$ weeks of menstrual age. **At this time, the serum level of the ß-subunit of human chorionic gonadotropin should be not less than 500 to 550 mIU/ml.**

°2) By $5\frac{1}{2}$ weeks, a yolk sac should be visible.

°3) **If the crown-rump length measures 5 to 6 mm, a heartbeat has to be detected. The heartbeat must be seen not later than $6\frac{1}{2}$ weeks.**

°4) The falx is complete by 9 to $9\frac{1}{2}$ weeks, and the highly echogenic choroid plexi should appear and be seen at this time.

°5) The appearance of body movements marks the gestational age of $8\frac{1}{2}$ weeks, whereas discrete limb movements do not appear before 9 weeks and 2 to 3 days.

°6) Indirect evidence points to the presence of a normal developmental midgut herniation into the cord. This becomes apparent at 9 weeks. This sudden thickening of the cord shortly before it enters the abdomen is not present after week 11.

°7) Starting in week 12, structural studies of the hand and foot can be undertaken.]

---

3. Which of the following can be used to monitor patients who are being superovulated and will undergo intrauterine insemination, so that multiple gestation can be avoided?

    A. amount of hMG
    B. duration of hMG administration
    C. number of preovulatory sized follicles
    D. serum estradiol concentration on day of hCG
    *E.   none of the above

---

p.385   (Dodson WC, Hughes CL, Haney AF, "Multiple pregnancies conceived with intrauterine insemination during superovulation: An evaluation of clinical characteristics and monitored parameters of conception cycles," Am J Obstet Gynec   1988; 159:382)

3. [F & I:•Background: Superovulation increases fecundity and the probability of multiple gestation.

°Parameters predictive of multiple gestation include

°maximum estradiol concentrations,

°rate of rise of estradiol concentration, and

°number of preovulatory-sized follicles observed sonographically.

•Objective: to evaluate whether any clinical characteristics of patients undergoing intrauterine insemination with human menopausal gonadotropin stimulation or any monitored features of the conceptive cycles of the patients, were associated with muliple gestation.

•Intentional superovulation has yielded an overall cycle fecundity rate of 15% and a multiple gestation rate of 25% to 30%.

•The infertile couple's historical factors, such as the cause or duration of infertility, could be indicative of an increased risk of multiple gestation.

•Results:

°historic clinical characteristics

°daily individualized human menopausal gonadtropin administration and

°daily serum estradiol and pelvic ultrasound monitoring,

are **not** helpful in determining which patients, whether normally ovulatory or not, are more likely to conceive twins or triplets.]

---

4.   Viability of a pregnancy is quite likely if fetal heart activity is identified and the gestational sac is at least (cm)

    A. 1
    *B.   1.5
    C. 2
    D. 2.5
    E. 3

---

p.409   (ChdeCrespigny L, "Early diagnosis of pregnancy failure with transvaginal ultrasound," Am J Obstet Gynec   1988; 159:408)

4. [F & I:•Background: **Blighted ovum** is a pregnancy in which fetal heart movements could not be visualized when the gestation sac volume was >2.5 ml (approximately 1.7 cm mean diameter).

•The smallest mean diameter in which fetal heart movements can always be found is 2 cm or 2.5 cm.

•Objective: to investigate whether the advent of transvaginal ultrasound transducers, with their improved visualization of early pregnancy, would allow a definitive diagnosis of early pregnancy failure when the mean gestation sac diameter is smaller than is possible to detect with transabdominal equipment.

•Material and Methods: The vaginal transducer used was the 5 Mz phased array probe of the General Electric 3600 scanner (B mode only).

•Any patient with a mean gestation sac diameter >2 cm in whom fetal heart movements were not seen was described as having pregnancy failure.

•The mean gestational sac diameter was calculated by averaging the maximum diameters taken in three planes at right angles to one another from the interface of sac wall and chorionic fluid.

°With transvaginal ultrasound the fetal heart movements could frequently be visualized in a gestation sac in which the mean diameter was <1 cm.

•When the mean gestation sac diameter was between 1.0 and 2.0 cm and no fetal heart movement was demonstrable, a diagnosis could not be made.

•Results: Of the 182 patients with a mean sac diameter between 1.6 and 2.0 cm, fetal heart activity could not be demonstrated in 18; all of the 18 were subsequently shown to have a failed pregnancy.

•Only gestational sac size and the presence or absence of demonstrable fetal life were considered.

°Other criteria such as the presence or absence of a yolk sac, distorted or irregular gestation sac, the decidual reaction, low implantation in the uterus, placenta covering the internal os, and intrauterine hematomas were not considered.

•Fetal life could be demonstrated by transvaginal ultrasound in patients with an ongoing pregnancy in whom the mean sac diameter was >1.2 cm.]

---

5.   The risk of abortion in cases of IUD failure when the IUD is left in place is about (%)

    A. 85
    B. 75
    C. 67
    *D.   50
    E. 33

---

p.962   (Stubblefield PG, Fuller AF JR. and Foster SC, "Ultrasound-guided intrauterine removal of intrauterine contraceptive devices in pregnancy," Obstet Gynec   1988; 72:961)

5. [Facts and Issues:•Background: When an IUD is left in situ, there is an increased incidence of premature rupture of the membranes, preterm labor, septic abortion and maternal death from infection.

•Management when the string cannot be retrieved without invading the uterus is cavity is not clear.

•Intrauterine manipulation might successfully remove the IUD without interrupting the pregnancy.

•Objective: to determine whether retrieval of an IUD with an inaccessible tail could be successfully accomplished by instrument.

•Material and Methods: A 3 mm diameter alligator forceps (IUD retrieval forceps) was introduced through the cervical canal into the lower uterine segment where it could be seen with ultrasound.

°The forceps were gently advanced to contact the IUD, opened and closed on the IUD and then with gentle traction, forceps and IUD were removed through the cervix.

°The patient was advised to take ampicillin, 500 mg four times a day for five days and was discharged.

•When the IUD was removed there was a total fetal wastage of 32.1%; when left in place there was a total fetal wastage of 52.3%.

•The best chance for removal occurs when the IUD lies in the lower uterine segment caudal to the pregnancy.

•Pregnancy with an IUD calls for urgent and expert management.

°**Ectopic pregnancy** is present in 3-5% of such cases.

°The string is usually accessible in early pregnancy but may soon be pulled up into the uterine cavity with the growth of an intrauterine gestation, necessitating intrauterine manipulations for removal.

•Real time ultrasound can confirm the relative location of the IUD and the pregnancy and whether the IUD can be removed without damaging the pregnancy.

•If the patient wishes to continue the pregnancy, the IUD should be removed.

•If the string is accessible, gentle, steady traction is advised and ultrasound guidance to avoid distortion of the gestational sac.]

---

6. A 19 year old patient with primary amenorrhea, sexual infantilism (46 XX) and a normal pelvic examination, developed hirsutism and clitoromegaly over a one year period. The next best step in management is

    A. dexamethasone suppression test
    *B.   exploratory laparotomy
    C. pelvic ultrasound
    D. serum CA 125 determination
    E. serum FSH and LH determination

---

p.679 (Rosen GF, Kaplan B, and Lobo RA, "Menstrual function and hirsutism in patients with gonadal dysgenesis" Obstet Gynecol 1988;71:677)

6. [F & I:•Background: Gonadal dysgenesis, or ovarian dysgenesis, is a rare form of infertility associated with primary amenorrhea, hypergonadotropic hpogonadism, and streak ovaries.

°This diagnosis includes patients with Turner's syndrome (45,X) 46,XY gonadal dysgenesis, and patients with 46,XX pure gonadal dysgenesis; as well as patients with structural rearrangements and/or mosaicism of the sex chromosomes.

°Not all patients with karyotypic findings of Turner's syndrome or with mosaicism of the sex chromosomes present with primary amenorrhea and sexual infantilism.

°Some of these patients present with secondary amenorrhea, secondary infertility, or hirsutism.

•Objective: to determine the prevalence of patients with gonadal dysgenesis and a history of spontaneous menses, previous pregnancies, or hirsutism.

•Women with gonadal dysgenesis have bilateral fibrous streak gonads rather than ovaries.

°They lack normal ovarian follicles because of an accelerated loss of follicles before puberty.

°°Possible etiologies include

°°°an inability of the germ cells to migrate to the fetal gonad,

°°°a failure of genital ridge formation, or

°°°genetically determined failure of division limited to the fetal germ cells.

•Most women with gonadal dysgenesis have an abnormal karyotype involving the sex chromosomes.

°50% of women with gonadal dysgenesis have **45,X;**

°25% exhibit **mosaicism** of the sex chromosomes, and

°25% have either a **structurally abnormal sex chromosome** or have no demonstrable chromosomal abnormality (**46,XX**).

°°An **autosomal recessive** mode of inheritance has been postulated as the etiology of 46,XX gonadal dysgenesis.

•Some women with gonadal dysgenesis can have a limited number of follicles that persist until puberty and sometimes beyond.

°This explains why some patients with gonadal dysgenesis have spontaneous development of secondary sexual characteristics, spontaneous menses, and even pregnancies.

•Up to 3% of patients with Turner's syndrome menstruate at least twice.

•Results: The prevalence of menses with gonadal dysgenesis was 20%, but occurred in 33% of patients who were not 46,XX.

•Patients with gonadal dysgenesis have become pregnant after estrogen replacement therapy for premature ovarian failure.

•The lack of granulosa cells for estrogen production, the absence of both theca and ovarian stromal cells leads to a decrease in serum **androgen** levels to ≈ 50% of the normal female concentration.

°The decreased concentration of serum testosterone and androstenedione primarily reflects **adrenal** production, but **dehydroepiandrosterone sulfate** levels may be low in patients with gonadal dysgenesis.

°A low androgen milieu in a **hirsute** patient with gonadal dysgenesis could indicate the presence of a Y chromosome, or a portion thereof, with its 15% risk for the development of gonadal tumors or the presence of another androgen-secreting tumor.

•Virilization occurs in both 46,XX and 46,XY gonadal dysgenesis and is commonly associated with gonadal tumors.

°Testicular tissue may be found even in the presence of normal androgens and the absence of either an intact or a portion of a Y chromosome .

»An exploratory laparotomy is advised in all patients with gonadal dysgenesis and hirsutism when no other etiology can be identified.]

---

7. Which of the following is increased in patients using a 50 µg/day transdermal estradiol patch after 4 weeks of use:

   A. Plasma renin substrate
   B. serum aldosterone
   C   serum HDL cholesterol
   *D.   superficial cells in maturation index
   E. systolic blood pressure

---

p.674 (Haas S, Walsh B, Evans S, Krache M, Ravnikar V, and Schiff I, "The effect of transdermal estradiol on hormone and metabolic dynamics over a six-week period." Obstet Gynecol 1988;71:671)

7. [F & I:•Background: Loss of ovarian estradiol (E2) secretion after the menopause causes vasomotor flushes, osteoporosis, and urogenital atrophy.

•Oral preparations pass first through the liver and increase hepatic protein sythesis.

°Orally ingested E2 is poorly absorbed and is metabolized in the gastrointestinal tract and the liver to **estrone.**

•By contrast, E2 in transdermal patch is well absorbed across the skin, with little conversion to estrone and no first-pass hepatic effects.

•Objective: to compare the effects of transdermal E2 and placebo on the number and severity of both subjective hot flashes and objective vasomotor flushes over six weeks.

°to define the immediate pharmacokinetics of application and removal of transdermal E2 on plasma levels of E2 and luteinizing hormone (LH).

°to evaluate the drug's effect on blood pressure, serm lipids, renin, and aldosterone, as well as on vaginal cytology and endometrial histology.

•Material and Methods: 17 patients completed the 12-week study protocol.

•Results: Transdermal E2 significantly decreased both subjective hot flashes and objective vasomotor flushes in severely symptomatic postmenopausal women.

°No significant differences in reported hot flashes between the transdermal E2 and placebo groups until the **fourth week.**

•There was a significant reduction in serum LH in transdermal E2 subjects, as compared with placebo subjects, beginning in the fifth hour after patch application.

•There was an increase in superficial vaginal epithelial cells.

•The ability of the transdermal E2 to cause endometrial proliferation was confirmed.

•There was no significance between the systolic or diastolic blood pressure, plasma renine substrate or activity, aldosterone or HDL cholesterol.]

---

8.   What percent of couples with recurrent fetal wastage have major chromosomal abnormalities?

*A.   5
B.   20
C.   22
D.   50
E.   67

---

p.32   (Portnoi M-F, Joye N, Van den Aker J, Morlier G, and Taillemite J-L,"Karyotypes of 1142 couples with recurrent abortion" Obstet Gynecol 1988;71:31)

8 [F & I:•Background: Balanced chromosome rearrangements occur with an increased frequency in couples with pregnancy wastage, especially recurrent spontaneous abortions.

•Objective: to investigate the frequency of different types of chromosomal abnormalities found in 1142 couples, karyotyped because of recurrent fetal loss.

•Results: Among 1142 couples, 55 major chromosomal rearrangements and 40 chromosomal variants were found.

°The major chromosomal abnormalities were of three different types: reciprocal translocations, Robertsonian translocations, and inversions.

°The reciprocal translocation group was the largest, and all chromosomes except 9, 12, X and Y were involved.

•4.8% were found to have major chromosomal abnormalities.

•The birth of a normal child before or in between the miscarriages is not a reason for canceling karyotyping.

°The highest rate of chromosome rearrangement was in the group of 256 couples having had abortions and a normal child.

°A possible explanation could be that the birth of at least one healthy child decreases the probability of an unknown extrachromosomal origin of these recurrent abortions, as a balanced translocation in one parent should allow birth of normal children.

•Chromosome analysis is also necessary in couples who have had abortions and a malformed child who died at birth or who was stillborn , whose karyotype was not studied.

•More male than female carriers were found.

°This may reflect an association between structural abnormalities and male hypofertility.

•There was a high frequency of reciprocal translocations (2.8%) among the observed chromosomal rearrangements, a rate 17.5 times higher than that of the general population.

°chromosomes 1, 2, 6, and 7 were the most frequently involved.

•Robertsonian translocations, less frequent than reciprocal translocations, was found with the frequency that was 4.4-fold more frequent than in the general population.

•Inversions, which are rare in couples with only abortions, were found especially in those with at least one live-born child.

°Their frequency is 52 times greater than that of the general population.

---

9. The pathogenesis of retroperitoneal endometriosis involves

    A. coelomic metaplasia
    B. endorphin deficiency
    C. hematogenous spread
    *D.   lymphatics
    E. tubal regurgitation

---

p.1295 (Moore GJ, Binstock MA, and Growdon WA, "The clinical implications of retroperitoneal endometriosis," Am J Obstet Gynecol 1988;158:1291)

9. [F & I:•Background: The pathogenesis of endometriosis is by vascular spread, coelomic metaplasia, and tubal regurgitation.

°Menstrually shed endometrium is viable.

•The general consensus has been that each of the classic proposals or a combination of the three may be operative in a given patient.

•Objective: to review the clinical course of 5 patients with retroperitoneal but little or no intraperitoneal endometriosis.

•Endometriosis seen only in the retroperitoneal areas of the pelvis probably is **not** the product of tubal regurgitation or coelomic metaplasia.

°De novo development of retroperitoneal endometriosis is unlikely, but could be induced by endometrium delivered by lymphatic vascular channels.

•All five patients had clinically symptomatic retroperitoneal endometriomata and only one had even minimal ovarian endometriosis.

°Four of the five patients were older than 40 years of age.

•Although such lesions were described as early as 1860 or even 1819, it was not until Sampson's publications beginning in 1921 that endometriosis was recognized as a disease and received clinical attention and scientific investigation.

•The etiology of endometriosis is not certain, but is almost always limited to women who have had menstruating endometrium.

°Endometriosis may improve after the removal of the uterus.

°Endometriosis may occur in the bladders of men and of postmenopausal women with prior hysterectomy.

°A **higher** incidence in **Japanese women** may be attributed to different estrogen metabolism,

°A **lower** incidence in women of **low socioeconomic class** may result from differences in steroidogenesis consequent to deficient diet.

•**Implantation secondary to surgical trauma** to the endometrium may have importance both directly and indirectly, e.g., endometriosis in wounds and rare distant sites after surgery.

•**Heredity** may have a causal significance

•**Immune mechanisms** may be altered in patients with endometriosis.

•**Vascular spread of endometrial fragments** first proposed by Halban, be a better explanation than tubal regurgitation for rare and distant sites of endometriosis.

•Fully 30% of reported cases of **ureteric endometriosis** has occurred as the sole evidence of endometriosis.

•**Sciatica** can result from endometriosis in the sacrosciatic notch (3 cases reported).

•Endometriosis of the **pleura** occurs in patients with prior **pelvic endometriosis,**

°Transportation occurs directly from the peritoneum across the diaphragm.

•Involvement of **parenchyma, bronchus, or heart** occurs in older patients usually without a history of coexisting pelvic disease but with a history of prior **pelvic surgery.**

°Transportation occurs by vascular transport as a result of surgical trauma.

•A patient with cyclic **paraplegia** resulting from **subarachnoid hemorrhage due to endometriosis in the spinal canal** has been reported.

•Fragments a residues of ß-endorphin, which has opioid effects, greatly enhance the cytotoxicity and the cytolytic activity of the lymphocytes called **natural killer cells.**

°These endorphins also **increase interferon and interleukin levels.**

•Opioid hormones may play a significant role in the **destruction** of displaced endometrial tissue.

•Endometriosis occurs more frequently in people with type A personalities (those who tend towards ulcerative colitis and coronary occlusions) and other aggressive types.

°**This may well be related to endorphins, which are secreted in or above the hypothalamus.**

°The activation of the macrophages and the production of prostanoids, which is associated with the pathogenesis of endometriosis are also associated with endorphin secretion.]

---

10. A change in electrical resistance of saliva consistently occurs how many days before ovulation?

    A. 3
    B. 5
    C. 7
    D. 9
    *E.   none of the above

---

p.49 (Roumen FJME and Dieben TOM.Ovulation prediction by monitoring salivary electrical resistance with the Cue fertility monitor: Obstet Gynecol 71:49,1988)

10. [F & I: •Background: There is a peak in the electrical resistance of saliva **five to six** days before the luteinizing hormone (LH) peak.

°Monitoring salivary electrical resistance and vaginal electrical resistance could provide the basis for a simple method of predicting and confirming ovulation.

•Objective: to evaluate the potential relationship between the salivary electrical resistance and ovulation.

•Results: There was no statistically significant salivary electrical resistance peak during the menstrual cycle.]

---

11. HLA B locus homozygosity in a mating couple is a cause of infertility because of maternal

    A. cumulus resistance to hydrolytic enzymes of sperm
    *B.   failure to recognize trophoblastic antigens
    C. IgG antibodies to sperm antigens
    D. IgM antibodies to sperm antigens
    E. antibodies which interfere with capacitation

---

p.1317 (Coulam CB, Moore SB, and O'Fallon W, "Investigating unexplained infertility," Am J Obstet Gynecol 1987;158:1374)

11. [F & I:•Background: Basic infertility evaluation consists of documenting egg and sperm availability and ensuring two gametes can meet.

•Techniques used to document egg **availability** include basal body temperature records, luteal phase endometrial biopsy, and serum progesterone level determinations.

•Sperm availability has been assessed with **semen analysis.**

•**Hysterosalpingography and laparoscopy** have been used to ascertain whether the sperm and egg could meet unimpaired by **tubal or peritoneal factors.**

•The prevalence of **unexplained infertility** in clinic based studies ranges from 6% to 60% and is generally accepted to average around 20%.

•Based on life table analysis to provide a prognostic guide for pregnancy in such couples, about 34% of those with primary infertility and 21% of those with secondary infertility remain infertile after 9 years of attempting to conceive.

°In contrast 10% of unselected nulliparous women and 3% of multiparous women remain undelivered for 3 1/2 years after stopping nonhormonal contraception.

•Objective: to assess the usefulness of ultrasonography, major histocompatibility testing, sperm antibody assay, and hamster egg penetration assay in the evaluation of **unexplained infertility.**

•Material and Methods: Fifty-seven couples with the diagnosis of unexplained infertility were studied.

•All of the **women** had the following normal or negative test results:

°history of regular, **predictable menses;**

°**biphasic basal body temperature** charts;

°normal luteal phase concentrations of **progesterone;**

°in-phase **endometrial biopsy** results;

°normal serum levels of **thyroxine** and **prolactin;**

°**hysterosalpingogram** indicating normal uterine contour and bilateral tubal patency; and

°**laparoscopic documentation** of bilateral tubal patency, absence of pelvic adhesions and absence of endometriosis.

•All of the **men** had normal semen analysis characterized by sperm concentrations $>20 \times 10_6$ sperm/ml with >50% displaying grade 3 or grade 4 motility and >60% normal morphology.

•All of the women had folliculogenesis monitored throughout the cycle with serial **ultrasound** examinations as well as serial drawing of serum for sperm and antibody testing.

•All of the men had a **hamster egg penetration assay** performed on a semen specimen.

•Both partners were typed for **major histocompatibility antigens.**

•**Ultrasound monitoring of folliculogenesis.**

°A number of follicles appear as small fluid filled spaces, measuring from 0 to 5 cm in diameter, and one follicle becomes dominant on approximately day 6 of the cycle.

°The dominant follicle accumulates antral fluid at a more rapid rate than the nondominant follicles, until it attains a diameter of 1.7 to 2.5 cm before follicular rupture.

°Rupture is characterized by a pronounced decrease in follicular size and the appearance of free fluid in the cul-de-sac.

°Ultrasound evidence for luteinization is present within 12 hours of follicular rupture and includes a loss of the clear demarcation of the follicular cyst wall and the appearance of intrafollicular echoes.

•**Sperm antibodies.**

•Serum specimens were screen for sperm antibodies by radiolabeled antiglobulin assay.

•When positive, this was confirmed by immunofluorescence to identify the immunoglobulin isotype.

•**Hamster egg penetration assay.**

•The fertile range for the sperm penetration assay is defined as **13%** of the ova penetrated.

•**Major histocompatibility antigens.**

•The standard complement-dependent microlymphocytotoxicity technique was used for human leukocyte antigen typing for regions A, B, DR, or DQ or peripheral blood lymphocytes.

•Results: **Ultrasound monitoring of folliculogenesis.** Three women (5%) of the patients with unexplained infertility demonstrated ultrasonic evidence of **luteinized unruptured follicle.**

•**Sperm antibodies:** three women (5%) demonstrated circulating antibodies directed toward sperm. This was confirmed by immunofluorescence.

°Two of the patients had antibodies of the IgG type and one patient demonstrated IgM antibody directed toward sperm.

•**Hamster egg penetration assay.** Six men (11%) had semen specimens in which the sperm penetrated <13% of the hamster eggs on at least two occasions.

•**Major histocompatibility antigens.** Homozygosity at the B locus occurred **more frequently** among couples with unexplained infertility than among fertile controls.

•Conclusion: by adding the use of ultrasound to monitor folliculogenesis, sperm antibody tests, hamster egg penetration assay, and major histocompatibility typing, the number of patients with no explanation for the infertility can be reduced by **60%**.

•Antigens bound to spermatozoa have the ability to induce specific autoimmunity with resulting infertility.

°The presence of antisperm antibody has been shown to inhibit binding of sperm to zona pellucida and hence prevent fertilization.

•There is evidence that **histoincompatibility** confers a **selective reproductive advantage.**

•The trophoblast lymphocyte cross-reactive antigen locus may be closely linked to the B locus.

°B locus homozygosity could reflect trophoblast lymphocyte cross-reactive antigen homozygosity, and the mechanism for reproductive failure would be similar to that reported for **unexplained recurrent abortions.**

•Data from couples experiencing unexplained recurrent abortions support the concept that trophoblast lymphocyte cross-reactive antigen **compatibility** between mating partners results in failure of maternal recognition of trophoblast antigens with consequent lack of immunologic protection and recurrent reproductive failure.

•One of the patients with the diagnosis of luteinized unruptured follicle underwent in vitro fertilization and embryo transfer and has delivered a baby.

•All three of the women with circulating antibody directed toward sperm produced eggs that were capable of being fertilized in vitro when fetal cord serum was used in the culture media, but not when the patient's serum was used.

•If B locus homozygosity turns out to be related to trophoblast lymphocyte cross-reactive antigen locus homozygosity, immunization with third party trophoblast lymphocyte cross-reactive antigen, which has been successful in treating women with primary recurrent abortions, may be appropriate treatment for those individuals.

»It would be inappropriate to diagnose unexplained infertility unless tests such as postcoital tests, in vitro sperm cervical mucus studies, and comprehensive immunologic tests to detect sperm antibodies in male and female sperm, serum and cervical mucus have been performed and cervical factor anomalies, immunologic factors, and other factors such as uterine anomalies have been ruled out.

•The presence of sperm antibodies in **cervical mucus** is a much better predictor of infertility than that of **serum** antibodies.]

---

12. A patient had undergone tubal plastic surgery by means of microsurgical technique through a Pfannenstiel incision. A 32% solution of dextran 70 was placed and the peritoneum was not closed. Corticosteroids, antibiotics, and antihistamines were not used. What would be most likely involved in abdominal wall adhesions at subsequent laparoscopy?

    A. adnexa
    B. large intestine
   *C.   omentum
    D. small intestine
    E. uterus

---

p.537   (Tulandi T, Hum HS, Gelfand MM, "Closure of laparotomy incisions with or without peritoneal suturing and second-look laparoscopy " Am J Obstet Gynecol 1988;158:536)

12. [F & I:•Objective: to examine the safety of laparotomy closure without peritoneal suturing and the incidence of adhesions to the laparotomy incision as assessed by second-look laparoscopy.

•Material and Methods: 333 healthy women, 21 to 38 years of age, who had undergone reproductive operations by laparotomy.

°Pfannenstiel incision was used for the laparotomy in all patients.

•Between January 1983 and June 1984, the peritoneum was loosely closed with a continuous suture of 000 plain cat gut, and between July 1984 and December 1985 , the peritoneum was left unsutured.

•In all patients, 150 ml of 32% solution of dextran 70 was instilled into the pelvic cavity before the abdominal cavity was closed.

•The rest of the wound closure was similar in the two groups of patients. The anterior rectus sheath was closed with a continuous suture of No. 0 Vicryl, and the skin was closed with a subcuticular suture of 4-0 polyglactin. The fatty layer was left unsutured.

•120 women who did not achieve pregnancy 6 months after the initial reproductive surgery agreed to undergo second-look laparoscopy.

•Results: **There is no difference in the early and late postoperative complication after abdominal closure with or without peritoneal suturing.**

•The postoperative complication rate and the incidence of wound dehiscence and incisional hernias were no different.

•Laparoscopic findings of adhesions to the anterior abdominal wall were encountered in 14 patients in the group with peritoneal closure (22.2%) and in 9 patients in the group without peritoneal closure (15.8%).

°**Omental adhesions were the type found in most patients.**

•No difference was found in the incidence of adhesions to the anterior abdominal wall after abdominal closure with or without peritoneal suturing.

•Conclusion: There is no difference in postoperative complications, wound healing, and adhesions to the previous laparotomy incisions after laparotomy closure with or without peritoneal suturing.]

---

13. Which mechanism is likely operative in explaining the effectiveness of progesterone in the treatment of the premenstrual syndrome?

    A. enhancer of adrenocorticotropic hormones
    *B.   suppressor of central nervous system activity
    C. suppressor of hepatic production of sex hormone binding globulin
    D. suppressor of ovarian steroid hormones
    E. suppressor of prolactin

---

p.10   (Rubinow ER, Hoban C, Grover GN, Galloway DS, Roy-Byrne P, Andersen R, and Merriam GR, "Changes in plasma hormones across the menstrual cycle in patients with menstrually related mood disorder and in control subjects" Am J Obstet Gynecol 1988;158: 5)

13. [F & I:•Background: Premenstrual syndrome is a group of disorders characterized by somatic, affective, cognitive, and behavioral disturbances that appear during the post-ovulatory phase of the menstrual cycle and then resolve rapidly at or near the onset of menses.

•A popular biochemical hypothesis is that of gonadal steroid dysequilibrium in the form of too little progesterone, too much estrogen, or an imbalance in the estrogen/progesterone ratio.

•Approximately 50% of women presenting with a history of premenstrual syndrome do not show evidence of menstrually related symptom variation when followed longitudinally.

•Objective: to study morning plasma levels of sex steroids and related hormones throughout the menstrual cycle in patients and controls who were well characterized by prospective longitudinal rating methods with respect to the presence or absence of major changes in mood in relation to the phase of the menstrual cycle.

•Results: Examination of **gonadotropins and gonadal steroids** in patients with premenstrual syndrome or control women whose diagnoses were confirmed by several months of daily mood ratings before study entry revealed no diagnosis-related differences in the amount of pattern of hormonal secretion.

•The premenstrual syndrome may not be a product of abnormal circulating levels of gonadotropins or gonadal steroids.

•Results: No diagnosis -related difference in the secretion of **prolactin** was noted.

•Conclusion: It appears unlikely that the therapeutic effect of bromocriptine in patients with premenstrual syndrome is in any way due to suppression of abnormally elevated plasma prolactin levels.

•Result: No diagnosis of menstrual cycle phase-related differences in **cortisol** secretion, was noted.

•Results: No diagnosis related alteration in the concentrations or pattern of secretion of **DHEAS or dihydrotestosterone** was seen.

•Conclusion: Failure to observe abnormal amounts or patterns of secretion of gonadotropins, gonadal steroids, androgens, prolactin, or cortisol across the menstrual cycle in women with carefully defined premenstrual syndrome and in control subjects suggests that prior attempts to ascribe menstrually related mood symptoms to simple excesses or deficits of these hormonal factors are simplistic and inaccurate.

•The effectiveness of progesterone and its metabolites may be related to its physicoactive and sedative properties.

•Premenstrual syndrome may represent an abnormal response in normal endocrine levels.

•The premenstrual cycle may serve as a synchronizer of endogenous mood rhythms or may function like an unconditioned stimulus in the conditioned recurrence of dysphoric mood states.]

---

14. Which of the following conditions is the basis for infertility associated with the inadequate corpus luteum?

    A. congenital absence of the uteroovarian ligament
    B. cystic fibrosis
    *C.   deficiency of immunosuppressive factors
    D. deficient cervical mucus
    E. XXX/XX karyotype

---

p.636   (Wang HS, Kanzaki H, Tokushige M, Sato S, Yoshida M,and Mori T, "Effect of ovarian steroids on the secretion of immunosuppressive factor(s) from human endometrium " Am J Obstet Gynecol 1988;158:629)

14. [F & I:•Background: Human nondecidualized endometrium releases soluble factor(s) capable of blocking the in vitro lymphocyte proliferation induced by allogeneic cells and phytohemagglutinin stimulation.

•the suppressive activity by the supernatants from secretory phase endometrial cultures is higher than that from proliferative ones.

•Progesterone concentrations are higher in the secretory than proliferative endometrium and is essential for promoting a decidual response capable of blocking the afferent arm of the immunologic reflex.

•**Progesterone** exerts either a direct immunosuppressive effect on lymphoproliferation or an indirect effect by inducing synthesis or secretion of endometrial immunosuppressive proteins in nonpregnant animals.

•**Estrogens** enhance the survival time of allografts and inhibit the activation of human lymphocytes to phytohemagglutinin; moreover, the progesterone-binding capacity in human endometrium is increased by estrogen priming.

•Ovarian steroids may be indispensable for the implantation of a genetically alien fetus by a direct immunosuppressive effect on the lymphocyte as well as an indirect effect by stimulating the secretion of immunosuppressive factor(s) from the cyclic endometrium.

•Objective: to determine the effect of ovarian steroids on the endometrial secretions of immunosuppressive factors

•Methods: Supernatants from human endometrial cultures with or without the addition of progesterone or estrogen were compared for their affects on mixed lymphocyte reaction and phytohemagglutinin-induced lymphocyte reactivity.

•Results:

°The immunosuppressive effect of secretory endometria on mixed lymphocyte reaction and phytohemagglutinin responsiveness of lymphocytes was **higher** than that of proliferative endometria;

°the addition of progesterone significantly enhances the inhibitory activity of supernatants when added to the explant cultures in proliferative but not in secretory endometria.

•The addition of estrogen showed no significant influence on the suppressive activity of either proliferative endometria or secretory endometria.

•Conclusion: There is a certain threshold concentration of progesterone for stimulating the endometrium to release the immunosuppressive factor(s) exceeding which little or no additional effect can be seen.

•The in vivo secretion of progesterone-inducible immunosuppressive factor(s) into the uterine lumen during periovulatory periods might work for the protection of allogeneic sperm migration in the genital tract and might be a great aid in the implantation of a semiallograftic fetus on the secretory phase endometrium.

•It could explain why the abnormalities of progesterone secretion in women with **corpus luteum defect** are associated with a high rate of infertility, since this defect may cause inadequate secretion of immunosuppressive factor(s) from the cyclic endometrium and consequently failure of implantation or early embryonic loss.]

---

15. Pregnancy wastage is LEAST likely with

    A. uterus bicornis
    B. uterus bicomplete
  *C.   uterus didelphys
    D. uterus septus
    E. uterus subseptus

---

p.29   (Ashton D, Amin HK, Richart RM, and Neuwirth RS,"The incidence of asymptomatic uterine anomalies in women undergoing transcervical tubal sterilization" Obstet Gynecol 1988;71:28)

15. [F & I:•Background: The embryologic development of the female genital system begins around the fifth to sixth week and continues through the fifth month of fetal life.

•The various müllerian system malformations can be described under four major categories.

°1. Failure of one or both müllerian ducts to develop.

°2. Failure to fuse or abnormal fusion of the ducts.

°3. Failure of the ducts to canalize.

°4. Failure of reabsorption of the midline uterine septum.

°The respective resulting anomalies are agenesis or unicornuate uterus; complete or partial duplication of the uterus, vagina and/or cervix (didelphic, duplex, or bicornuate uteri); rudimentary uterine structures without proper cavities; and septate or subseptate uteri.

•Identification of these anomalies has been made by hysterosalpingography.

•Objective: to report the incidence of congenital uterine anomalies based on the following criteria for a normal radiographic uterine configuration.

°1. A generally triangular shape.

°2. An internal os-to-fundus length of 7-8 cm.

°3. A fundal breadth of 7-8 cm.

°The bicornuate/septate anomaly appeared as a midline, triangle-shaped symmetric filling defect extending toward the internal os for 50% or more of the vertical uterine length, as measured from the internal os to the midpoint of a line drawn between the apices of the uterine horns.

°Filling defects of a lesser degree were considered normal varieties of the arcuate uterine configuration.

•The majority of uterine anomalies are asymptomatic and probably cause no reproductive difficulties, with the obvious exceptions of agenesis and duct obstructions.

•In this study 16 women had multiple successful pregnancies and unrecognized congenital uterine anomalies.

•**Complications of pregnancy appear to be more common in association with uteri of dual müllerian origin (uterus bicornis, septus, and subseptus) than with uteri of single müllerian origin (uteri didelphys and unicornis).**

•The spontaneous abortion rate among women with subseptate/bicornuate uterine anomalies-16% in this study-is not different from that generally quoted in the literature.]

Directions: Each group of numbered words or phrases is preceded by a list of lettered statements. MATCH the lettered item most closely associated with the numbered word or phrase. Each item may be used once, more than once, or not at all.

    A. intrauterine synechiae
    B. polycystic ovarian disease
    C. hyperthyroidism
    D. prolactinoma
    E. hypothalamic hypogonadism

16. hirsutism and insulin resistance   Ans: B

17. anosmia   Ans: E

18. galactorrhea   Ans: D

---

p.178   (Reid R, Fretts R, and Van Vugt D,, "The theory and practice of ovulation induction with gonadotropin-releasing hormone" Am J Obstet Gynecol 1988;158: 176)

16-18. [F & I: •Theoretical basis of GnRH treatment.

°The pulsatile pattern of gonadtropin secretion of the normal menstrual cycle is probably the result of intermittent delivery of hypothalamic GnRH to the pituitary.

°In the normal menstrual cycle, neurotransmitters, including endogenous opiates and catecholamines, modulate the pulsatile release of GnRH from the hypothalamus.

°GnRH, a decapeptide, is released as discrete pulses into the hypophyseal-portal venous system and is delivered to the anterior pituitary where it bathes the cells responsible for gonadotropin secretion.

°Coincident with the arrival of the GnRH pulse at the pituitary, luteinizing hormone and follicle-stimulating hormone are released from the gonadotropes and travel through the peripheral circulation to the ovary.

    °°Factors, including the amplitude and frequency of GnRH pulses, the influence of steroidal and nonsteroidal feedback signals to the pituitary, and the differing half-lives of luteinizing hormone (20 minutes) and follicle-stimulating hormone (3 hours), influence the relative concentrations of these two gonadotropins in circulation.

°Initially, **follicle-stimulating hormone** acts to recruit primary oocytes for the coming reproductive cycle.

°**Estradiol**, increases linearly as ovarian follicular development proceeds, feeds back in concert with other nonsteroidal products from the developing follicle to inhibit the release of follicle-stimulating hormone and augment luteinizing hormone secretion through actions at hypothalamic and pituitary sites.

°GnRH treatment, in theory, when properly administered, should lead to increased release of pituitary gonadotropins without influencing the negative feedback system between the developing ovarian follicles and the pituitary.

°Large doses of GnRH may, in fact, override innate control mechanisms and lead to second critical determinant of successful GnRH therapy.

•**Patient assessment:**

°In the amenorrheic woman a history of recent weight loss or of other significant physical, psychological, or nutritional stresses should focus attention on the possibility of **suppressed hypothalamic GnRH secretion** as the underlying pathophysiologic mechanism.

°Evidence of **anosmia** or of a midline facial defect in a woman with primary amenorrhea should suggest a **congenital absence of GnRH production**.

°Acne, hirsutism, and oligomenorrhea, particularly if associated with recent weight gain or long-standing obesity, point toward a pattern of chronic anovulation associated with **polycystic ovary disease.**

°Hyperandrogenism with polycystic ovary disease in the nonobese individual is often associated with **insulin resistance.**

°The presence of galactorrhea and/or amenorrhea should suggest the likelihood of **hyperprolactinemia** while hot flushes and inadequate vaginal lubrication would point toward amenorrhea on the basis of **ovarian failure.**

°Minimum evaluation of the amenorrheic patient should include a determination of luteinizing hormone, follicle-stimulating hormone, and prolactin levels and thyroid function tests.

•**Selection of patients for GnRH therapy:**

°Indications for GnRH therapy:

°°congenital GnRH deficiency

°°acquired GnRH deficiencies resulting from organic hypothalamic-pituitary disease

°°suppression of GnRH release as a result of physical, psychological, or nutritional stresses often have extremely low circulating gonadotropin levels and clinical features of hypoestrogenism.

°Delayed pubertal development because of complete or partial congenital deficiency of GnRH, appropriate steroid hormone replacement is first indicated to complete the pubertal transition.

°°When acquired GnRH deficiency has resulted in prolonged hypoestrogenism, endometrial priming with cyclic estrogen and progestin for several cycles before GnRH therapy is probably warranted.

°**Experimental uses of GnRH therapy:**

°**Polycystic ovary syndrome:** The most common pattern of chronic anovulation is that associated with polycystic ovary disease.

°°Elevated luteinizing hormone/follicle stimulating hormone ratios suggest excessive hypothalamic GnRH secretion and/or increase pituitary sensitivity to GnRH occasioned by tonic elevation in circulating estrogen concentrations.

°°**Clomiphene citrate**, which functions as a very weak estrogen, occupies the estrogen receptors of the hypothalamus and pituitary and thereby blocks the follicle-stimulating hormone inhibiting property of circulating estrogen.

°°There is a rise in circulating concentrations of follicle-stimulating hormone and resumption of follicular maturation.

°°Blockade of the negative feedback signal of estradiol carries with it the attendant risk of follicle-stimulating hormone oversecretion with the result that the number of mature follicles occasionally exceeds the normal ovulatory quotient for man.

°°The risk of multiple pregnancy in women treated with clomiphene citrate is reported to approximately 8%.

°°The antiestrogenic property of clomiphene citrate may impair cervical mucus production.

°In theory GnRH therapy should not be of benefit polycystic ovary syndrome.

°The luteinizing hormone/follicle-stimulating hormone ratio is partly attributed to the exaggerated pulsatile release of GnRH by the hypothalamus and increased pituitary sensitivity to pulses of GnRH.

°Excesses in either amplitude or frequency of GnRH pulses will lead to an increase in the luteinizing hormone/follicle stimulating hormone ratio, hence the addition of exogenous GnRH pulses when endogenous activity is already increased, in theory, should do nothing to improve the unfavorable gonadotropin profile unless the exogenous program overrides the natural one.

°Pregnancy rates in patients with polycystic ovary disease have been considerably lower than those reported for other patients receiving GnRH therapy.

°**Hyperprolactinemia**

°GnRH restores fertility in anovulation secondary to hyperprolactinemia.

°The euprolactinemic state is best restored by the use of **bromocriptine**.

°**Luteal phase defects and cervical mucus deficiency:**

°There are other simpler means to correct these problems.

°**Induction of multiple ovulation for in vitro fertilization**

°Large doses of intravenous GnRH can induce multiple follicles.

°**Resistant ovary syndrome.**

°Women with amenorrhea resulting from ovarian failure with premature depletion of oocytes should not respond to exogenous GnRH.

•**Practical application of GnRH therapy**

°Before the initiation of GnRH therapy an ultrasonogram should be obtained to assess the pretreatment status of the endometrium and ovaries.

°°endometriosis, can, on ultrasound, be confused with a developing follicle; hence, a baseline scan is valuable.

°Baseline determinations of luteinizing hormone, follicle-stimulating hormone, prolactin, and estradiol are worthwhile before treatment is initiated.

°Education of patients about the purpose of therapy, how to charge or refill the pump, and signs of symptoms of local or systemic infection is vital to the success and safety of outpatient GnRH therapy.

°Patients are initially started on subcutaneous GnRH therapy at a dosage of 5 μg every 2 hours.

°A first follow-up visit should be scheduled for 1 week after the initiation of therapy.

°Pelvic examination is conducted to determine whether estrogenic changes are developing in cervical mucus.

°If these changes are evident, ultrasound examination is scheduled to document the number and size of developing follicles.

°There is a close correlation between follicular diameter and peripheral plasma estradiol levels.

°Although 15 mm follicles may, on occasion, rupture, indicating ovulation, such follicles usually grow by 2 to 3 mm/day and reach diameters of 20 to 25 mm before ovulation occurs.

°As a rough "rule of thumb" ovulation can be expected to occur approximately 3 to 5 days after the follicle has reached 15 mm in diameter.

°When the follicle approaches 18 to 20 mm the patients are advised to have intercourse daily.

°If patients have shown no evidence of response by 10 days with subcutaneous therapy, the dosage is increased to 20 μg per pulse for a further 10 days.

°If the patient still has shown no evidence of response by 20 days the dosage may be increased 10 μg every 5 days until day 30; if no response is observed at this dosage, intravenous therapy should be initiated.

°Intravenous therapy is conducted by use of the basilic vein of the forearm with a long connecting tubing to the pump that is worn in a brassiere or about the waist, depending on the model.

°A dosage of 2.5 to 5 μg (approximating 75 to 100 ng/kg) every 90 minutes is used initially with increments every 10 days as indicated by clinical response.

°The average time from initiation of treatment of ovulation ranges from 10 to 20 days for intravenous infusion but may be as long as 15 to 30 days with subcutaneous treatment.

°In contradistinction to the situation in patients undergoing therapy with menopausal gonadotropins, in which case a spontaneous luteinizing hormone surge occurs infrequently, the experience with GnRH therapy indicates that a spontaneous luteinizing hormone surge is the norm for this treatment.

•Complications of GnRH therapy

°Subcutaneous delivery has been asssociated with hematomas at the site of subcutaneous needle or catheter insertion.

°°heparin is not necessary and is not used for delivery of GnRH.

°Local inflammation at the site of subcutaneous needle insertion is usually avoided by attention to proper sterile technique.

°Superficial phlebitis has been reported.

°Antibodies to exogenous GnRH have been found in patients born with a congenital deficiency of GnRH.

°°Both urticaria and an overt anaphylactic reaction have been reported in isolated cases after treatment cycles with exogenous GnRH.

°A search for anti-GnRH antibodies should be conducted if resistance to high dosages of GnRH becomes apparent in an individual who formerly responded to GnRH or in the presence of obvious allergic manifestations when GnRH is restarted.

°Ovarian hyperstimulation has been associated with large intravenous dosages of GnRH.

°°The incidence of multiple pregnancies resulting with GnRH therapy is estimated to be approximately 7%, with most of them being twins but with occasional reports of triplets.

°The rate of spontaneous abortion with GnRH therapy is approximately 20%, and compares favorably with the spontaneous abortion rate in the general population.]

Directions: Each set of lettered headings below is followed by a list of numbered words or phrases. For each numbered word or phrase select:

  A. if the item is associated with *(A) only*
  B. if the item is associated with *(B) only*
  C. if the item is associated with *both (A) and (B)*
  D. if the item is associated with *neither (A) nor (B)*

  A. ampullary tubal ectopic pregnancy
  B. isthmic tubal ectopic pregnancy
  C. both
  D. neither

19. salpingitis principal etiology   Ans: A

20. implantation more often intraluminal   Ans: A

21. absence of decidual reaction   Ans: D

---

p.941 (Sentermann M, Jibodh R, and Tulandi T, "Histopathologic study of ampullary and isthmic tubal ectopic pregnancy" Am J Obstet Gynecol 1988;159:939)

19-21. [F & I:•Background: Ampullary and infundibular pregnancies account for 85% to 95% of all tubal pregnancies; approximately 5% to 15% of tubal pregnancies occur in the isthmus.

   •Objective: to evaluate the effects of ampullary and isthmic pregnancies on the wall of the fallopian tube and detail the histopathologic changes.

  •Results: Most tubal ectopic pregnancies occur in the ampullary portion of the fallopian tube.

    °Isthmic pregnancies account for only 7.7% of all tubal pregnancies.

•In **ampullary** ectopic pregnancy, the implantation tends to be either intraluminal or mixed.

    °The mucosal layer is usually destroyed in both of these situations, although the destruction often involves only a small portion of the circumference of the mucosa.

    °The muscularis layer is usually preserved.

    °Blood vessels in the lamina propria and subserosa are invaded by trophoblast cells early in the gestation.

    °The resulting hemorrhage into the wall and lumen of the tube causes much more of the distortion of tubal anatomy than the products of conception.

    °Careful evacuation of these blood clots and the products of conception may allow such a tube to anatomically return to its prepregnancy state.

    °The disruption of the tubal wall in ampullary pregnancy is less severe than in isthmic pregnancy.

 •In **isthmic** ectopic pregnancy the implantation is usually extraluminal or mixed.

    °The muscularis is destroyed in more than half the cases.

•Mixed implantation, such as in ampullary pregnancy, is particularly destructive to both the mucosa and muscularis layers.

•**Decidual change**, which occurs in the tubal mucosa, is usually focal and much less developed than that seen in the endometrium of early pregnancy.

°The relative lack of a decidualized mucosa and the small-caliber lumen in the isthmus may allow earlier trophoblast invasion into the tubal wall and adjacent blood vessels.

•Chronic salpingitis is found in half of the cases of ampullary pregnancy and in only one third of isthmic pregnancies.

•**Delay in ovum transport** caused by external transmigration or factors inherent in the embryo itself, might be more important in the pathophysiology of isthmic pregnancy.

•In most ampullary pregnancies trophoblastic growth takes place **within** the tubal lumen, whereas in isthmic pregnancy, the trophoblast penetrates the tubal wall relatively early.

•Conclusion: Linear salpingostomy can be done for ampullary pregnancy without jeopardizing luminal integrity.]

    A. foremilk
    B. hindmilk
    C. both
    D. neither

22. primarily for hydration   Ans: A

23. primarily for energy   Ans: B

24. prolactin content significantly affects newborn fluid and electrolyte exchange   Ans: B

---

p.585   (Yuen BH, "Prolactin in human milk: The influence of nursing and the duration of postpartum lactation " Am J Obstet Gynecol 1988;158:583)

22-24. [F & I:•Background: **Prolactin** in milk is biologically potent and is absorbed by the newborn.

•In the intestine, prolactin influences fluid, sodium, potassium, and calcium transport.

°Intraductal application of prolactin stimulates milk formation locally in alveoli exposed to the hormone.

•Objective: to determine if prolactin concentrations varied in the milk of postpartum lactating mothers, from the initiation of lactation to weaning.

•Results: The levels of prolactin in milk varied with duration of puerperal lactation.

°The milk prolactin content was highest in the early transition milk immediately after the colostrum phase, then steadily declined but remained detectable in the mature milk until weaning occurred in lactating women observed up to 40 weeks post partum.

•The finding that **foremilk contained significantly higher prolactin concentrations** than the hindmilk indicates that prolactin enters the intra-alveolar mammary secretion **early** in the process of milk formation.

°Replenishment of milk removed from the breast during nursing occurs as a continuous process from the secretion of the mammary alveolar cells between episodes of milk removal.

°**The foremilk is low in fat but high in water as compared with the hindmilk.**

•The fat content as determined by the **creamatocrit** method confirms that the samples obtained were consistent with foremilk and hindmilk.

•Prolactin can influence intestinal fluid and solute transport, including that of calcium.

•Prolactin transmitted in the milk is absorbed by the newborn.

•Substances enter the intra-alveolar space by either the paracellular or the transcellular pathways.

°The former may account for the presence of prolactin in the intraalveolar secretions during the colostrum phase.

°The paracellular pathway is operative in the colostrum phase, when the junctions between alveolar cells are leaky.

•With the onset of lactogenesis, the copious phase of milk secretion by the mammary alveolar cells, the junctions between these cells become tight, and substances enter the alveolar secretions via the transcellular pathway.

°Thus, according to the data, the most likely explanation for the passage of prolactin into the intra-alveolar milk is via the transcellular pathway.

•Prolactin is present in milk secreted by women with the galactorrhea-amenorrhea syndrome.

°The prolactin content in milk in these abnormal states of lactation declines after treatment with bromocriptine, which suppresses the pituitary secretion of prolactin.

•The presence of higher prolactin levels in foremilk in breast-feeding women may simply reflect its pattern of excretion during milk formation.

°**Foremilk serves mainly to provide hydration to the newborn rather than caloric energy, which is concentrated in the high fat content of hindmilk.**

•Prolactin physiologic action on the intestine of the human neonate is unknown.

•Conclusion: The release of prolactin into the intra-alveolar milk was maximal during lactogenesis, the phase of copious milk secretion in the first week of the postpartum interval, then declined as lactation was established, but remained detectable in all milk samples studied until weaning occurred.

°Prolactin entered the milk with maximal release occurring in the aqueous foremilk.

°Transmission of prolactin to the suckling newborn occurred in the aqueous phase of the foremilk early in the course of nursing.

•The release of prolactin into the intra-alveolar secretions plays some role in the establishment and maintenance of lactation.

•The early transmission of prolactin in the aqueous foremilk to the suckling newborn infant has an obligatory effect on intestinal fluid and electrolyte exchange in the human newborn.]

Gynecologic Oncology

Directions: Each of the questions or incomplete statements below is followed by several suggested answers or completions. Select the BEST answer in each case.

1. Which of the following chemotherapeutic agents used for the treatment of advanced ovarian cancer is associated with the highest risk of recurrence after a negative second-look laparotomy?

    A. chlorambucil
    B. cisplatinum
    C. cyclophosphamide
    D. cytoxan
    E. doxorubicin

2. The role of human papilloma virus in carcinogenesis is one of

    A. activator
    B. blocker
    C. converter
    D. initiator
    E. promotor

3. In the absence of regional node metastases, what is the 5 year survival rate of early stage vulvar squamous cell carcinoma?

    A. 67
    B. 75
    C. 90
    D. 95
    E. 99

4. Which of the following is the most important factor ensuring success in the use of the split thickness graft in vaginal reconstruction following exenteration?

    A. concurrent versus delayed reconstruction
    B. no previous radiation therapy
    C. nulliparity
    D. preparation of graft bed
    E. type of obturator

5. The principle difference between vaginal lesions which resemble condylomata but are **not** associated with detectable human papilloma virus DNA and those that **are** associated with human papilloma virus DNA is

    A. acanthosis
    B. cellular disorganization at the basal zone
    C. increased mitotic activity
    D. koilocytotic atypia
    E. papillomatosis

6. Which of the following is most useful in the evaluation of cervical or uterine tumor spread?

    A. cystography
    B. cystoscopy
    C. cystosonography
    D. cytology of urine sediment
    E. intravesical endosonography

7. The most common site of metastasis of **adenocarcinoma** of the cervix is

    A. intraabdominal
    B. liver
    C. lung
    D. lymphatic
    E. vulva

8. After initial surgery and systemic chemotherapy, a patient has a reassessment laparotomy. In the presence of residual intraperitoneal ovarian cancer, what is the approximate % of peritoneal cytologic washings that will be positive?

    A. 10
    B. 30
    C. 50
    D. 70
    E. 90

9. What is the most active single chemotherapeutic agent in the treatment of leiomyosarcoma?

    A. actinomycin D
    B. adriamycin
    C. cisplatin
    D. doxorubicin
    E. methotrexate

10. Verrucous vulvar carcinoma is associated with papilloma virus type

    A. 6
    B. 11
    C. 16
    D. 18
    E. 33

11. Which complication precludes the use of abdominopelvic radiation in advanced ovarian carcinoma patients after appropriate chemotherapy and a negative second-look laparotomy?

    A. intestinal obstruction
    B. leukopenia
    C. thromboembolism
    D. urothelial fistula
    E. vomiting and diarrhea

12. What percentage of lymph node involvement in bulky (> 4 cm) locally advanced invasive squamous cell carcinoma of the cervix can be expected?

    A. 25
    B. 33
    C. 50
    D. 67
    E. 80

13. What is the most favorable prognostic factor in melanoma of the vulva?

    A. depth of invasion < 2 mm
    B. medial vulvar occurrence
    C. melanoma of the nodular type
    D. mode of therapy
    E. patient age > 50 years

14. The most prominent side effect of hydroxyurea when used in conjunction with radiation in the treatment of bulky cervical carcinoma is

    A. cardiotoxicity
    B. hematuria
    C. leukopenia
    D. nausea
    E. pulmonary fibrosis

15. The most common pure malignant germ cell tumor of the ovary is

    A. choriocarcinoma
    B. dysgerminoma
    C. embryonal cell tumor
    D. gonadoblastoma
    E. malignant teratoma

16. A patient with malignant trophoblastic disease is cured with chemotherapy. With regard to future childbearing she should be told that there is an increased

    A. chance of fetal wastage.
    B. chance of her getting lymphoma.
    C. incidence of congenital anomalies.
    D. incidence of placenta accreta.
    E. none of the above

17. Which papilloma virus type appears to be a marker for more rapid progression to cervical epithelial neoplasia?

    A. 6
    B. 11
    C. 16
    D. 18
    E. 31

18. Which preoperatively assessed factor is significantly associated with a poor prognosis in the surgical treatment of stage IB/IIA carcinoma of the cervix?

    A. tumor cell type
    B. cell differentiation
    C. channel invasion
    D. age > 50
    E. tumor size

19. When (weeks) during normal pregnancy is free serum β-hCG highest?

    A. 5
    B. 10
    C. 20
    D. 30
    E. 40

20. Which of the following factors has the LEAST effect on survival for endometrial adenocarcinoma?

    A. age
    B. clinical stage
    C. depth of myometrial invasion
    D. histopathologic grade
    E. presence of estradiol receptors

21. The LEAST critical outcome variable in superficially invasive squamous cell carcinoma of the cervix is

    A. depth of invasion
    B. lymph node metastases
    C. lymphvascular invasion
    D. number of quadrants of the cerix involved
    E. tumor grade

22. Positive cytologic washings in patients with endometrial carcinoma are associated with all of the following EXCEPT.

    A. adnexal involvement
    B. depth of myometrial invasion
    C. grade
    D involvement of the lower uterine segment
    E. para-aortic and pelvic node metastases

Directions: Each group of numbered words or phrases is preceded by a list of lettered statements. MATCH the lettered item most closely associated with the numbered word or phrase. Each item may be used once, more than once, or not at all.

    A. laminin
    B. plasma cholinesterase
    C. plasma urokinase-type plasminogen activator antigen
    D. serum 5-nucleotidase
    E. sulpiride

23. invasive squamous cell carcinoma of cervix

24. intact basement membrane

Directions: Each set of lettered headings below is followed by a list of numbered words or phrases. For each numbered word or phrase select:

A. if item is associated with (A) only
B. if item is associated with (B) only
C. if item is associated with both (A) and (B)
D. if item is associated with neither (A) nor (B)

In treating stage III/IV intraperitoneal ovarian epithelial malignancy:

    A. cisplatinum
    B. recombinant alpha-2 interferon
    C. both
    D. neither

25. response predicted by peritoneal malignant cell count

26. creates intense mesothelial reaction

27. induces a brisk influx of macrophages

In the diagnosis of endometrial adenocarcinoma:

    A. office curettage
    B. operating room curettage
    C. both
    D. neither

28. grade will be increased in more than 10% of patients post-hysterectomy

29. more than 95% of uteri will have residual disease found after curettage

30. findings can obviate need for node sampling

    A. ovarian carcinoma
    B. fallopian tube carcinoma
    C. both
    D. neither

31. prognosis depends on residual disease

32. survival depends on tumor grade

33. survival improved with cis-platinum multiagent therapy

34. associated with low parity and infertility

    A. placental site trophoblastic tumor
    B. hydatidiform mole
    C. both
    D. neither

35. sensitive to chemotherapeutic drugs

36. fatal if untreated

37. hCG serves as a tumor marker

Gynecologic Oncology- References

Directions: Each of the questions or incomplete statements below is followed by several suggested answers or completions. Select the BEST answer in each case.

1. Which of the following chemotherapeutic agents used for the treatment of advanced ovarian cancer is associated with the highest risk of recurrence after a negative second-look laparotomy?

    A. chlorambucil
    *B.   cisplatinum
    C. cyclophosphamide
    D. cytoxan
    E. doxorubicin

p.1094   (Rubin SC, Hoskins WJ, Hakes TB, Markman M, Cain JM, and Lewis JL Jr., "Recurrence after negative second-look laparotomy of ovarian cancer: Analysis of risk factors ," Am J Obstet Gynec   1988; 159:1094)

1. [Facts and Issues:•Background: The likelihood of being free of disease at second-look laparotomy is related to initial stage of disease, histologic grade of tumor, and the amount of tumor remaining after primary surgery.

•Lack of detection of ovarian cancer at second look laparotomy is not synonymous with a cure.

•Recurrence of disease after negative second look laparomtomy with recurrence rates approximately 25%.

•Objective: to review patients having negative second look laparotomy.

•Results: A negative second look laparotomy after platinum-based chemotherapy has much different significance than that after nonplatinum chemotherapy.

°In patients with stage II, III and IV disease treated with platinum-based chemotherapy, the overall recurrence rate was 50%, with a median interval to recurrence of 14 months compared with a recurrence rate of 25% and a median interval to recurrence of 23 months in the nonplatinum group.

•The reasons for this higher recurrence rate after platinum based treatment probably relate to the **higher response rates and shorter duration of administration** of this type of chemotherapy compared with single agent or nonplatinum combintion regimens.

•Because platinum based regimens are generally given for a shorter duration than a single agent or nonplatinum combination regimens, patients are required to remain clinically free of disease for a shorter period of time before second look laparotomy.

•There is no clear difference in the likelihood of negative findings at second look lapartomy with platinum regimens compared to nonplatinum regimens.

•If the risk of recurrence by chemotherapy type beginning at 24 months for each group, the likelihood of relapse would be about equal.]

2. The role of human papilloma virus in carcinogenesis is one of

    A. activator
    B. blocker
    C. converter
    D. initiator
    *E.   promotor

p.1255   (Iwasaka T, Yokoyama M, Hayashi Y, and Sugimori H, "Combined herpes simplex virus type 2 and human papillomavirus type 16 or 18 deoxyribonucleic acid leads to oncogenic transformation," Am J Obstet Gynec   1988; 159:1251)

2. [Facts and Issues:•Objectives:

    °1) to test the tumorogenic activity of HPV 16 and HPV 18 on normal diploid cells, and

    °2) to observe whether carcinogenesis would occur by combining HSV 2 as the initiator and HPV 16 or HPV 18 as a promotor.

•Results: The role of HPVs in carcinogenesis is one of promoter.

°Carcinogenesis might be mediated by the combination of HSV 2 and HPV DNA.

•The **hit and run theory:**

°When the HPV 18 DNA is incorporated into cellular DNA, expression or insertion of HPV sequences induces cellular oncogene amplification or expresion and consequently the immortalized cell line is converted to a tumorigenic one.

•Different events related to the viral oncogenesis between HPV 16 and HPV 18 might result from differences in affinity to cellular DNA or to differences in the facility to delete from the transformed cells.

•HPV 16 DNA sequences are detected more frequently in cervical cancer tissue than of those of HPV 18 DNA.]

3. In the absence of regional node metastases, what is the 5 year survival rate of early stage vulvar squamous cell carcinoma?

    A. 67
    B. 75
    *C.   90
    D. 95
    E. 99

p.715   (Burrell MO, Franklin EW III, Campion MJ, Crozier MA, and Stacy DW, "The modified radical vulvectomy with groin dissection: An eight-year experience " Am J Obstet Gynecol 1988;159:715)

3. [F & I:•Background: Surgery is the standard managment of squamous cell carcinoma of the vulva.

•Primary invasive vulvar carcinoma is often detected as a small, early stage tumor.

•In the absence of regional node involvement, early-stage vulvar carcinoma has a 90% 5-year survival rate.

•Lymph node metastases have not been reported with squamous vulvar carcinoma with <1 mm of invasion.

°Such lesions are described as microinvasive and lymphadenectomy is not considered necessary.

°For tumor with >1 mm of invasion, there is a risk of nodal involvement, including carcinoma with 2 to 5 mm of invasion, which has been classified "microinvasive."

•A treatment modification of vulvar carcinoma of >1 mm depth of invasion, incorporates a full bilateral inguinofemoral lymphadenectomy but local dissections less than a full radical vulvectomy.

•Objective: to review experience with 51 cases of vulvar squamous cell carcinoma >1 mm of invasion.

•Surgical approach: In 35 cases, separate groin incisions involving a skin bridge were used and in 40 patients the inguinofemoral lymph nodes were removed en bloc bilaterally with ligation of the lumphatics at the medial edge of the wound.

•Sartorius muscle transfer to cover the femoral vessels and sump drainage was used bilaterally.

•The presence of positive lymph nodes in stage I disease with minimal invasion of 4 and $2\frac{1}{2}$ mm reflects the belief that patients with depth of invasion between 1-5 mm are at risk for lymph node metastases.

°The lack of contralateral involvement without ipsilateral involvement suggests that dissection can be limited to a unilateral lymphadectomy.]

---

4. Which of the following is the most important factor ensuring success in the use of the split thickness graft in vaginal reconstruction following exenteration?

    A. concurrent versus delayed reconstruction
    B. no previous radiation therapy
    C. nulliparity
    *D.   preparation of graft bed
    E. type of obturator

---

p.913   (Beemer W, Hopkins MP, and Morley GW, "Vaginal reconstruction in gynecologic onocology," Obstet Gynec   1988; 72:911)

4. [Facts and Issues: •Objectives: to update experience with the split-thickness skin graft, vaginoplasty after pelvic exenteration and to study the use of this type of vaginal reconstruction after other therapies for gynecologic malignancies.

•Surgery can be performed successfully at varying intervals relative to extirpative surgery.

°There is no increase in technical difficulty; surgery is actually easier because of a smaller cavity when performed sometime after the extirpative procedure.

•In patients undergoing hysterectomy and vaginectomy, the split thickness skin graft is favored because the cavity is not large and a myocutaneous graft may narrow the vagina unnecessarily.

•There is no difference in the rate of infection or the eventual outcome in patients for whom **glass obturators** were used as compared with cotton packs.

°The obturator type may not be as important as the proper preparation of the graft bed and fitting of the obturator.

•There was no significant difference in the **graft take** between women with an eventual satisfactory outcome versus and unsatisfactory result.

•**Previous radiation** therapy did not appear to be a contraindication to successful vaginal reconstruction; satisfactory results were achieved at comparable rates in patients with and without previous radiation therapy.

•In patients with a poor outcome, the interval betweeen procedures, percent graft take, obturator choice, or presence of infection did not seem to dictate eventual degree of success.]

---

5. The principle difference between vaginal lesions which resemble condylomata but are **not** associated with detectable human papilloma virus DNA and those that **are** associated with human papilloma virus DNA is

    A. acanthosis
    B. cellular disorganization at the basal zone
    C. increased mitotic activity
    *D.   koilocytotic atypia
    E. papillomatosis

---

p.771   (Nuovo GJ, Blanco JS, Silverstein SJ, and Crum CP, "Histologic correlates of papillomavirus infection of the vagina" Obstet Gynecol 1988;72:770)

5. [F & I:•Background: Human papillomavirus is in most condylomata from the cervix, vagina and vulva.

°These lesions which often regress frequently contain HPV viruses type 6 and 11.

•HPV types which predominate in in carcinoma of the female genital tract, include HPV 16, 18, 31, 33, and 35.

°There is not an absolute correlation between histology, viral type, and biologic behavior.

•The colposcopic appearance of HPV-associated lesions is highly variable.

°The diagnosis depends on the presence of koilocytotic atypia, characterized by superficial cells with perinuclear halos and marked nuclear atypia, including frequent bi- and multinucleate forms.

•Higher-grade lesions (vaginal intraepithelial neoplasias) are differentiated from condylomata by increased mitotic activity, atypical mitotic forms, and a greater degree of nuclear atypia and cellular disorganization toward the basal zone.

•Clinically lesions that resemble condyloma may contain histologic findings such as acanthosis, papillomatosis and perinuclear halos, the degree of nuclear atypia may be insufficient for precise diagnosis of condyloma.

°Terms such as early condyloma, mild condyloma or borderline condyloma are used to describe these lesions

•Epithelial changes that do not fulfill the conventional histologic criteria for diagnosis for condyloma or intraepithelial neoplasia may or may not be actually related to HPV infection.

•Material and Methods: 39 women referred because of abnormal Papanicolau smears and had vaginal lesions clinically resembling condylomata.

•Results: Some vaginal lesions that resemble condyloma are not associated with detectable HPV DNA.

•Histologically the principal difference between this group of vaginal lesions and those associated with HPV DNA was an absence of clear-cut **koilocytotic atypia and multinucleation.**

•The **tissue** changes associated with HPV infection overlap with non HPV associated changes.

•These include papillary mucosal excrescences; **histologic** changes include acanthosis, papillomatosis, and cytoplasmic halos with mild nuclear changes.]

---

6.   Which of the following is most useful in the evaluation of cervical or uterine tumor spread?

    A.   cystography
    B.   cystoscopy
    C.   cystosonography
    D.   cytology of urine sediment
    *E.   intravesical endosonography

---

p.952   (Koelbl H and Bernaschek G, "Cystosonography: A diagnostic adjunct for the staging of advanced gynecologic malignancies," Obstet Gynec   1988; 72:951)

6. [Facts and Issues:•Background: Cystoscopy is essential for pretherapeutic assessment of bladder wall invasion or displacement.

°Even though tumor invasion of the bladder wall may be optically and bioptically diagnosed, the mere evidence of mucosal edema is not a reliable indicator of bladder wall invasion.

•Cystosonography is a transurethral endosonographic technique routinely used in urology for the diagnosis of bladder tumors.

•Objective: to compare the cystoscopic and cystosonography findings in patients with advanced gynecologic malignancies.

•Negative cytstoscopic findings probably do **not** exclude bladder involvement of the outer layers in patients with gynecologic malignancies.

•Cystoscopic and cystosonographic findings were normal in three patients with advanced gynecologic malignancies.

•Intravesical endosonography can detect tumor invasion of the external layers of the bladder even in cases of clinically defined early staged disease.

•Cystoscopy should precede intravesical endosonography to exclude intraurethral or intravesical pathology and to avoid hemorrhage or inadvertant damage to anatomical structures.]

---

7.   The most common site of metastasis of **adenocarcinoma** of the cervix is

    A.   intraabdominal
    B.   liver
    *C.   lung
    D.   lymphatic
    E.   vulva

---

p.795   (Hopkins MP, Schmidt RW, Roberts JA, and Morley GW, "Gland cell carcinoma (adenocarcinoma) of the cervix" Obstet Gynecol 1988;72:789)

7. [F & I:•Background: Gland cell carcinoma has been replaced by the term adenocarcinoma.

°There are a variety of adenocarcinoma subtypes, each having a different survival.

°There may be a varying prognosis based on the histologic subtype.

•Objective: to determine the prognostic features of adenocarcinoma.

•Material and Methods: Cervical adenocarcinomas: endovervical (adeniform), adenosquamous, papillary, mucoid, and clear cell were classified.

°Tumor grades were assigned using histologic and cytologic features: the endocervical or **adeniform** subtype was the least difficult to grade.

°Tumors of **adenosquamous** type contained definite foci of both squamous and glandular diggerentiation, generally within any single low-power field.

°**papillary** tumors were characterized by prominent delicate papillation with little stroma; they were graded according to cytologic features and were generally well-differentiated.

°**mucinous** tumors generally contained large lakes of mucin that contained, or were surrounded by, large mucin-containing cells that often produced papillations.

•**Clear-cell** tumors were variable in appearance with tubular, microcystic, and solid patterns; the cells either contained abundant clear cytoplasm that was periodic acid-Schiff-positive or had a typical hobnail configuration.

•Results: The distribution of clinical parameters associated with the various adenocarcinoma subtypes showed no significant difference when the following features were evaluated: stage of disease, size of lesion, age, lymph node status, parity, obesity, hypertension, diabetes, symptoms of bleeding, or oral contraceptive usage.

•Stage for stage, there was no significant difference in survival by adenocarcinoma subtypes.

•**Lung was the most common site of distant disease.**

•There was no significant difference in survival between the various subtypes of disease.

•The histologic grade of the malignancy in adenocarcinoma of the cervix influences prognosis, with the poorly differentiated lesions having the worst prognosis.

•The stage of disease is a critical factor influencing survival.

°Unlike squamous cell carcinoma, in which a percentage of patients with advanced stage III disease can be expected to survive, advance stage adenocarcinoma of the cervix appears to carry a very poor prognosis regardless of subtype with few patients surviving.

•The advanced stage adenocarcinomas were treated by conventional radiation therapy.

°There is an improved survival over radiation therapy alone for stages II and III lesions with adjuvant hysterectomy.

°Only a small percentage of patients had local recurrence which would suggest that adjuvant surgery would benefit only a small number of patients.

•The age of the patient was a predictor of survival.

°The older age group was more likely to have advance stage of disease in an extended interval between pelvic examinations contributing to their decreased survival.

•Symptoms of bleeding may also occur late after the disease has spread beyond the cervix.

°This highlights the importance of endocervical sampling which may be difficult in the post-menopausal cervix.

•The decreased survival in the elderly patients with adenocarcinoma of the cervix appears to contrast with squamous cell disease for which there is a decreased survival in the younger patients.]

---

8. After initial surgery and systemic chemotherapy, a patient has a reassessment laparotomy. In the presence of residual intraperitoneal ovarian cancer, what is the approximate % of peritoneal cytologic washings that will be positive?

     A. 10
     *B.   30
     C. 50
     D. 70
     E. 90

---

p.852   (Rubin SC, Dulaney ED, Markman M, Hoskins WJ, Saigo PE and Lewis JL, "Peritoneal cytology as an indicator of disease in patients with residual ovarian carcinoma" Obstet Gynecol 1988;71:851)

8. [F & I:•Background: Ovarian cancer spreads primarily by exfoliation of cells within the peritoneal cavity.

°Cytologic assessment of ascitic fluid or peritoneal washings are important in evaluating patients with ovarian cancer, and is a standard procedure used during second-look laparotomy.

•The major drawback to cytologic assessment of ovarian cancer has been **uncertainty over the technique's reliability.**

°Cytology at second-look laparotomy fails to detect malignancy in 47- 86% of patients with residual disease.

•Objective: to determine the reliability of peritoneal cytology in the detection of residual ovarian cancer during surgical reassessment.

•Materials and Methods: Ascitic fluid or peritoneal washings were obtained during 96 reassessment laparotomies that were biopsy positive for residual ovarian cancer.

•Results: Cytologic studies performed on specimens obtained at reassessment laparotomy after initial surgery and systemic chemotherapy **fail to detect malignancy in approximately 70% of laparotomies with residual intraperitoneal ovarian cancer.**

•Size of residual tumor, cell type, histologic grade, and initial stage of disease did **not** influence the reliability of cytologic assessment.

•Ascitic fluid cytology may be more reliable than those done on peritoneal washings.

•Cytologic studies done at surgical reassessment may be **less** reliable than those done at primary surgery.

•Conclusion: The most significant finding of the study is that peritoneal cytology does **not** reliably detect ovarian cancer in patients undergoing surgical reassessment.]

---

9.   What is the most active single chemotherapeutic agent in the treatment of leiomyosarcoma?

    A.   actinomycin D
    B.   adriamycin
    C.   cisplatin
    *D.   doxorubicin
    E.   methotrexate

p.849   (Berchuck A, Rubin SC, Hoskins WJ Saigo, PE, Pierce VK and Lewis JL, "Treatment of Uterine Leiomyosarcoma" Obstet Gynecol 1988;71:845)

9. [F & I:•Background: Leiomyosarcomas are rare tumors that account for approximately 25% of uterine sarcomas and 1% of all uterine malignancies.

•The histologic hallmarks of malignancy in these uterine smooth-muscle tumors are an **increased frequency of mitoses and cellular atypia.**

•The treatment of uterine leiomyosarcoma is primarily **surgical** and clinical trials designed to evaluate the effect of multimodal therapy, including radiation and chemotherapy, do not show any improvement in survival.

•Material and Methods: Uterine leiomyosarcoma was defined histologically as any tumor of uterine smooth-muscle origin with cytologic atypia and **5** or more mitoses per **ten** high-power fields.

•Uterine leiomyosarcoma is usually confined to the uterus at the time of diagnosis, but is a highly lethal disease.

•An overall disease-free survival rate of 22% was found in this study.

    °All survivors initially had stage I disease.

•Survival rates for patients with stage I and stage II disease was 29%.

•The poor prognosis of uterine leiomyosarcoma is due to its propensity to recur both locally in the pelvis and at distant sites, most notably the lungs, even when the initial surgical resection is apparently complete.

•Because of this pattern of widespread recurrence, **radiation therapy has not been appropriate** for treatment of recurrent disease.

•Uterine leiomyosarcoma may be the least radiosensitive of the three common histologic types of uterine sarcoma.

•**Doxorubicin** has proved the most active single agent in these tumors, with response rates up to 40%.

    °Several drugs including dimethyltriazenoimidazole, methotrexate,dactinomycin, and cyclophosphamide have produced response rates of 10-20% as single agents in the treatment of advanced and recurrent uterine and adult soft-tissue sarcomas.

•Combination chemotherapy regimens are **not** significantly superior to single-agent therapy.

•Reasons why uterine sarcomas have been considered appropriate malignancies in which to use adjuvant chemotherapy.

°1. Although gross disease in confined to the uterus, most patients have microscopic metastatic disease at the time of surgery.

°2. Most patients develop widespread recurrent disease and die rapidly.

°3. Chemotherapeutic agents with moderate activity are available.

•For patients with advanced or recurrent leiomyosarcoma, chemotherapy and/or radiation must be considered palliative, and it is often ineffective even for palliation.]

---

10. Verrucous vulvar carcinoma is associated with papilloma virus type

*A.   6
B. 11
C. 16
D. 18
E. 33

---

p.605   (Buscema J, Naghashfar Z, Sawada E, Daniel R, Woodruff JD, Shah K, "The predominance of human papillomavirus type 16 in vulvar neoplasia " Obstet Gynecol 1988;71:601)

10. [F & I: Background: Approximately 12 of the 45 known human papillomaviruses infect the genital tract.

•Among these, type 6 and type 11 are largely responsible for benign exophytic condylomas and are associated with flat cervical condylomas, atypical condylomas and milder grades of cervical intraepithelial neoplasia.

•Type 16 and 18 exist in some benign lesions and constitute the main virus types of high-grade cervical intraepithelial neoplasia and invasive epidermoid lesions of the cervix.

°Human papillomavirus 31 has been described in a spectrum of cervical lesions.

•A high proportion of intraepithelial neoplasia in the lower tract is multicentric.

•Objective: to examine the association of human papillomaviruses with vulvar and vaginal lesions.

°Types 6 and 11 were the predominant viruses of condyloma acuminata; type 16 was also identified in some condylomata.

°Type 16 was associated with vulvar intraepithelial neoplasia lesions; type 6 or type 11 were never recovered from these lesions.

•Conclusion: There is a possibility that an "atypical condyloma" harboring type 16 is the precursor of vulvar malignancy.

•The association of individual human papillomavirus types with lesions of specific histopathology suggests a causative role of papillomaviruses in lower genital tract neoplasia.

•Multicentric epidermoid neoplasia in the lower genital tract is best explained by a field effect of a carcinogen.

°The exposure of many sites in the genital tract to viral agents that routinely cause benign papillomatous proliferation may contribute to carcinogenesis.

°The cervical transformation zone, with its rapid turnover of metaplastic epithelium, makes this site vulnerable to virally induced proliferation.

°°The susceptibility of the transformation zone explains the relatively large numbers of intraepithelial and invasive neoplasms of the cervix as compared with other sites in the lower genital tract.

•Type 6 and 11 are associated with benign condylomas and milder forms of intraepithelial neoplasia. Types 16 and 18 are consistently associated with more severe dysplasia.

°Type 16 and 18 are the most frequently identified papillomaviruses in invasive cervical neoplasms.

°In many invasive cervical cancers, viral DNA is integrated within the host cell chromosomes.

°°The integration site on the viral genome is specific.

°°The early viral genes are transcribed and early proteins are expressed in malignant cells.

•Among the vulvar and vaginal lesions studied, most were identified in condyloma acuminatum as type 6/11.

°21% of DNA positive condylomas contained type 16 or type 18.

°The inability to detect human papillomaviruses in 19% of histopathologically proved condylomas may be because bisection of small colposcopically derived tissue yields minimal diseased epithelium for virologic diagnosis.

•Among vulvar intraepithelial lesions type 6 and 11 could not be identified, and type 16 predominated.

°The invasive neoplasms harbored type 16 with the exception of a verrucous carcinoma, which contained type 6/11.

°**Verrucous carcinoma** is a locally invasive neoplasm with no propensity for dissemination; its association with type 6 has been reported.

•Conclusion: Human papillomavirus type 16 appears to be the predominant type in vulvar neoplasia.

°Its presence in most high-grade vulvar intraepithelial neoplasia lesions and in invasive squamous cancers, and the exclusion of type 6/11 in these lesions, suggests that type 16 may be the oncogenic virus at this location.]

---

11. Which complication precludes the use of abdominopelvic radiation in advanced ovarian carcinoma patients after appropriate chemotherapy and a negative second-look laparotomy?

    *A.   intestinal obstruction
    B. leukopenia
    C. thromboembolism
    D. urothelial fistula
    E. vomiting and diarrhea

---

p.329   (Shelley WE, Starreveld AA, Carmichael JA, O'Connell G, Roy M, Swenerton K, "Toxicity of abdominopelvic radiation in advanced ovarian carcinoma patients after Cisplatin/Cyclophosphamide therapy and second look laparotomy " Obstet Gynecol 1988;71:327)

11. [F & I: •Objective: to determine the effectiveness of abdominopelvic radiation in patients with advanced ovarian carcinoma who had minimal residual disease after cisplatin-based therapy and second-look laparotomy.

•Results: It proved feasible to deliver the radiotherapy dosage planned for this series in patients who had been previously treated with cyclophosphamide and cisplatin and who had at least two previous laparotomies.

°Nineteen (70%) of the 27 patients received the full dose of treatment without interruption, and only three were unable to complete treatment.

•The incidence of serious late toxicity was of concern.

•After a median duration of follow-up of 17 months since the completion of radiotherapy, 14 (48%) of 27 patients experienced **bowel obstruction,** ten (37%) requiring surgery.

•Thirteen of 27 patients developed clinically detectable progressive cancer, and five (38%) of the thirteen required surgery for bowel obstruction.

•Previous radiation therapy increases the risk of bowel obstruction requiring surgery in patients with recurrent ovarian cancer.

•Conclusion: The curative potential of this treatment modality at this dosage is not as great as initially anticipated.

•The treatment has been modified by eliminating the pelvic boost, so the the entire abdominopelvic field receives a maximum dose of 2250 cGy.]

---

12. What percentage of lymph node involvement in bulky (> 4 cm) locally advanced invasive squamous cell carcinoma of the cervix can be expected?

    A. 25
    B. 33
    C. 50
    D. 67
    *E.   80

p.347   (Panici PB, Scambia G, Greggi S, Roberto PD, Baiocchi G, and Mancuso S, "Neoadjuvant chemotherapy and radical surgery in locally advanced cervical carcinoma: A pilot study. " Obstet Gynecol 1988;71:344)

12. [F & I: •Background: Using combined aggressive surgery and radiotherapy, prognosis of patients with locally advanced cervical carcinoma (tumor volume greater than 4 cm) is poor.

°The two-year disease-free survival ranges from 10-50%.

°Treatment failures occur from local and regional recurrence, and from distant recurrence.

•Distant metastases are present at diagnosis in 10-15% of patients at all stages, and the percentage is higher for locally advanced disease.

•Cisplatin-containing regimens are effective in primary untreated cervical carcinoma and recurrent disease in areas not previously irradiated.

•Objective: to evaluate the toxicity and efficacy in terms of clinical response, operability, and pathologic response in 33 consecutive patients with locally advanced primary cervical carcinoma treated with cisplatin, bleomycin, and methotrexate neoadjuvant chemotherapy followed by radical surgery.

•The mean duration of surgery was 380 minutes, with an average blood loss of 700 mL.

•Intraoperative complications arose in only two cases:

°hemorrhage (blood loss about 3000 mL) because of a lesion of the left common iliac vein, and

°a lesion of the lower tract of the left ureter which was repaired by surgical reimplant.

•Results: cisplatin, bleomycin, and methotrexate combination is feasible in a neoadjuvant setting in patients with locally advanced cervical cancer.

°A remarkable clinical and pathologic response rates observed, 75.7 and $54\frac{1}{2}$%, respectively, indicate that cervical cancer is a chemosensitive tumor.

•Cisplatin, bleomycin, and methotrexate therapy permitted surgical treatment in a high percentage of patients (75.7%) despite initial bulky tumor.

°Vaginal disease had the highest regression rate at histologic examination (80%), followed by cervical (72%) and parametrial disease (63.1%).

•**Lymph node involvement in bulky disease is expected in up to 80%.**

°Less than 20% lymph node involvement suggests a beneficial role of neoadjuvant chemotherapy.

•The toxicity was limited to nausea and vomiting.

•Radical surgery was not compromised by chemotherapy, but was challenging because the entire site of original invasion had large tumor extension.

•Postoperative complications included lymphocysts and deep venous thromboses, which occurred despite prophylactic heparin therapy.

•Surgery permitted histologic evaluation which providedthe basis for postoperative treatment.

°Four complete responders had no further treatment, the four with lymph node metastases had further chemotherapy, and the one patient with positive surgical resection margins had radiation therapy.]

---

13. What is the most favorable prognostic factor in melanoma of the vulva?

    *A.   depth of invasion < 2 mm
    B.   medial vulvar occurrence
    C.   melanoma of the nodular type
    D.   mode of therapy
    E.   patient age > 50 years

---

p.55   (Rose P, Piver S, Tsukada Y, and Lau T. "Conservative therapy for melanoma of the vulva," Am J Obstet Gynec 1988; 159:52)

13. [F & I:•Background: For vulvar lesions less radical surgical resection of melanoma is equally as effective as a traditional radical approach.

°This is true for both early lesions without nodal involvement and advanced lesions for which metastatic nodal or distant disease precludes benefit from extensive local resection.

•**The most significant pathologic variable is the depth of tumor invasion,** which is highly correlated with lymph node metastasis.

°The presence of regional nodal metastasis dramatically decreases 5-year survival from 76% to 31%.

•Objective: to report the results of patients treated with less radical surgery who had favorable prognostic variables.

•Material and Methods: Pathologic slides were reviewed and evaluated for melanoma histology, depth of invasion according to Brelow, mitotic count per 10 high-power fields, vascular invasion, lymphocytic infiltration, and the presence of ulceration.

•Radical therapy consisted of classic Basset's vulvectomy.

•Recurrences were classified as local, regional nodal, distant, or none.

•36 patients with primary vulvar melanoma were studied.

°10 patients were excluded, 8 of whom were treated with radiation therapy in combination with local therapy, one who had stage IV disease with lung metastasis at presentation, and one was not treated because of advanced age (94 years old).

•Results: For all patients survival correlated with **depth of invasion**.

°Younger patient age resulted in improved patient survival but was not dependent on depth of invasion.

•Survival was not worsened by mode of therapy when local and radical treatment groups were compared.

•8 patients who received conservative therapy via local excision (with 2 cm margins) for early lesion (<2 mm) have a high disease free survival rate (75%).

•Age was statistically correlated with increased survival but not with depth of invasion.

•Younger age is associated with more frequent superficial spreading melanoma and overall less melanoma invasion.]

---

14. The most prominent side effect of hydroxyurea when used in conjunction with radiation in the treatment of bulky cervical carcinoma is

    A. cardiotoxicity
    B. hematuria
    *C.   leukopenia
    D. nausea
    E. pulmonary fibrosis

---

p.92   (Stehman FB, Bundy BN, Keys H, Currie JL, Mortel R, and Creasman WT. "A randomized trial of hydroxyurea versus misonidazole adjunct to radiation therapy in carcinoma of the cervix," Am J Obstet Gynec 1988; 159:87)

14. [F & I:•Background: Bulky carcinoma of the cervix contains hypoxic cells that are more resistant to radiation than oxygenated cells.

°This could account for failure of treatment in the pelvis in patients receiving radiation therapy.

•Techniques used to enhance the effect of radiation therapy include: hyperthermia, hyperbaric oxygen, hyperfractionation, and concurrent chemotherapy.

•The administration of hydroxyurea to a standard radiation therapy regimen in advanced cervical cancer gave a statistically significant improvement of survival.

•The nitroimidazoles appear to have the pharmacologic characteristics of selectively sensitizing hypoxic tumor cells to radiation injury.

°Misonidazole, the first of this group of drugs put into clinical trials, has an oxygen enhancement ratio of 1.2 to 2.4.

•Material and Methods: to be eligible for study patients were required to have biopsy-proved untreated invasive carcinoma of the cervix, clinical stages (FIGO) IIB, IIIA, IIIB, or IVA.

°All patients had normal renal, hepatic, and marrow function and were free of infection, sepsis, or medical contraindications to surgery.

•Patients with metastatic disease involving the periaortic nodes or intra-abdominal contents were ineligible for this study.

•All patients were treated with standardized radiation therapy irrespective of randomization arm.

°Total dose was determined by clinical stage.

°Patients with stage IIB lesions received 40.00 Gy external therapy over 4 to 5 weeks and 40.00 Gy to point "A" from either one or two intracavitary implants.

°A minimum dose of 55.00 Gy to point "B" was delivered by the use of a parametrial boost.

•Patients with stages III or IVA lesions received 50.00 to 60.00 Gy over 50 to 8 weeks and 20.00 to 35.00 Gy to point "A" from either one or two intracavitary applications.

°A minimum dose of 55.00 Gy to point "B" was delivered by the use of parametrial boost.

•External therapy was delivered by radiation sources with a peak energy 1 MeV Cobalt-60 irradiator.

•Hydroxyuria in 500 mg capsules was administered in a single oral dose of 80 mg/kg body weight rounded to the nearest 500 mg (not to exceed 6000 mg) at least 2 hours before external radiation each Monday and Thursday for the duration of external therapy.

°Drug was withheld if the white blood cell count was <3000 cells/mm or platelets <100,000 cells/mm.

•Misonidazole was provided in 100 and 500 mg capsules and administered as a single oral dose of 1 gm/mm^3 rounded to the nearest 100 mg 4 hours before external radiation each Monday and Thursday and continued through external therapy to a maximum cumulative dose of 12 gm/m^2.

°Blood samples for measurement of serum misonidazole levels were drawn 24 hours after the first dose to assess initial metabolism of the drug.

•The accrual goal of 135 patients per regimen was determined to detect a 15% increase in survival by the misonidazole regimen relative to the hydroxyurea regimen (estimated to be 65% at 2 years).

•The principle evaluation parameters were:

°**progression-free interval,** defined as the time from date of entry into protocol to the date of reappearance of disease;

°**survival**, defined as observed length of life from entry into protocol or, for living patients, the date of last contact; and adverse effects, as scored by the Gynecologic Oncology Group adverse effects criteria.

•296 patients were studied.

°139 were randomized to receive hydroxyurea and 157 were randomized to receive misonidazole.

•Marrow suppression (predominantly total white blood cell count <2000 cells/mm^3) was more common among the patients receiving hydroxyurea as was gastrointestinal toxicity (predominantly nausea or vomiting leading to dehydration or requiring hospitalization).

•Central and peripheral neurologic adverse effects occurred more frequently among the patients receiving misonidazole.

•Control of pelvic disease is a significant component of cure on which improved survival in cervical carcinoma depends.

•Bulky carcinoma of the cervix can contain central nests of poorly vascularized, necrotic, and hypoxic cells that are more resistant to the effects of ionizing radiation than are well-oxygenated cells.

•Innovative attempts to improve local control will fail when periaortic nodes are positive.

•Hydroxyurea's mechanism of action is not certain.

°Hydroxyurea probably kills cells in the S phase of the cell cycle, and prevents cells in G_1 from entering the S phase.

°This leads to a synchronization at the sensitive G_1/S interface when radiation is delivered.

°Hydroxyurea might prevent the repair of sublethal radiation damage.

•There was no increase in radiation-associated complications such as skin injury, fistula formation, or bowel obstruction.

•Although hydroxyurea does not appear to sensitize normal tissues to radiation injury, it does have adverse effects.

°The most prominent of these is **leukopenia**.

•Misonidazole sensitizes hypoxic tumor cells through its **electron affinity,** thus stabilizing the radiation effect upon the cells.

°These drugs are highly lipid soluble, which permits adequate tissue levels in poorly vascularized hypoxic and necrotic tumors.

•The incidence of peripheral sensory neuropathy limited the cumulative dose, with an incidence of 36% below 12 gm/m^2 and 74% above 12 gm/m^2.

•Misonidazole appears not to be an ideal radiosensitizer.

•The differences in median survival appear to be attributable to an excess number of extrapelvic failures in the misonidazole arm rather than poorer pelvic control.

•Results: There is no statistically significant difference in progression-free interval or survival between the two regimens.

°The subset of patients with more advanced disease who received hydroxyurea had a better progression-free interval than their counterparts who received misonidazole, although there was no difference between the regimens for patients with stage II disease.

•There was better pelvic control with the hydroxyurea regimen.

°Failure limited to the pelvis occurred in 18% of patients receiving misonidazole.

•Conclusion: Hydroxyurea is the more appropriate potentiator in patients with bulky cervix cancers.]

---

15. The most common pure malignant germ cell tumor of the ovary is

    A. choriocarcinoma
    *B.   dysgerminoma
    C. embryonal cell tumor
    D. gonadoblastoma
    E. malignant teratoma

---

p.591   (Gallion HH, Van Nagell JR, Donaldson ES, and Powell DE, "Ovarian dysgerminoma: Report of seven cases and review of the literature " Am J Obstet Gynecol 1988;158:591)

15. [F & I:•Background: **Dysgerminoma** which is analogous to seminoma of the testis, **is the most common pure malignant germ cell tumor of the ovary.**

°Although it is the most frequent ovarian malignancy in children and young adults, this tumor is relatively rare, representing only 2% of all ovarian malignancies.

°In contrast to surface spread, which is typical of epithelial ovarian tumors, ovarian dysgerminoma has a propensity for early lymphatic spread to the pelvic, para-aortic, mediastinal, and supraclavicular lymph nodes.

°Biologically, dysgerminoma is extremely **radiosensitive** and even in the presence of metastatic disease, cure rates with radiotherapy have been excellent.

•Total abdominal hysterectomy and bilateral salpingo-oophorectomy followed by postoperative radiation therapy has been the standard therapy for ovarian dysgerminomas.

°Unilateral adnexectomy alone is an effective therapeutic alternative in young women with disease confined to one ovary.

°Primary adjuvant chemotherapy may be as effective as radiation therapy in the treatment of patients with advanced or recurrent dysgerminoma.

•Objective: to review the treatment of dysgerminoma and the summarize the recent literature concerning the optimal method of therapy.

•Dysgerminoma is composed of germ cells that are not differentiated into embryonic or extraembryonic structures.

°These tumor cells are morphologically and immunohistochemically identical to primordial germ cells.

°The concept of origination from primordial germ cells is strengthened by the occurrence of homologous neoplasms in the testes and along the route of migration of the primordial germ cells from the yolk sac of the embryo to the primitive gonad.

•Although ovarian dysgerminomas may occur at any age, most occur in children and young adults.

°Due to their extreme **radiosensitivity** and their predictable pattern of spread to the retroperitoneal lymph nodes, surgery and adjuvant radiation has been the standard therapeutic approach when disease has spread beyond one ovary.

°Surgery in combination with radiation therapy had a 100% survival rate in the current series.

•The optimal method of therapy for patients with disease confined to one ovary remains controversial.

•Conservative surgery should be offered only to those patients with unilateral encapsulated tumors < 10 cm in diameter.

°There is some limited data to suggest that **tumor diameter is a critical factor** in predicting recurrence after unilateral surgery.

•Conclusion: Unilateral salpingo-oophorectomy should be limited to patients with unilateral, encapsulated tumors and no histologic evidence of pelvic or para-aortic lymph nodal metastases.

•Both **LDH** and **hCG** are potentially useful markers in the diagnosis and management of patients with pure dysgerminoma.

°In contrast to LDH isoenzyme patterns typical of other malignant neoplasms, Serum LDH_1 and LDH_2 fractions are characteristically elevated in patients with seminoma and dysgerminoma.

•Immunohistochemical evidence suggests that hCG is produced by syncytial-like giant cells that can be present in pure dysgerminomas.

°An elevated serum hCG level in patients with pure dysgerminoma does not appear to worsen the prognosis.

°If serum levels of either LDH or hCG are elevated preoperatively, serial determinations should be performed after therapy to monitor disease status.

•**At least 15%** of ovarian dysgerminomas contain other malignant germ cell elements.

°In those cases, the **prognosis** is that of the **most malignant germ cell element** present.

•Conclusion: Properly evaluated patients with stage IA ovarian dysgerminoma who desire further childbearing can be safely treated with unilateral adnexectomy.

•Total abdominal hysterectomy and bilateral salpingo-oophorectomy with para-aortic lymph node sampling followed by radiation therapy is the accepted treatment for all other patients.

•Preliminary reports indicate that dysgerminoma is very sensitive to **platinum-based combination chemotherapy.**]

---

16. A patient with malignant trophoblastic disease is cured with chemotherapy. With regard to future childbearing she should be told that there is an increased

    A. chance of fetal wastage.
    B. chance of her getting lymphoma.
    C. incidence of congenital anomalies.
    *D.   incidence of placenta accreta.
    E. none of the above

---

p.544   (Song HZ, Wu PC, Wang Y, Yang X, and Dong S, "Pregnancy outcomes after successful chemotherapy for choriocarcinoma and invasive mole: Long-term follow-up " Am J Obstet Gynecol 1988;158:538)

16. [F & I:•Background: Standard treatment for gestational trophoblastic neoplasms has been hysterectomy with subsequent loss of fertility.

•Chemotherapy is successful in the treatment of gestational trophoblastic disease.

•All chemotherapeutic agents have mutagenic and teratogenic potential.

•Objective: to present the long term results of patients and their children born after successful chemotherapy for gestational trophoblastic neoplasms.

•Results: Of 265 women with 355 pregnancies there was no increase in the incidence of fetal wastage and congenital anomalies.

•The only remarkable obstetrical complication was an increased incidence of placenta accreta.

•Long term follow-up of mothers for 5 to 26 years revealed no increase in the rate of recurrence of the diseases.

•Conclusion: The treatment of malignant trophoblastic neoplasms with chemotherapy alone, without removal of the uterus, is feasible for the preservation of fertility in most women.

°As 54% of the patients in this series had metastases of various organs, including those of the central nervous system; metastasis was not a contraindication for the preservation of fertility of young women, provided that the treatment response was satisfactory.

•Most mutations are recessive and therefore may not be easily detected in the first generation of the patients.]

---

17. Which papilloma virus type appears to be a marker for more rapid progression to cervical epithelial neoplasia?

    A. 6
    B. 11
    *C.   16
    D. 18
    E. 31

---

p.933   (Peters RK, Thomas D, Skultin G and Henderson BE, "Invasive squamous cell carcinoma of the cervix after recent negative cytologic test results-A distinct subgroup? " Am J Obstet Gynecol 1987;158:926)

17. [F & I:•Background: Cervical cancer is a slow-growing tumor with between 8 and 20 years of preinvasion.

•The proportion of invasive cancer that appears within 3 years after negative cytologic test results range from 8% to 30%.

•Reasons for the failure of screening to detect tumors before they become invasive are:

°screening errors.

°sampling errors.

°tumors may fail to shed characteristic abnormal cells, or at least not all the time or in the usual quantities.

°some tumors may progress too rapidly through the preinvasive stages to be detected.

•When smears originally reported as negative within 3 years of invasive cervical cancer have been reexamined, **25% to 60%** are found to contain abnormal cells or at least a few atypical cells.

•Objectives:

°(1)   to determine if invasive cervical cancer that occur shortly after negative cytologic test results represent a distinct subgroup of these tumors.

°(2)   to determine if the risk factors for women with such tumors differs from those for other women with invasive cervical cancer.

•Material and Methods: This was a case-controlled study in which 200 women with histologically confirmed invasive squamous cell carcinoma of the cervix were prospectively identified by the tumor registry.

•Three groups were established on the basis of available information about cytologic histories.

•Group 1 had had at least one verified **negative** smear during the 5 year reference period and no history of ever having an abnormal smear before the reference date.

•Group 2 had had at least one **abnormal** smear during or before the reference period.

°A smear was classified as abnormal if it was originally reported or reclassified as classes II through V or if the presence of atypical or abnormal cells was noted in words on the report.

•Group 3 had either never had a Papanicolaou test before the reference date or had had at least one cervical smear before the reference period but none during these 5-year periods.

•Results: Women with cancers occurring suddenly did **not** appear to represent a distinctive subgroup in terms of either demographic characteristics or specific risk factors.

•The cancers in group 1 **did** appear to progress more rapidly than those in group 2.

°The cancers in group 1 were twice as likely as group 2 cancers to have progressed beyond the microinvasive stage by diagnosis.

•The average transition period from grade 3 cervical intraepithelial neoplasia to invasive cancer is 20 to 30 years, a small percentage of patients have progression to the invasive stage in ≤1 year.

°Most estimates of the proportion of invasive tumors that appear within 1 to 3 years after negative cytologic results range from 4% to 22%.

•Conclusion: **Rapidly progressing cancers do not occur more often in younger or in older women.**

•Human Papillomavirus (HPV) types 16, 18 and 31 have been linked to cervical cancer while HPB types 6, and 11 are more often associated with condyloma and minor dysplasia.

°HPV-16 appears to be a marker for more rapid progression to more severe forms of dysplasia (grade 3 cervical intraepithelial neoplasia), while HPV-6 is associated with persistent mild disease.

•Patients in group 1 had a more frequent history of **genital herpes** than in group 2, but were not statistically significant.

•**The use of oral contraceptives does not accelerate the rate of progression.**

•Cancers in women with recent cervical screening, whether positive or negative, were less likely to have extension to adjacent tissues than those in women who had not been screened, emphasizing that regular screening does shift detection of invasive cervical cancer to the earlier stages.

•More than 20% of the invasive cancers followed abnormal smears that did not result in a final positive diagnosis.

»colposcopic evaluation should be mandatory after one abnormal smear, regardless of the degree of the cytologic abnormality.

°Colposcopic follow-up of smears showing minimal dysplasia would increase the number of negative (and therefore unnecessary) cervical biopsies, since between 1% and 7% of all smears show at least some atypical cells.

•In the presence of carcinoma in situ, a repeat smear within 12 weeks of the first smear can be negative 30% to 40% of the time.]

---

18. Which preoperatively assessed factor is significantly associated with a poor prognosis in the surgical treatment of stage IB/IIA carcinoma of the cervix?

    A. tumor cell type
    B. cell differentiation
    C. channel invasion
    *D.   age > 50
    E. tumor size

p.253   (O'Brien D, and Carmichael JA, "Presurgical prognostic factors in carcinoma of the cervix, Stages IB and IIA," Am J Obstet Gynecol 1988;158:250.)

18. [F & I:•Background: Radical hysterectomy and pelvic lymph node dissection is primary treatment for early stage carcinoma of the cervix.

•Surgery offers the benefits of preserved ovarian and sexual function.

•Factors affecting results include: patients age, tumor cell type, size, and differentiation, and lymphatic or vascular invasion.

•Objective: to demonstrate

°(1) which of these factors can be accurately evaluated before definitive surgery and

°(2) which of these factors are significantly associated with a poor prognosis in patients treated by radical surgery.

•Methods: During the period of this study, radical surgery was the primary choice of treatment of stage IB and IIA cervical cancer in the gynecologic oncology service.

°Surgery continued in the presence of clinically positive pelvic nodes, as long as they were not fixed to surrounding structures.

°This aggressiveness is reflected by the relatively high incidence of nodal metastases (19%) compared with other surgical series, which average 14% positive nodes.

°The overall outcomes of 90% disease-free survival at 2 years and 85% at 5 years are similar to other reports.

•Results: Only **patient age > 50** and **large tumor size** were statistically significant.

°2-year disease free survival in those women < 50 years 93%, compared with 73% in those >50 years.

°Large tumor size was associated with 42% positive nodes, compared with only 11% in the case of medium or small lesions.

•Only surgical patients were considered and a decreased survival in patients > 50 years is clearly evident, age was not associated with an increase in nodal metastases.

•Various criteria define a large tumor size from 2 to 4 cm.

°all these have a poor prognosis and increased nodal metastases with large lesions.

°Even if no nodal metastases are present, large tumors may be associated with a significant increase in recurrence.

°One possible explanation is that a significant percentage of stage IB and IIA large tumors are **understaged,**

°°it is difficult to differentiate between inflammatory changes in the parametria or extension of a large irregular cervical lesion.

•Results: Tumor size assessed in the presurgical staging under anesthesia correlates well with the size in the final pathologic specimen.

°Large tumor size was not associated with poorer **differentiation.**

•Large tumor size was associated with an increase node metastases yet not with decreased survival.

°**Prognosis for patients with node metastases appears to be independent of tumor size.**

•**Channel invasion** by tumor has been widely held to be associated with poor prognosis.

°channel invasion is assessed on the final pathologic specimen, which is not helpful in selecting patients for surgery.

°Channel invasion as determined from the cone biopsy or multiple cervical biopsy specimens was **not** a prognostic indicator of survival or node metastases.

°°**This suggests that channel invasion at the time of staging need not be a contraindication to primary surgical management.**

•Channel invasion as assessed at the time of staging did not agree with the assessment based on the final pathology.

•**Poor tumor differentiation was not associated with large tumor size.**

•While adenocarcinoma and adenosquamous carcinomas recur earlier, there is no increased frequency of recurrence of lymph node metastases.

°There is no difference in survival or incidence of node metastases between tumors of various cell type.

°Cell type was not associated with patient age or lesion size.

•Results: 100 consecutive patients with stage IB and IIA cervical cancer, in an aggressive radical surgical series, followed for at least 2 years, are reviewed.

•Findings of possible prognostic significance including patient age, tumor size, differentiation, and cell type, and presence of channel invasion were assessed based only on the prelaparotomy staging and biopsies.

•Only patient age > 50 years and large tumor size were found to be indicators of poor outcome and increased node metastases.

•Channel invasion, tumor differentiation, and tumor cell type did **not** affect survival or node metastases.

»These factors should not be a contraindication to primary surgical management.]

---

19. When (weeks) during normal pregnancy is free serum β-hCG highest?

    *A.   5
    B. 10
    C. 20
    D. 30
    E. 40

---

p.195   (Ozturk M, Berkowitz R, Goldstein D, Bellet D, and Wands J , "Differential production of human chorionic gonadotropin and free subunits in gestational trophoblastic disease" Am J Obstet Gynecol 1988;158: 193)

19. [F & I:•Background: Placental human chorionic gonadotropin shares structural homology with pituitary glycoprotein hormones, and is composed of noncovalently bound α and ß subunits.

°The α-subunit gene is expressed in both the pituitary gland and placenta.

°In contrast the ß subunit genes are expressed only in the placenta.

•Dimeric hCG is the major species secreted during pregnancy.

•Objective: to determine the free subunits and intact hormone serum levels in normal nonpregnant populations, during pregnancy, and in patients with gestational trophoblastic disease.

•Results: In 70% women over 45, levels of hCG of 0.02 to 0.40 ng/ml.

°Luteinizing hormone, follicle-stimulating hormone, thyroid-stimulating hormone, and free α and ß subunits would not be identified by this immunoradiometric assay.

•During normal gestation there is a dissociation of free subunit production according to gestational age.

°There is an excess of free ßhCG in early pregnancy.

°Subsequently, equal molar ratios of ßhCG and αhCG are reached between 12 to 15 weeks followed by an excess of free αhCG thereafter.

°When expressed as a percentage of total hCG, free α and ßhCG are low.

°For example, free ßhCG is about 1% of total hCG in early gestation but subsequently falls to a remarkably constant value of approximately 0.5% throughout the next 17 weeks.

°Since the production of ßhCG relative to hCG is under stringent physiologic control in normal gestation, ßhCG to hCG and ßhCG to αhCG ratios may be assessed under pathologic states such as hydatidiform mole and choriocarcinoma.

•The normal trophoblast differentiates predominantly from the cytotrophoblast in early gestation and the syncytiotrophoblast (hCG-producing cells) at term.

°The higher ßhCG to hCG ratio observed in early pregnancy suggests that the cytotrophoblast readily produces ßhCG.

°Molar pregnancy and choriocarcinoma are composed in part of increased cytotrophoblastic elements.

°Levels of ßhCG may reflect differentiation of the trophoblast.

°Serum concentrations of ßhCG in hydatidiform mole and choriocarcinoma often exceed values of normal pregnancy.

°Absolute levels of hCG and αhCG are not useful in distinguishing normal pregnancy from trophoblastic disease.

•ßhCG to hCG ratio and ßhCG serum concentration can differentiate hydatidiform mole from normal pregnancy.

°ßhCG to hCG ratios in molar pregnancy were intermediate between normal pregnancy and choriocarcinoma.

°Malignancy was characterized by an even higher ßhCG to hCG ratio, and mole can be distinguished from choriocarcinoma with high probability.

•The ratio adjusts for the quantity and differentiation of the trophoblast.

•Quantitative measurements of hCG levels are vitally important to monitor the treatment of patients with gestational trophoblastic disease.

•There is a good correlation between the volume of viable trophoblastic tumor cells and absolute serum hCG levels.

•Conclusion: The clinical management of patients with gestational trophoblastic disease may be improved by the increased sensitivity of hCG assays.

°hCG serum levels > 0.02 ng/ml strongly suggest the presence of trophoblastic tumor cells, particularly in those women < 45.

•A rising hCG level even if < 0.5 to 1 ng/ml signifies the presence of recurrent tumor; such patients developed hCG concentrations in the detectable range of the polyclonal RIA.

°Detection of recurrent tumor at the earliest possible time allows for the initiation of chemotherapy when tumor burden is minimal.]

20. Which of the following factors has the LEAST effect on survival for endometrial adenocarcinoma?

    A. age
    B. clinical stage
    C. depth of myometrial invasion
    D. histopathologic grade
    *E.   presence of estradiol receptors

p.803   (Ehrlich CE, Young PCM, Stehman FB, Sutton GP and Alford WM, "Steroid receptors and clinical outcome in patients with adenocarcinoma of the endometrium " Am J Obstet Gynecol 1987;158:796)

20. [F & I:•Objective: to report experience with progesterone and estradiol receptors in endometrial adenocarcinomas.

•Results: When receptor status was correlated with early (stages I and II) versus advanced (stages III and IV) clinical stage, **no statistically significant trend** was observed with **advancing stage.**

•Statistically **significant** association between **increasing tumor anaplasia and decreasing progesterone receptor,** but no estradiol receptor, in the cancers.

    °This statistically significant difference was observed for lack of estradiol and progesterone receptor binding in the adenosquamous, clear cell, and papillary adenocarcinomas as compared with the adenocarcinoma-adenocanthoma group.

•There was a statistically **significant** relationship between **adnexal metastases and lack of progesterone receptor and estradiol receptor in all stages and in stage I cases.**

•There was **no** association between **myometrial invasion, positive peritoneal cytology, and retroperitoneal lymph node metastasis and receptor status of the cancers.**

•**Advancing age is associated with a worsening prognosis in patients with endometrial cancer.**

    °There was a statistically significant trend toward lack of progesterone receptor but not estradiol receptor binding with advancing patient age.

    »This may be related to a trend for older patients to have a higher percent of **anaplastic** tumors compared with younger patients.

•A statistically significant association between **recurrence rate and negative receptor status** for both progesterone receptor and estradiol receptor.

•Where the receptor status correlated with clinical histopathologic variables the level of significance was always higher for progesterone receptor status than for estradiol receptor status.

•There was no relationship between estradiol receptor status and survival, although one was found for progesterone receptor status and survival.

°Survival was superior for all stages of progesterone receptor-positive tumors over progesterone receptor-negative tumors.

•The variables of age, clinical stage, histopathologic grade, and depth of myometrial invasion significantly affected survival.

    °Estradiol receptor did **not** affect survival.

°**Age and clinical stage were the strongest prognostic variables.**

°°This effect persisted in clinical stages I and II for age, histopathologic grade, and depth of myometrial invasion, and progesterone receptor status.

•Approximately **one-third** of unselected patients with advanced or recurrent endometrial carcinomas respond to progestin therapy.

•A statistically significant relationship exists between progesterone receptor-positive tumors and response to progestin therapy.]

---

21. The LEAST critical outcome variable in superficially invasive squamous cell carcinoma of the cervix is

    A. depth of invasion
    B. lymph node metastases
    C. lymphvascular invasion
    D. number of quadrants of the cerix involved
    *E.   tumor grade

---

p.402   (Maiman MA, Fruchter RG, DiMaio TM and Boyce JG, "Superficially invasive squamous cell carcinoma of the cervix " Obstet Gynecol 1988;71:399)

21. [F & I:•Background: Superficially invasive squamous cell cervical carcinoma has an unknown malignant potential.

°The morbidity associated with radical therapeutic measures must be weighed against the probability of lymph node metastases, recurrence, and death from cancer.

•Material and Methods: 117 women with histologically defined, superficially invasive squamous cell carcinoma of the cervix, with 5 mm or less of invasion.

•Histologic evaluation included several parameters:

°depth of stromal invasion (100% evaluable),

°lateral spread (defined as the number of quadrants of the cervix with tumor; 92% evaluable),

°grade of tumor,

°involvement of paremetrial tissue, and

°status of pelvic lymph nodes (81% evaluable).

•The maximum depth of stromal invasion was measured from the basement membrane of the surface epithelium by means of an ocular micrometer.

°Microscopic lymphvascular invasion was diagnosed when tumor cells were found within lymphatic capillary spaces lined by flattened endothelial cells.

•Overall, 77% of patients had either modified radical hysterectomy or radical hysterectomy with pelvic node dissection (an additional five subjects had node sampling).

•Results: In superficially invasive squamous cell carcinoma of the cervix, specific histomorphologic variables can be identified that place patients at higher risk.

°Recurrence is rare, and pelvic lymph node metastasis is the critical outcome variable.

°**Depth of stromal invasion** is the most critical factor in predicting pelvic node metastases.

°The overall incidence of metastases was 5%.

°depth of invasion correlated well with other risk factors.

•The prognostic significance of **lymph-vascular space involvement** is controversial.

°Invasion of lymph-vascular spaces was a definite poor prognostic factor in stage I patients.

°The overall incidence of lymph-vascular space involvement was 8%.

°There was a trend toward increasing incidence of pelvic node metastases with the presence of lymph-vascular invasion.

°Only 3% of patients **without** lymph-vascular invasion had positive nodes, 25% with lymph-vascular space invasion had pelvic node metastases.

•Tumor grade in cervical carcinoma may not have the same prognostic significance as it does in endometrial or ovarian carcinoma.

•Conclusion: Pelvic lymph nodes should be sampled in all patients with superficial invasion, except for those with 1 mm or less of invasion and without lymph-vascular invasion.

•The cure rate can approach 100% when radical or modified radical surgery is used for all patients, except for those with 1 mm or less of invasion and without lymph-vascular invasion.]

---

22. Positive cytologic washings in patients with endometrial carcinoma are associated with all of the following EXCEPT.

    A.   adnexal involvement
    B.   depth of myometrial invasion
    *C.   grade
    D   involvement of the lower uterine segment
    E.   para-aortic and pelvic node metastases

---

p.397   (Harouny VR, Sutton GP, Clark SA, Feisler HE, Stehman FB, and Ehrlich CE, "The importance of peritoneal cytology in endometrial carcinoma " Obstet Gynecol 1988;71:394)

22. [F & I:Background: The importance of peritoneal cytology in endometrial carcinoma is unclear.

•Objective: to review peritoneal washings in patients with endometrial carcinoma.

•Material and Methods: Peritoneal washings were obtained for cytologic examination in 340 patients.

•All patients had endometrial carcinoma diagnosed by endometrial biopsy or fractional D&C.

•Stage I:

°75 patients received preoperative pelvic radiotherapy with or without an implant.

°57 patients received postoperative pelvic or extended-field radiotherapy.

•Stage II and III disease patients received radiotherapy;

•Stage IV disease patients were treated with adjunctive hormonal therapy, radiotherapy, or chemotherapy when appropriate.

•Peritoneal washings were obtained at the time of initial exploration by instilling 100 mL or sterile balanced salt solution over the pelvic viscera after manually elevating the small bowel.

°The solution was aspirated from the posterior cul-de-sac and sent directly to the cytology laboratory, where volume was measured before the sample was divided into two centrifuge tubes and spun down.

•Results: Among the group of 340 patients, 75 were reported to have contained malignant cells.

•Positive cytologic washings were found to correlate directly with the **depth of myometrium invasion, adnexal involvement, para-aortic and pelvic node metastases, and involvement of the lower uterine segment.**

°No correlation with stage or grade was identified.

•A greater risk of recurrence and subsequent death from endometrial cancer in all stages for patients with malignant peritoneal cytology was found.

°Patients with surgical stage I endometrial cancer had superior disease-free survival when cytology was negative.]

Directions: Each group of numbered words or phrases is preceded by a list of lettered statements. MATCH the lettered item most closely associated with the numbered word or phrase. Each item may be used once, more than once, or not at all.

    A. laminin
    B. plasma cholinesterase
    C. plasma urokinase-type plasminogen activator antigen
    D. serum 5-nucleotidase
    E. sulpiride

23. invasive squamous cell carcinoma of cervix   Ans: C

p.252   (Koelbl H, Kirchheimer J, Tatra G, Christ G, and Binder Bernd. "Increased plasma levels of urokinase-type plasminogen activator with endometrial and cervical cancer" Obstet Gynecol 1988;72:252)

23. [F & I:•Background: In the fibrinolytic system, the inactive precursor plasminogen is converted into its active form, plasmin, by plasminogen activators, serine proteases exhibiting common structures.

    °There are two different types of plasminogen activators:

        °°a **urokinase-type** plasminogen activator produced and secreted by several mammalian cells and found in different body fluids, and

        °°a **tissue-type** plasminogen activator, synthesized mainly by endothelial cells and exhibiting its function as an antithrombotic agent.

    •Plasminogen activator inhibitors, capable of inhibiting the effects of both plasminogen activators, are found in endothelial cells and the placenta, and are released by several stimuli, such as **endotoxins, hypoxia, or interleukin-1.**

    •Plasminogen activators, acting via plasmin, focus on the local effect of the serine proteases on the cell membrane to induce firbronectinolysis and collagenolysis.

    •Objective: to study plasma levels of urokinase-type plasminogen activator antigen, tissue-type plasminogen activator antigen, and plasminogen activator inhibitor antigen in patients with uterine malignancies.

    •Results: Plasma urokinase-type plasminogen activator antigen levels was significantly **increased** in patients with cervical and endometrial cancer.

    •Exceedingly high plasma urokinase-type plasminogen activator antigen levels in women with advanced cervical cancer (FIGO stages III and IV disease), which is of particular interest whether or not the malignant tumor itself causes an increase in plasma urokinase-type plasminogen activator antigen levels.

    •Increased urokinase-type plasminogen activator from the gastrointestinal tract, the breast, the respiratory tract, and the prostate, and in melanomas.

    •Plasma tissue type plasminogen activator antigen levels were **not** elevated in patients of either carcinoma group.

    •Plasma levels of plasminogen activator inhibitor activity, representing an acute-phase protein, were **not different** in both the cervical and endometrial cancer groups.

    •In uterine malignancies, the only fibrinolytic parameter is plasma affected significantly by the malignant disease is urokinase-type plasminogen activator, although its origin is unclear.

24. intact basement membrane

Ans: A

p.257   (Ehrmann RL, Dwyer IM, Yavner D, and Hancock WW. "An immunoperoxidase study of laminin and type IV collagen distribution in carcinoma of the cervix and vulva" Obstet Gynecol 1988;72:257)

24 [F & I:Objective: to see whether immunoperoxidase staining of basement membrane components would help in the identification of early stromal invasion (ie, microinvasion) arising from vulvar and cervical squamous cell carcinoma in situ.

•Total keratinization or necrosis of an invasive tumor nest is accompanied by loss of surrounding basement membrane, suggesting that the previous **laminin** covering was metabolized and that the maintenance of a basement membrane requires viable epithelial cells.

•Laminin with varying defectiveness surrounded invasive foci, whereas adjacent carcinoma in situ and normal epithelial had intact laminin.

•The tendency of laminin gaps and tumor buds to contain large malignant cells of pleomorphic nuclei support the concept of a change in tumor cell metabolism during active invasion.]

Directions: Each set of lettered headings below is followed by a list of numbered words or phrases. For each numbered word or phrase select:

> A. if the item is associated with (A) only
> B. if the item is associated with (B) only
> C. if the item is associated with both (A) and (B)
> D. if the item is associated with neither (A) nor (B)

In treating stage III/IV intraperitoneal ovarian epithelial malignancy

> A. cisplatinum
> B. recombinant alpha-2 interferon
> C. both
> D. neither

25. response predicted by peritoneal malignant cell count   Ans: C

26. creates intense mesothelial reaction   Ans: B

27. induces a brisk influx of macrophages   Ans: B

---

p.787   (Sagae S, Berek JS, Fu YS, Chang N, Dauplat J, and Hacker NF, "Peritoneal cytology of ovarian cancer patients receiving intraperitoneal therapy: Quantitation of malignant cells and response" Obstet Gynecol 1988;72:782)

25-27. [F & I:•Background: Patients with advanced-stage epithelial ovarian cancer treated by cytoreductive surgery and combination chemotherapy have a 60-70% rate of persistent disease at second-look laparotomy.

•Intraperitoneal chemotherapy and immunotherapy have been used as salvage treatment for patients with persistent ovarian cancer.

°Phase I-II trials of intraperitoneal therapy have demonstrated histologically and cytologically confirmed complete responses in patients with persistent ovarian cancer after chemotherapy.

°Responses have been limited to those with minimal residual disease, ie, less than 5 mm in maximum tumor dimension.

•A careful distinction must be drawn between host cells that are frankly malignant and "reactive" mesothelial cells, a cellular pattern that may be confused by the cytologist.

•Objective: to describe a quantitative cytologic analysis of malignant and nonmalignant host cells found in peritoneal fluid obtained before and during the intraperitoneal administration of cisplatin or recombinant alpha-2 interferon in patients with persistant epithelial ovarian cancer.

•Material and Methods: Twenty-three patients with stages III and/or IV epithelial ovarian carcinoma of the ovary.

•No patient had clinical ascites.

•Twenty patients had serous histology, two mucinous, and one endometrioid.

•Cisplatin (Platinol; Bristol Myers Co.) was adminstered intraperironeally into a total of 2 L of dialysis solution, which was instilled intraperitoneally via peritoneal dialysis catherters.

•Human alpha-interferon (SCH 30500; Shering Corp. Kenilworth, NJ) was administered into 2 L of dialysis solution and instilled intraperitoneally via peritoneal dialysis catherters.

°Before each treatment and 24 hours after treatment, 2 L of warmed dialysis fluid were instilled into the perioneal cavity and recovered for cytologic assays.

°The exposed ends of the Tenckhoff catheters were resealed aseptically.

•One to six weeks after the final course of the drug, an operation was performed to evaluate the response.

•Response was defined as follows:

°1) Complete response-no evidence of disease at the completion of therapy, including the absence of malignant cells in the peritoneal fluid in those patients whose cytologies had been positive;

°2) partial response-the presence of positive cytoogy only at the completion of therapy in those patiens who had had macroscopic disease, or the regression of mactoscopic disease vy at least 50% in tumor dimension;

°3) stable disease-persistnet pos8itive cytology and/or no change in the rumor dimenstion; and

°4) progressive disease-evidence of tumor growth during or by completion of treatment.

•Results: Among twelve patients treated with intraperitoneal cisplatin, 5 responded to treatment and 7 did not.

•Of the eleven patients treated with intraperitoneal alpha-interferon, five responded, and six progressed.

•No patient with a malignant cell count over $10^3/cm^2/dL$ responded.

•The concentration of malignant cells in the peritoneal cytology before therapy correlates with the surgically documented response.

•The malignant cell concentration at the initiation of treatment predicted response in all but one patient.

•Alpha-interferon induced a pronounced **mesothelial reaction** particularly in those who responded to treatment.

°The mesothelial response is suppressed by intraperitoneal cisplatin.

•Alpha-interferon may affect an anti-tumor response by inducing endogenous lymphocytes and macrophages where intraperitoneal cisplatin exerts a direct cytotoxic on the malignant and mesothelial cells.

•Alpha-interferon induced a brisk influx of interperitoneal white cells predominantly lymphocytes and macrophages, a phenomenon suppressed by intraperitoneal cisplatin.

•Reactive mesothelial cells especially in women with previous abdominal surgery, radiotherapy and chemotherapy may be associated with nuclear atypisms and psammoma bodies.]

In the diagnosis of endometrial adenocarcinoma:

    A. office curettage
    B. operating room curettage
    C. both
    D. neither

28. grade will be increased in more than 10% of patients post-hysterectomy   Ans: C

29. more than 95% of uteri will have residual disease found after curettage   Ans: A

30. findings can obviate need for node sampling   Ans: D

p.614   (Daniel Ag,m and Peters WA III, "Accuracy of office and operating room curettage in the grading of endometrial carcinoma " Obstet Gynecol 1988;71:612)

28-30. [F & I: Background: Current recommendations for the treatment of stage I adenocarcinoma of the endometrium includes initial hysterectomy with surgical staging.

°Adjuvant radiation therapy may be recommended for patients with high tumor grade, deep myometrial invasion,cervical involvement, or extrauterine disease.

•The indications for lymph node evaluation was based upon pre-operative curettage if grade 2 and 3 tumors were found.

°The assumption was that curettage can reliably predict tumor grade.

•Objectives:

°to determine whether pre-operative curettage can accurately determine tumor grade in stage I endometrial carcinoma and

°whether office aspirate curettage is accurate as operating room curettage in the determination of grade.

•Less than half of the uterine cavity was curetted in 60% of patients who have operating room curettage.

°Examination under anesthesia showed a 21% variance with the findings of laparotomy.

•Results: There was no significant difference in the ability of either procedure to predict tumor grade.

•There was a substantial **increase** in grade at hysterectomy after both techniques of curettage (20% after office curettage and 15% after operating room curettage).

°Upgrading implies incomplete tumor sampling by the curette and downgrading results from aggressive tumor removal.

•The curettage under anesthesia sampled the greater depth or greater surface area of endometrium in that tumor residual was significantly less than after office curettage.

°A 15 to 20% discrepancy in grade is generally **not** acceptable in medical diagnosis.

°Only 5% of grade 1 tumors had greater than 50% invasion.

°°Previously the incidence had been 15-20% with deep myometrial invasion in grade 1 disease.

•Conclusion: Intraoperative gross evaluation, with possible frozen section of the uterus, should be used to assess grade and depth of invasion in cases for which node sampling is not already indicated.]

    A. ovarian carcinoma
    B. fallopian tube carcinoma
    C. both
    D. neither

31. prognosis depends on residual disease   Ans: C

32. survival depends on tumor grade   Ans: A

33. survival improved with cis-platinum multiagent therapy   Ans: C

34. associated with low parity and infertility   Ans: C

---

p.760 (Peters WA III, Andersen WQ, Hopkins MP, Kumar NB, and Morley GW, "Prognostic features of carcinoma of the fallopian tube" Obstet Gynecol 1988;71:757)

31-34. [F&I:•Background: **Carcinoma of the fallopian tube** has an incidence of 0.24-0.5% of gynecologic malignancies.

°It is associated with low parity and the high incidence of histological or gross evidence of old **pelvic inflammatory disease.**

»One or more sexually transmitted agents may be an etiologic factor for both the infertility and the tubal carcinoma.

•Carcinoma of the fallopian tube is similar to carcinoma of the endometrium or colon because it arises in a hollow organ and because the depth of invasion of the muscularis is a strong prognostic feature in patients with disease limited to the fallopian tube.

•Although its spread via the the peritoneal cavity is similar to ovarian carcinoma, a much higher percentage of patients have disease limited to the tube alone.

•The association between survival and the amount of residual disease after surgery is quite similar to that of ovarian carcinoma.

•Unlike ovarian carcinoma, the **grade** in fallopian tube carcinoma does **not** appear to be an important prognostic feature.

•Nodal evaluation should be performed at the time of initial surgery in patients without obvious extratubal spread as the findings of uniform nodal involvement in autopsies and a large number of patients with isolate nodal metastasis.

•Results: No major impact on survival with either single alkylating-agent cheomtherapy and/or pelvic irradiation was found.

•Because cis-platinum-based multiagent chemotherapy appears to be active with advanced disease, it may also be an appropriate form of adjuvant therapy in stage I.

•For surgical stage II it would appear that the majority of women treated with surgery alone or surgery and pelvic irradiation will die from their disease.

»A multiagent chemotherapy and/or whole abdominal irradiation might benefit these patients.

•There appears to be improvement in the survival for patients receiving aggressive multiagent chemotherapy containing cis-platinum.

•Cis-platinum containing combination therapy would appear to be the optimal treatment for women with stage IV disease.]

    A.   placental site trophoblastic tumor
    B.   hydatidiform mole
    C.   both
    D.   neither

35. sensitive to chemotherapeutic drugs   Ans: B

36. fatal if untreated   Ans: C

37. hCG serves as a tumor marker   Ans: C

p.857   (Finkler NJ, Berkowitz RS, Driscoll RG, Goldstein DP and Berstein MR, "Clinical experience with placental site trophoblastic tumors at the New England trophoblastic disease center" Obstet Gynecol 1988;71:854)

35-37. [F & I:•Background: **Placental site trophoblastic tumor** is characterized by mononuclear and occasional multinuclear trophoblastic cells that infiltrate the uterus and its blood vessels.

°Chorionic villi are very **rarely** present.

ᵁ**Unlike** gestational choriocarcinoma, placental site trophoblastic tumor is composed almost entirely of intermediate trophoblast and is associated with little necrosis and hemorrhage.

°Immunohistochemical studies demonstrate a variable reactivity and relatively few cells that stain for human chorionic gonadotropin (hCG); however, the majority stain for human placental lactogen (hPL).

•Objective: to describe the clinical characteristics of placental site trophoblastic tumor.

•Placental site trophoblastic tumor is malignant and sometimes fatal.

°It may develop after any type of gestation, and symptoms may develop from weeks to months after termination of the pregnancy.

•Most patients present with **irregular bleeding**, but some unusual presentations have been reported, including amenorrhea,virilization, and nephrotic syndrome.

•Placental site trophoblastic tumors produce low levels of serum hCG.

•Metastases occur mainly in the **lung**, and also in the lymph nodes, brain, liver, kidney, vagina, stomach, and spleen.

°Placental site trophoblastic tumors with high mitotic counts have a greater risk of developing metastases.

•The presence of metastatic placental site trophoblastic tumor is an **ominous** sign.

•**Unlike** gestational choriocarcinoma, placental site trophoblastic tumor is **relatively insensitive to aggressive cytotoxic chemotherapy.**

•**Radiation therapy** may successfully provide local control of tumor and palliate the symptoms.

•Serial hCG levels should be carefully measured over long intervals because metastases occur as late as ten years after initial treatment.

•These tumors usually secrete low levels of hCG, and a large tumor burden may be present before hCG levels are detectable.

•**The diagnosis of nonmetastatic placental site trophoblastic tumor should be followed by prompt hysterectomy.**]

Obstetrics

Directions: Each of the questions or incomplete statements below is followed by several suggested answers or completions. Select the BEST answer in each case.

1. Which of the following hormones depresses lung surfactant production?

   A. corticosteroids
   B. epidermal growth factor
   C. estrogen
   D. mullerian inhibiting substance
   E. thyroid hormone

2. The mechanism of fetal heart rate acceleration after vibroacoustic stimulation is

   A. catecholamine mediation
   B. reflex increase in fetal cardiac preload
   C. umbilical vein engorgement
   D. uterine artery spasm
   E. vagal responsiveness

3. Relaxin inhibits uterine contractions by

   A. ß-adrenergic stimulation
   B. binding calmodulin
   C. decreasing intracellular Ca^{+2}
   D. increasing phosphodiesterase concentration
   E. increasing progesterone receptors

4. Low dose aspirin used in the treatment of preeclampsia

   A. increases intracellular calcium
   B. inhibits angiotensin II production
   C. inhibits production of atrial natriuretic peptide
   D. inhibits thromboxane production
   E. stimulates prostacyclin production

5. Which of the following tests is most sensitive for the detection of iron depletion in pregnancy?

   A. serum iron
   B. serum ferritin
   C. serum transferrin
   D. mean corpuscular volume
   E. red cell distribution width

6. Approximately what percentage of women with a retained dead fetus will have laboratory evidence of abnormal coagulation?

   A. < 1
   B. 5
   C. 10
   D. 25
   E. 50

7. When does the switchover from fetal to adult hemoglobin synthesis begin?

   A. 30 weeks gestation
   B. 36 weeks gestation
   C. 7-10 days post-natal
   D. 3 weeks post-natal
   E. 6 months post-natal

8. Which of the following is the best modality for diagnosing acute puerperal ovarian vein thrombosis?

   A. abdominal sonography
   B. computed tomography
   C. femoral venography
   D. intravenous pyelography

9. A 30 year old para 0-0-0-0, LMP 17.5 weeks ago, has a maternal serum alpha-fetoprotein 0.4 multiples of the median. Ultrasound shows a single fetus with dimensions consistent with a 15 week gestation.

The next best step in the patient's management is

A. determine the fetal karyotype
B. no further testing until the third trimester
C. repeat the maternal serum alpha-fetoprotein in 2 weeks
D. repeat the maternal serum alpha-fetoprotein now
E. repeat the ultrasound in 2 weeks

10. A patient at risk for preterm labor is self-monitoring her hourly uterine activity while at home. What is the fewest contraction per hour after which treatment should be initiated?

A. 2
B. 4
C. 6
D. 8
E. 10

11. Which of the following is significantly associated with systemic tocolysis and pulmonary edema?

A. age of gestation at the time of treatment
B. multiple gestation
C. presence of infection
D. previous reproductive history
E. type of pharmacologic therapy for preterm labor

12. What percentage of children with long-term handicaps are the product of entirely normal pregnancies and uneventful deliveries?

A. 1-2%
B. 5-10%
C. 20-25%
D. 33%
E. > 50%

13. Which of the following when detected in utero ultrasonographically has the best prognosis?

A. coarctation of the aorta
B. Ebstein's anomaly
C. endocardial fibroelastosis
D. tetralogy of Fallot
E. transposition of the great arteries

14. What is the minimum predonation hematocrit required of a pregnant patient in anticipation of autologous transfusion at delivery?

A. 36
B. 34
C. 32
D. 30
E. 28

15. The most important element initiating the active management of labor is

A. parity
B. regular uterine contractions
C. rupture of the membranes
D. station of presenting part
E. the dilation of the cervix

16. Which of the following conditions has the greatest effect on accelerating fetal lung maturity?

A. insulin dependent diabetes mellitus
B. intrauterine growth retardation
C. pregnancy-induced hypertension
D. premature rupture of the membranes
E. second trimester uterine bleeding

17. What is the platelet count (x 10^9/L) at term, above which an epidural anesthetic can safely be administered?

A. 20
B. 50
C. 67
D. 75
E. 100

18. For which fetal condition would maternal serum alpha-fetoprotein values be the highest?

    A. diaphragmatic hernia
    B. Down syndrome
    C. gastroschisis
    D. omphalocele
    E. spina bifida occulta

19. "Toe jam" refers to abuse of

    A. marijuana
    B. cocaine
    C. toluene
    D. glue
    E. PCP

20. The drug of choice for treating typhoid fever in pregnancy is

    A. ampicillin
    B. chloramphenicol
    C. clindamycin
    D. gentamicin
    E. metronidazole

21. Meconium aspiration syndrome can best be prevented by

    A. awaiting spontaneous amniorrhexis.
    B. direct treacheobronchial suctioning via laryngoscope below the levels of the cords.
    C. nasopharyngeal and oropharyngeal suctioning with a DeLee suction catheter before delivery of the chest followed by chest physiotherapy and postural drainage.
    D. nasopharyngeal and oropharyngeal suctioning with a DeLee suction catheter before delivery of the chest followed by direct treacheobronchial suctioning via laryngoscope below the levels of the cords.
    E. averting fetal hypoxia.

22. Which of the following is the earliest sign of fetal hydrops accompanying severe Rh isoimmunization?

    A. ascites
    B. blunting of fetal heart rate variability
    C. dilation fo the umbilical vein
    D. pericardial effusion
    E. sinusoidal fetal heart rate pattern

23. The most common finding in patients who develop post-partum **hypo**thyroidism is

    A. cold intolerance
    B. depression
    C. goiter
    D. lack of concentration
    E. weight gain

24. At 36 weeks of completed gestation, the chance of a breech presentation spontaneously converting to a vertex presentation is (%)

    A. < 20
    B. 33
    C. 50
    D. 67
    E. 75

25. The most common systemic side effect of the intravaginal application of prostaglandin gel used for the induction of labor is

    A. bronchospasm
    B. diarrhea
    C. headache
    D. hypotension
    E. none of the above

26. Which of the following studies is most sensitive for the detection of amniotic fluid bacterial colonization?

    A. Gram stain
    B. lactic acid dehydrogenase test
    C. leukocyte esterase test
    D. limulus amebocyte lysate test
    E. neutrophile count

27. An asymptomatic patient has a unilocular 6 cm ovarian cyst at 16 weeks gestation. The next best step in her management is

    A. biweekly ultrasonogram for cyst growth
    B. culdocentesis for cytological study of peritoneal fluid
    C. laparoscopy with aspiration of cyst
    D. ovarian cystectomy
    E. reevaluation in one month

28. The underlying pathophysiology of hemorrhagic endovasculitis of the placenta is

    A. diabetes mellitus
    B. graft versus host reaction
    C. ischemia
    D. mycoplasma infection
    E. systemic lupus erythematosus

29. The principle hemodynamic alteration in amniotic fluid embolism is

    A. "shock lung"
    B. acute reflexive adrenal insufficiency
    C. impaired left ventricular function
    D. increased pulmonary vascular resistance
    E. splanchnic pooling of effective circulatory volume

30. The leading infectious cause of congenital deafness in the United States is

    A. Coxackie B virus
    B. cytomegalovirus
    C. haemophilus influenzae
    D. mumps
    E. syphilis

31 In the management of Rh isoimmunization, what is the most accurate method of determining whether a non-hydropic fetus would benefit from a transfusion in utero before 26 weeks gestation?

    A. amniotic fluid ΔOD_{450}
    B. Doppler determination of umbilical artery end diastolic flow
    C. serial maternal antibody titers
    D. ultrasound surveillance of fetus
    E. umbilical cord hematocrit

32. At 27 weeks an ultrasound examination made because of polyhydramnios shows a distended stomach but no other abnormality. What karyotype is most commonly associated with this condition?

    A. 45, XO
    B. 46, XX, p5-
    C. 46, XX
    D. 47, XX, 21+
    E. 47, XYY

33. What is the most common X-linked **lethal** disease in man?

    A. agammaglobulinemia
    B. Duchenne muscular dystrophy
    C. glucose-6-PD deficiency
    D. hemophilia
    E. vitamin D resistant rickets

34. The overall accuracy of the L/S ratio and phosphatidylglycerol level in predicting respiratory difficulty is (%)

    A. 75
    B. 80
    C. 85
    D. 90
    E. 98

35. Which factor is most predictive of therapeutic failure in the treatment of post-cesarean endomyometritis?

    A. parity
    B. infant weight
    C. wound infection
    D. type of uterine incision
    E. type of anesthesia

37. Which of the following symptoms of
cardiorespiratory distress in a heart transplant
recipient is LEAST likely to be manifested
during pregnancy?

    A. palpitations
    B. orthopnea
    C. edema
    D. dyspepsia
    E. chest pain

38. Which of the following antibiotics given in
the usual intravenous doses for intrapartum
sepsis would be LEAST concentrated in the
fetal membranes?

    A. ampicillin
    B. cefoxitin
    C. clindamycin
    D. gentamicin
    E. mezlocillin

39. Which of the following would be the
LEAST helpful in managing abnormalities
of the active phase of labor?

    A. ambulation
    B. expectant observation
    C. maternal sedation
    D. oxytocin stimulation
    E. x-ray pelvimetry

40. Clinically useful in the treatment of septic
shock during pregnancy, all of the following
EXCEPT

    A. dexamethasone
    B. dobutamine
    C. dopamine
    D. norepinephrine
    E. phenylephrine

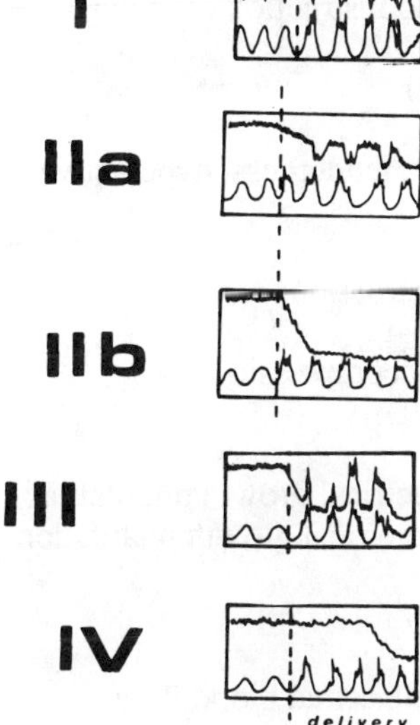

36. Which of the these tracings in the second
stage of labor most likely reflects fetal
acidosis?

    A. Type I
    B. Type IIa
    C. Type IIb
    D. Type III
    E. Type IV

Directions: Each group of numbered words or phrases is preceded by a list of lettered items. MATCH the lettered item most closely associated with the numbered word or phrase. Each item may be used once, more than once, or not at all.

For each drug listed below, MATCH the most likely fetal effect.

   A. lithium
   B. nitrofurantoin
   C. propanolol
   D. thiazide
   E. valproate

41. hypoglycemia

42. anemia

43. CNS malformation

44. thrombocytopenia

45. cardiac malformation

Obstetrical ultrasound findings:

   A. aortic root dilatation
   B. hypoplasia of the middle phalanx of the 5th digit
   C. periventriuclar hemorrhage
   D. pseudohydrocephalus
   E. ventriculomegaly

46. microcephaly

47. tetralogy of Fallot

48 osteogenesis imperfecta

49. trisomy 21

50. agenesis of corpus callosum

   A. laminin
   B. plasma cholinesterase
   C. plasma urokinase-type plasminogen activator antigen
   D. serum 5-nucleotidase
   E. sulpiride

51. abruptio placentae

52. intrahepatic cholestasis

Directions: Each set of lettered headings below is followed by a list of numbered words or phrases. For each numbered word or phrase select:

A. if item is associated with (A) only
B. if item is associated with (B) only
C. if item is associated with both (A) and (B)
D. if item is associated with neither (A) nor (B)

In a patient post-operative day 2 following cesarean section:

   A. cecal volvulus
   B. pseudoobstruction of colon
   C. both
   D. neither

53. abdominal pain, tenderness, hyperactive bowel sounds

54. mechanical obstruction

55. colonoscopic decompression

   A. symmetrical growth retardation
   B. asymmetrical growth retardation
   C. both
   D. neither

56. impaired uteroplacental blood flow

57. intrinsic fetal abnormalities

58. predicted by sonographic estimation of fetal weight

At 16 weeks gestation

    A. elevated maternal serum alpha-fetoprotein
    B. decreased maternal serum alpha-fetoprotein
    C. both
    D. neither

59. karyotyping from amniotic fluid indicated

60. increased incidence of congenital anomalies

61. increased incidence of fetal loss

    A. toxemia
    B. hypertension without toxemia
    C. both
    D. neither

62. increased incidence of pneumothorax

63. increased incidence of coagulopathy

64. increased incidence of germinal matrix hemorrhage

Directions: For each of the questions or incomplete statements below, ONE or MORE of the answers or completions given is correct. In each case select:

    A. if only 1, 2 and 3 are correct
    B. if only 1 and 3 are correct
    C. if only 2 and 4 are correct
    D. if only 4 is correct
    E. if all are correct

65. Effects of prolonged neonatal phototherapy include

    1. decreased unconjugated bilirubin
    2. hyperthermia
    3. increased insensible water loss
    4. retinopathy

66. Clinically useful in identifying patients at risk for pregnancy-induced hypertension

    1. rollover test
    2. isometric handgrip exercise
    3. calcium/creatinine ratio and microalbuminuria
    4. angiotensin II pressor response

67. The human yolk sac is the embryonic source of

    1. blood cells
    2. epithelia of the respiratory and digestive tracts
    3. primitive germ cells
    4. yolk

68. In considering vaginal delivery after cesarean section, conditions predisposing to uterine dehiscence include

    1. use of prostaglandin E suppositories to ripen unfavorable cervix
    2. use of oxytocin
    3. unknown scar
    4. single layer closure

69. Factors which decrease insulin sensitivity during pregnancy include

    1. hPL
    2. hCG
    3. hPRL
    4. glucagon

70. Criteria for diagnosing endomyometritis post-partum include

    1. oral T elevated >100.4° at least 6 hr apart
    2. uterine or parametrial tenderness
    3. negative urinalysis
    4. negative chest x-ray

71. Pregnant women with essential hypertension have an increased risk of developing

    1. acute renal failure
    2. coagulation disturbances
    3. pregnancy-induced hypertension
    4. increased peripheral insulin resistance

72. Useful in the management of a prolapsed cord at 26 weeks gestation when vaginal delivery is not imminent

    1. bladder distention
    2. elevation of presenting part out of pelvis
    3. ritodrine
    4. epidural anesthesia

73. True statements about premature rupture of the membranes with a cerclage in place include

    1. The risk of infection is not increased compared to patients who do not have a cerclage in place.
    2. Delivery will take place within 2 to 3 days.
    3. The risk of prematurity exceeds the risk of infection for the neonate.
    4. If the cerclage is left in place the pregnancy will be prolonged.

74. Clinically useful for establishing fetal karyotype in midtrimester

    1. amniocentesis
    2. cordocentesis
    3. transabdominal chorionic villus sampling
    4. transcervical chorionic villus sampling

75. Which of the following variables increase as term approaches in a normal pregnancy?

    1. fetal tone
    2. fetal breathing
    3. fetal movement
    4. fetal heart rate accelerations

76. A fetus is noted to have a heart rate of 200 bpm at 30 weeks gestation. Further evaluation of the pregnancy should include

    1. amniotic fluid L/S ratio
    2. fetal cardiac assessment
    3. fetal karyotype
    4. assessment of maternal thyroid function

77. Mothers carrying hepatitis B surface antigen can be expected to have

    1. more stillbirths.
    2. more infants with congenital anomalies.
    3. infants with lower birth weight.
    4. infants who have a 90% risk of contracting hepatitis.

78. Common central hemodynamic findings in severe preeclampsia include

    1. Hyperdynamic ventricular function
    2. Low central venous pressure
    3. Low colloid osmotic pressure
    4. No pulmonary hypertension

79. Microbes associated with endotoxin production

    1. fusobacterium
    2. mycoplasma
    3. E. coli
    4. Candida albicans

80. Types of human papilloma virus associated with squamous papillomas of the larynx and respiratory tract seen in infants delivered through a contaminated birth passage include

    1. 35
    2. 11
    3. 18
    4. 6

81. A pregnant patient complained of pain over the right portion of her lower back. Examination revealed a normal hip joint and no tenderness or contracture over the adductor muscles on the right. Findings corroborative of sacroiliac joint dysfunction include pain upon

    1. manually pressing the pelvis apart
    2. manually pressing the pelvis together
    3. placing the left heel on the right knee and rotating the leg outward
    4. palpation of the right sacrospinous ligament

82. Cystic fibrosis

    1. is an autosomal recessive disorder
    2. has a gene locus on chromosome 7
    3. carriers of the gene are asymptomatic
    4. cannot be detected in first trimester pregnancies

83. A gravida 2, para 1 is diagnosed as having a complete placenta previa, confirmed by ultrasound, at 24 weeks gestation after an episode of uterine bleeding requiring hospitalization. After 24 hours bleeding stops. Further management to prolong the pregnancy includes

    1. tocolysis
    2. bed rest at home
    3. cerclage
    4. alpha-hydroxyprogesterone

84. Indications for transabdominal cerclage for recurrent pregnancy loss include patients with

    1. congenitally short cervix
    2. T-shaped uterine cavity from DES exposure in utero
    3. penetrating forniceal lacerations
    4. subseptate uterus

85. A patient who is 16 weeks pregnant is found to have a breast mass which on needle aspiration is diagnosed as carcinoma. Indicated in her further management

    1. chemotherapy
    2. mammography
    3. mastectomy
    4. radiation therapy

86. Hypothyroidsim during pregnancy is associated with an increased risk for

    1. abruptio placentae
    2. anemia
    3. postpartum hemorrhage
    4. preeclampsia

87. Pregnancies in which there is elevated maternal serum alpha-fetoprotein and oligohydramnios are associated with

    1. deformations
    2. intrauterine growth retardation
    3. pulmonary hypoplasia
    4. renal agenesis

88. Twin zygosity can be determined prenatally by

    1. blood group antigens
    2. HLA typing
    3. oligonucleotide probes
    4. ultrasound

89. Intrapartum treatment of intraamniotic infection results in

    1. lower incidence of neonatal sepsis
    2. increased incidence of late neonatal sepsis
    3. shorter maternal hospital stay
    4. increased incidence of nosocomial infection

90. At 41 weeks, a patient has a non-reactive non-stress test after 40 minutes, adequate amniotic fluid, and satisfactory intrauterine physical assessment by ultrasound. The Bishop score is 9. Appropriate further management options include

    1. repeat NST in 2 hours
    2. medical induction of labor
    3. contraction stress test
    4. amniocentesis

91. Advantages of transvaginal ultrasound diagnosis of placenta previa include

    1. better visualization of a posterior placenta
    2. full bladder not necessary for the study
    3. increased image resolution
    4. more accurate in obese patients

Obstetrics-References

Directions: Each of the questions or incomplete statements below is followed by several suggested answers or completions. Select the BEST answer in each case.

1.   Which of the following hormones depresses lung surfactant production?

    A. corticosteroids
    B. epidermal growth factor
    C. estrogen
    *D.   mullerian inhibiting substance
    E. thyroid hormone

p.1302   (Catlin EA, Manganaro TF, and Donahoe PK, "Müllerian inhibiting substance depresses accumulation in vitro of disaturated phosphatidylcholine in fetal rate lung ," Am J Obstet Gynec 1988; 159:1299)

1. [Facts and Issues:•Background: Male neonates are at increased risk for newborn repiratory disress syndrome.

    °A deficiency of pulmonary surfactant (the major component of which is disaturated phosphatidycholine) is the cause of respiratory distress syndrome.

•Testosterone and **mullerian inhibiting substance** are the principal hormones directing genital development in the male fetus.

    °mullerian inhibiting substance:

        °°interacts with the urogenital ridge and causes regression of the mullerian duct and its surrounding mesenchyme.

        °°may antagonize the action of epidermal growth factor via inhibition of epidermal growth factor-induced receptor autophosphorylation.

    •Objective: to determine if mullerian inhibiting substance might inhibit biochemical lung maturation measured as disaturated phosphatidylcholine accumulation.

    •The fetal lung, which begins as a diverticulum of the ventral foregut, responds to several hormones.

    °**Corticosteroids** accelerate lung development and surfactant production

    °**thyroid hormone**, estrogen, and epidermal growth factor stimulate surfactant by **increasing** numbers of type II pneumonocytes and lamellar bodies,

    °**androgens** may depress surfactant production.

        °**Dihydrotestosterone** inhibits fibroblast-pneumonocyte factor-mediated synthesis of saturated phosphatidylcholine by fetal type II pneumonocytes.

    •Mullerian inhibiting substance is secreted by the fetal testis from week 6 throughout gestation and testes continue to produce mullerian inhibiting substance after birth

    •Mullerian inhibiting substance exerts its regressive effect at a distance from the testicular source; the effect of mullerian substance is enhanced by testosterone.

•Results: mullerian inhibiting substance may also exert a regulatory effect on fetal surfactant production.

•The fetal lung differentiated in in vitro organ culture and disaturated phosphatidylcholine accumulated.

•Testicular fragments, suppressed disaturated phosphatidylcholine production.

•Mullerian inhibiting substance suppressed disaturated phosphatidylcholine accumulation by an unknown mechanism.

•Mullerian inhibiting substance can block phosphorylation of the epidermal growth factor receptor of mullerian inhibiting substance-sensitive tumor cells by inhibiting tyrosine kinase.

°Conversely, epidermal growth factor inhibits mullerian inhibiting substance-induced regression of the mullerian duct in organ culture.

•Epidermal growth factor accelerates fetal lung maturation.]

---

2   The mechanism of fetal heart rate acceleration after vibroacoustic stimulation is

*A.   catecholamine mediation
B.   reflex increase in fetal cardiac preload
C.   umbilical vein engorgement
D.   uterine artery spasm
E.   vagal responsiveness

---

p.625   (Polzin GB, Blakemore KJ, Petrie RH, and Amon E, "Fetal vibro-acoustic stimulation: Magnitude and duration of fetal heart rate accelerations as a marker of fetal health " Obstet Gynecol 1988;72:621)

2. [F & I:•Background: •Fetal heart rate (FHR) acceleration in response to external stimulation may be a reliable predictor of fetal well-being.

•When acoustic stimulation evoked and FHR acceleration exceeding 15 beats per minute, the subsequent contraction stress test (CST) was always negative.

°Suspicious or positive CSTs were frequently preceded by no response to auditory stimulation.

•A response to fetal scalp puncture or to a gentle pinch of the scalp with atraumatic clamp correlated uniformly with a fetal scalp blood pH 7.20 or higher.

•Objective: to evaluate whether there are significant differences in the intrapartum fetal acid-base status according to the magnitude and duration of FHR accelerations in response to fetal vibroacoustic stimulation.

•The most frequent indication was moderate and/or severe variable FHR decelerations followed by loss of FHR variability or an abnormal baseline FHR.

•A tiny umbilical cord with fetal growth retardation was noted in half of those fetuses from the nonacceleration group who responded with a variable deceleration.

•Results: The fetal heart rate response to noninvasive fetal vibroacoustic stimulation reliably predicted an acidotic state in the fetus with a nonreassuring FHR tracing during labor or who, for other reasons, was determined to be at increased risk of intrapartum compromise.

•Using the cutoff pH value of 7.20, the overall ability to identify the acidotic fetus using fibro-acoustic stimulation was 90%.

•Of the 20 patients in the group with an FHR response of 10-15 beats per minute and 10-15 seconds, no fetus had a pH value of less than 7.20, indicating that this magnitude and duration of FHR acceleration is as highly sensitive in detecting the acidotic fetus as is the more marked response.

•Results: An accleration of at least ten beats per minute and 10 seconds will reliably predict at fetal pH of 7.20 or higher, but not always one that is above 7.25.

•The mechanism of FHR acceleration is probably related to a burst of fetal activity and/or an intact fetal nervous system reflex response, mediated perhaps through **catecholamines**.

•The magnitude and duration of the FHR change after acoustic stimulation are diminished intrapartum as compared with antepartum, and diminished further with the progression of labor.]

---

3. Relaxin inhibits uterine contractions by

     A. ß-adrenergic stimulation
     B. binding calmodulin
     *C.   decreasing intracellular Ca^{+2}
     D. increasing phosphodiesterase concentration
     E. increasing progesterone receptors

---

p.1399 (Ginsburg RW, Rosenberg CR, Schwartz M, Colon JM, and Goldsmith LT, "The effect of relaxin on calcium fluxes in the rat uterus" Am J Obstet Gynecol 1988;159:1395)

3. [F&I:•Background: •Objective: to determine whether relaxin inhibits uterine muscle contractility by affecting uterine muscle Ca^{2+} flux.

•Smooth muscle contraction is the end result of a cascade of events that results in the cross-linking of actin and myosin.

°Contraction is associated with an increase in cytosolic free calcium concentrations.

°Relaxation of muscle is associated with a decrease in cytosolic free calcium.

°If the action of relaxin is a calcium-mediated event, the hormone may cause increased calclium efflux from muscle cells, decreased calcium uptake, or both.

•Results: Relaxin inhibition of uterine contractions is associated with a decrease in intracellular free calcium levels.

°Relaxin appears to do this at least in part by promoting calcium efflux from uterine cells.

•Although the mechanisms by which calcium regulates smooth muscle contraction and relaxation is complex, presently available evidence suggests the following chain of events occurs:

°1) Excitation of the muscle results in an increase in intracellular calcium concentration;

°2) this results in calcium binding to calmodulin;

°3) the calcium calmodulin complex binds to myosin light chain kinase;

°4) this complex catalyzes phophorylation of the 20,000 dalton myosin light chain, resulting in actin activation of its magnesium adenosine triphosphatase activity initiating the contractile process;

°5) when the calcium level decreases, myosin light chain kinase becomes inactive due to its dissociation from the calcium calmodulin complex;

°6) The myosin phosphatase is active under these low calcium conditions, resulting in myosin dephosphorylation and relaxation.

•Relaxin may modulate smooth muscle contraction by other mechanisms in addition to affecting calcium fluxes.

°Activation of adenylate cyclase may result in a rise in cyclic adenosine monphosphate levels and activation of a cyclic adenosine monophosphate-dependent protein kinase, which catalyzes phophorylation of myosin light-chain kinase.

°Since the calcium calmodulin complex binds more weakly to the phosphorylated than to the nonphosphorylated mysoin light-chain kinase, myosin light-chain kinase becomes less active, favoring the dephosphorylated form of myosin and causing relaxation.

•Relaxin may have a crucial role in early pregnancy in the inhibition of uterine contractions.

°Relaxin may play a role in the promotion of labor later in pregnancy by means of a softening effect on human cervical connective tissue.

•Relaxin is present in large quantities in human seminal fluid and has been demonstrated to increase the motility of human sperm.]

---

4.   Low dose aspirin used in the treatment of preeclampsia

    A.   increases intracellular calcium
    B.   inhibits angiotensin II production
    C.   inhibits production of atrial natriuretic peptide
    *D.   inhibits thromboxane production
    E.   stimulates prostacyclin production

---

p.1383   (Throp JA, Walsh SW, and Brath PC, "Low-dose aspirin inhibits thromboxane, but not prostacyclin, production by human placental arteries" Am J Obstet Gynecol 1988;159:1381)

4. [F&I:•Background: Preeclampsia with intrauterine growth retardation is associated with increased vascular resistance and decreased placental blood flow.

•Thromboxane is a potent vasoconstrictor and stimulator of platelet aggregation, whereas prostacyclin (PGI$_2$) is a potent vasodilator and inhibitor of platelet aggregation.

•Thus, the imbalance of increased thromboxane/decreased PGI$_2$ production by preeclamptic placentas is clinically relevant.

•Low dose aspirin can selectively inhibit thromboxane production by fetal platelets without affecting PGI$_2$ production by umbilical vessels in vitro.

•Cyclooxygenase metabolites might be involved in the vasoconstrictive effect of angiotensin II.

°Low dose aspirin therapy may alter thromboxane/PGI$_2$ ratio in favor of PGI$_2$.

•Objective: to assess the effect of low dose aspirin on placental arterial production of thromboxane and PGI$_2$ in the presence and absence of a vasoconstricting dose of angiotensin II.

•Low dose aspirin selectively inhibits thromboxane production in human placental arteries, both with and without vasoconstricting doses of angiotensin II.

•Results: The effect on antiotensin II in placental vasculature is not mediated by changes in thromboxane and/or PGI_2 production rates.

•The possible mechanism of action of low dose aspirin in preventing or treating preeclampsia appears to be the **selective inhibition of thromboxane**.

•Conclusion:

°1) Normal placental arteries produce significantly more PGI_2 than thromboxane;

°2) low dose aspirin significantly decreases production of thromboxane but not PGI_2 in isolated human placental arteries and;

°3) addition of angiotensin II in a dose sufficient produce vasoconstriction does not significantly alter thromboxane or PGI_2 production by placental arteries nor does angiotensin II alter the effect of low-dose aspirin to selectively inhibit thromboxane.]

---

5.   Which of the following tests is most sensitive for the detection of iron depletion in pregnancy?

A.   serum iron
*B.   serum ferritin
C.   serum transferrin
D.   mean corpuscular volume
E.   red cell distribution width

---

p.1132   (Thompson WG, "Comparison of tests for diagnosis of iron depletion in pregnancy," Am J Obstet Gynec   1988; 159:1132)

5. [Facts and Issues:•Background: Iron deficiency is common in pregnant women for three reasons:

°1) many women of childbearing age are in precarious iron balance (33% to 50% of women between the ages of 23 and 30 years have no bone marrow iron),

°2) the erythrocyte volume increase in pregnancy requires iron, and

°3) fetal iron requirements are satisfied before maternal iron needs.

•Absent bone marrow iron is an extremely common finding in pregnancy.

•A low ferritin level in pregnancy correlates with absent bone marrow iron stores, indicating that a low ferritin level represents true iron deficiency.

•Approximately half the patients in the present study had a hemoglobin value >12 gm/dl (120 gm/L), so **iron depletion** may be a more appropriate term than iron deficiency for these patients.

•Women with iron deficiency have babies with lower cord ferritin levels.

°The difference in infant iron stores can persist for at least as long as six months.

•The red cell distribution width is superior to the mean corpuscular volume but neither is sufficiently sensitive to screen for iron depletion and deficiency.

•The mean corpuscular volume and transferrin saturation are poor markers for iron deficiency and pregnancy.

•Iron depletion is defined by a low **serum ferritin levels** and are extremely common in pregnancy.

•Other tests such as a red cell distribution width, mean corpuscular volume and transferrin saturation are not sufficiently sensitive to diagnose iron depletion and deficiency.]

---

6. Approximately what percentage of women with a retained dead fetus will have laboratory evidence of abnormal coagulation?

    A. < 1
    B. 5
    C. 10
    *D.   25
    E. 50

---

p.1182 (Chescheir NC, and Seeds JW, "Spontaneous resolution of hypofibrinogenemia associated with death of a twin in utero: A case report ," Am J Obstet Gynec 1988; 159:1183)

6. [Facts and Issues:•Background: Maternal coagulation defects associated with a retained dead fetus rarely develop less than 4 weeks after fetal death.

°Only 25% of women with a retained dead fetus will ever have laboratory evidence of abnormal coagulation and a few of these will have clinical complications.

•Chronic release of thromboplastin from the fetal unit into the maternal ciruclation with resultant chronic intravascular coagulation is the mechanism for this coagulopathy.

•Heparin therapy for clinical consumptive coagulatopathy may be efficacious.

•This case supports conservative management with close monitoring without heparin therapy in the presence of laboratory, but not clinical evidence of hyperfibrinogenemia.

•There was spontaneous resolution of hypofibrinogenimia related to a cessation of thromboplastin release into the maternal circulation; this may vary with the gestational age and somatic mass of the dead twin.]

---

7. When does the switchover from fetal to adult hemoglobin synthesis begin?

    *A.   30 weeks gestation
    B. 36 weeks gestation
    C. 7-10 days post-natal
    D. 3 weeks post-natal
    E. 6 months post-natal

---

p.1280 (Bard H, and Fouron JC, "The increase in fetal hemoglobin synthesis in the fetal lamb during hyperglycemic hypoxema ," Am J Obstet Gynec 1988; 159:1269)

7. [Facts and Issues:•Background: Elevated levels of fetal hemoglobin at birth can be caused by maternal hypoxia, intrauterine growth retardation, placental insufficiency and maternal diabetes.

•The period of rapid switchover from fetal hemoglobin to adult hemoglobin synthesis begins at about 28 weeks of postconceptional age and lasts around 22 weeks.

•Objectives:

°to evaluate the effect of hyperglycemia on myocardial function,

°to compare fetal and adult hemoglobin synthesis during hypoxemia induced by hyperglycemia.

•In the fetus of the diabetic mother, hypoxemia results from hyperglycemia.

°At birth, infants of diabetic mothers are hypoxemic, have higher levels of erythropoietin and immature red cells, and have increased fetal hemoglobin synthesis.

•Major effects of glucose excess are fetal hypoxemia resulting from stimulation of fetal oxidative metabolism that increases O2 consumption and O2 extraction, an increase in the concentration of erythropoietin and expanded erythropoises.

•Results: Fetal hypoxemia resulting from hyperglycemia increases fetal hemoglobin synthesis.

•Erthytroid progenitor cells can be prematurely committed and forced into terminal differentiation during stress erythropoiesis.]

---

8.   Which of the following is the best modality for diagnosing acute puerperal ovarian vein thrombosis?

    A.   abdominal sonography
    *B.   computed tomography
    C.   femoral venography
    D.   intravenous pyelography

---

p.907 (Khurana BK, Rao J, Freidman SA, and Cho KC, "Computed tomographic features of puerperal ovarian vein thrombosis " Am J Obstet Gynecol 1988;159:905)

8. [F & I:•Background: Puerperal ovarian vein thrombosis involves the right ovarian vein in 80% of cases, the left ovarian vein in 6%, and is bilateral in 14%.

•The diagnosis of puerperal ovarian vein thrombosis is difficult and has usually been presumed on the basis of late clinical findings or confirmed at operation, which carries with it a high mortality rate.

°In the past only 20% of the cases were diagnosed without operation.

°Postoperative pulmonary embolism was reported in 16.5% of these patients.

•Femoral venography and intravenous pyelography can suggest the diagnosis in a relatively late stage by demonstrating iliac vein thrombosis and proximal ureteral obstruction, but these findings are nonspecific.

•Abdominal sonography including duplex Doppler ultrasound is useful for imaging the inferior vena cava, but intervening bowel gas usually precludes adequate examination of the ovarian veins even with coronal and steep oblique approaches.

•Both **computed tomographic scanning** and magnetic resonance imaging can visualize the ovarian vein directly.

•The following features are helpful in making the diagnosis:

°1. A sausage shaped structure arising in the adnexa that becomes tubular in higher sections and disappears at the level of the renal veins.

°2. A dilated ovarian vein that may be even larger than the inferior vena cava.

°3. Associated thrombosis of inferior vena cava, iliac veins, and even femoral veins.

°4. Enhancement, on contrast injection, of the walls of the thrombosed bein, with the thrombus appearing as a low-density area.

°5. An inflammatory mass around the ovarian and iliac veins mimicking retroperitoneal lymphadenopathy.]

9. A 30 year old para 0-0-0-0, LMP 17.5 weeks ago, has a maternal serum alpha-fetoprotein 0.4 multiples of the median. Ultrasound shows a single fetus with dimensions consistent with a 15 week gestation.

The next best step in the patient's management is

    *A.   determine the fetal karyotype
    B. no further testing until the third trimester
    C. repeat the maternal serum alpha-fetoprotein in 2 weeks
    D. repeat the maternal serum alpha-fetoprotein now
    E. repeat the ultrasound in 2 weeks

p.370   (Albright SG, Lingley LH, Seeds JW, Lincoln-Boyea B, "Pitfalls of gestational age reassignment in evaluation of low maternal serum α-fetoprotein levels," Am J Obstet Gynec 1988; 159:369)

9. [F & I:•Background: There is an inverse relationship between maternal serum alpha-fetoprotein (AFP) concentrations and the risk of fetal trisomy including trisomy 21.

•Alpha-fetoprotein screening programs utilize maternal serum AFP level along with maternal age to identify the younger women who has a risk similiar to that of a 35 year old women for carrying a fetus with trisomy.

•A significant number of low maternal AFP levels are due to misdated (less advanced of non-viable pregnancies).

•Fetal trisomy may cause early severe growth retardation.

•Objective: to describe two cases of low maternal serum AFP that are illustrative of that point.

•Women carrying fetuses with trisomy 18 (uncomplicated by ventral wall and neural tube defects) have markedly decreased maternal serum AFP levels with a median of 0.6 multiples of the median.

•When ultrasound identifies the misdated pregnancy and a change in dates of greater than two weeks allows for reinterpretation of of maternal serum alpha-feto protein levels into the normal range; the patient should be carefully cautioned that revised interpretation of the maternal serum alpha-fetoprotein level based on mild discrepancies in fetal biometric data does not guarantee the absence of a chromosomal abnormality.]

10. A patient at risk for preterm labor is self-monitoring her hourly uterine activity while at home. What is the fewest contraction per hour after which treatment should be initiated?

    A. 2
    *B.   4
    C. 6
    D. 8
    E. 10

p.595 (Iams JD, Johnson FF, and O'Shaughnessy RW, "A prospective random trial of home uterine activity monitoring in pregnancies at increased risk of preterm labor. Part II " Am J Obstet Gynecol 1988;159:595)

10. [F & I:•Background: Early detection of uterine activity will improve the success rate of preterm labor treatment.

    •Objective: to report the results from the second year of a study comparing self palpation with electronic monitoring.

    •Methods: All patients were between 20 and 34 weeks' gestation.

    •Results: There was no improvement in pregnancy outcom´ **associated with electronic activity monitoring.**

    •Conclusion: Daily contact with the nurse whose only goal is the prevention of prematurity may be the feature of the electronic monitoring system most responsible for the successful reduction of prematurity previously reported.

    •The **Hawthorne effect** is the tendency of study subjects to behave as they believe they are expected to, thus confounding an experiment designed to test the intervention.

    •Both preterm labor and preterm rupture of the membranes may begin with alterations in cervicovaginal microflora.

        °The cervix and decidua may then be the first part of the uterus affected by these events, leading to symptoms of increased vaginal discharge, pelvic pressure, and backache before the development of uterine activity.

        °If this is so, then a contraction -based warning system for incipient preterm labor would not be timely.]

11. Which of the following is significantly associated with systemic tocolysis and pulmonary edema?

    A. age of gestation at the time of treatment
    B. multiple gestation
    *C.   presence of infection
    D. previous reproductive history
    E. type of pharmacologic therapy for preterm labor

p.725   (Hatjis CG, and Swain M, "Systemic tocolysis for premature labor is associated with an increased incidence of pulmonary edema in the presence of maternal infection " Am J Obstet Gynecol 1988;159:723)

11. [F & I:•Background: Premature onset of labor complicates approximately 7% to 10% of deliveries and may account for 60% to 70% of all perinatal mortality and morbidity.

•Objective: to determine if there is an infection underlying the development of pulmonary edema on patients undergoing tocolysis.

•Methods: Medical records review of all patients who developed pulmonary edema to determine if pulmonary edema was seen more frequently in patients with an infectious or inflammatory complication that occurred while they were received systemic tocolytic therapy.

•Sixteen patients were studied.

•Pulmonary edema was diagnosed on basis of clinical findings (primarily rales), chest x-ray films (evidence of pleural effucsion, fluid overload, cardiomegaly, increased vascularity), and arterial blood gases.

•An electrocardiogram was obtained in most cases.

•Invasive hemodynamic monitoring was not done because all patients responded to conservative management favorably in a short period of time.

•Once the diagnosis of pulmonary edema was established, the patients stopped receiving tocolytic therapy and were given intravenous furosemide (Lasix).

°The majority of patients received intramuscularly betamethasone therapy.

•Results: Sixteen patients developed pulmonary edema while receiving systemic tocolysis.

°In 11 of these 16 patients, there was evidence of maternal infection.

•There was a highly significant association between the occurrence of pulmonary edema and treatment with systemic tocolysis.

•Of the 527 patients receiving tocolysis, there was evidence of maternal infection in 52.

°The incidence of pulmonary edema was higher in the presence of maternal infection.

°Patients with urinary tract infections did not have the clinical picture of pyelonephritis.

•There was no significant fluid overload.

•Arterial blood gas levels in room air were uniformly abnormal in all cases but one.

°Electrocardiogram showed nonspecific STT wave abnormalities wave abnormalities either alone or in association with normal sinus tachycardia.

°There was no evidence of ischemia.

•There was no association between betamethasone treatment and the presence of maternal infection.

•The exact causes of pulmonary edema associated with treatment for preterm labor is not known.

•Despite the complication of pulmonary edema, six of these patients were successfully treated for preterm labor, achieved pregnancy prolongation without any further therapy, and were delivered at term.

°An additional nine mothers were delivered of infants weighing between >1500 and 2500 gm.

•Preexisting conditions should be ruled out: an electrocardiogram before the start of tocolytic therapy and (in selected cases) a chest x-ray film might be helpful.

•The major side-effects of ß-adrenergic drugs include hyperglycemia, hypokalemia, hypotension, cardiac dysrhythmias, myocardial ischemia, and pulmonary edema.

•Patients treated with ß-mimetics for bronchial asthma or cardiac insufficiency seldom have pulmonary edema.

•Observations:

°(1) Pulmonary edema occurs only in the first 3 days of intravenous therapy;

°(2) it is usually seen only in the third trimester, when there is a tendency toward water retention;

°(3) there is a frequent association with the use of other medications such as glucocorticoids, magesium sulfate, prostaglandin antagonists, or calcium antagonists; and

°(4) certain pregnancy conditions (multiple gestations, hydramnios, pregnancy-induced hypertension) are more frequently associated with pulmonary edema than is normal pregnancy.

»Pathophysiology of pulmonary edema during tocolysis:

°1) ß-mimetics cause an increase in hydrostatic pressure;

°2) there is a decrease in the colloid osmotic pressure from antidiu.ѹ and thirst;

°3) there is a concurrent increase in capillary permeability; and

°4) these effects lead to an increase of filtration of water into the interstitium of the lung.

•An infectious agent may release a toxic substance that has a direct effect on the uterus, causing labor, and also has an effect on the endothelial lining of the capillaries, increasing their permeability and allowing fluid to escape into the extravascular space.

•Or an infection causes an increase in the cardiac output that, compounded with increased cardiac output of the tocolytic agent, can lead to high output failure.

•Conclusions:

°1) Strict attention to fluid intake with the use of a high concentration of drug in a smaller volume of fluid so as not to overload the patient;

°2) strict attention to output, including the use of a Foley catherter to obtain hourly reoprts;

°3) the restriction of tocolysis to only one drug;

°4) the restriction of glucocosteroids; and

°5) frequent evaluation of the patient for signs and symptoms of respiratory compromise.

•Pulmonary edema can develop even in the presence of fairly low doses of oral terbutaline.]

12. What percentage of children with long-term handicaps are the product of entirely normal
    pregnancies and uneventful deliveries?

    A. 1-2%
    B. 5-10%
    C. 20-25%
    D. 33%
    *E.   > 50%

p.504   (Clapp JF, Peress NS, Wesley M, Mann LI, "Brain damage after intermittent partial cord
occlusion in the chronically instrumented fetal lamb," Am J Obstet Gynec   1988; 159:504)

12. [F & I:•Background: The incidence of late disability after ominous perinatal events remains <50%
and **>50% of children with long-term handicaps are the product of entirely normal
pregnancies and uneventful deliveries.**

    •Because of the redistribution of intracerebral blood flow, hemispheric white matter becomes
selectively vulnerable to injury when cerebral oxygenation is marginally compromised by
hemodynamic instability with or without superimposed hypoxia.

        °The mechanism underlying selective vulnerability is a regional imbalance between blood flow
        and metabolism, which is accentuated during late fetal and neonatal life by the metabolic
        demands of myelination.

    •Objective: to test the hypothesis that intermittent partial cord occlusion or its attendant
hemodynamic instability results in cerebral white matter injury without systemic evidence of protracted
hypoxia or progressive acidosis.

    •Results: Intermittent partial occlusion of the umbilical circulation for as little as 2 hours is a
causal factor in antenatal brain damage, with a pattern of injury almost entirely limited to a specific
area of the cerebral white matter.

        **°The consistent anatomic location of lesions in the tips of the tongues of
        the white matter suggests that this region may be the anatomic radial
        watershed area between the central and circumferential cerebral circulations.**

    •The specific pattern of injury occurs in the absence of progressive systemic acidosis or protracted
hypoxia and without hyperglycemia or a surge in fetal cortisol levels.

    •The pulsatile, intermittent, partial nature of the interference with umbilical flow, chosen to mimic
the pattern produced when the cord is intermittently partially occluded by uterine contractions, produced
defined evidence of fetal stress (baseline tachycardia and increased variability between occlusions) with
cyclic fluctuations in systemic arterial pressure without defined systemic evidence of fetal distress or
compromise as judged by arterial pH and lactate, glucose, and cortisol levels.

        °The interruption was not severe or prolonged enough to reduce oxygen availability below a
        critical level in most tissues, which is the case in the majority of clinical situations involving
        intermittent cord compromise for an equivalent period.

    •The presence of this central nervous system injury is associated with persistent abnormalities in
fetal heart rate and electrocortical activity in its acute stage.

    •Conclusion: There is selective cerebral white matter vulnerability during marginal tissue
oxygenation.]

13. Which of the following when detected in utero ultrasonographically has the best prognosis?

      *A.   coarctation of the aorta
      B.   Ebstein's anomaly
      C.   endocardial fibroelastosis
      D.   tetralogy of Fallot
      E.   transposition of the great arteries

p.355   (Crawford DC, Chita SK, Allan LD, "Prenatal detection of congenital heart disease: Factors affecting obstetric management of survival," Am J Obstet Gynec   1988; 159:352)

13. [F & I:•Background: •Objective: to present the experience and diagnosis and management of fetal congential heart disease.

•Patients and methods: All pregnancies were referred for fetal electrocardiography that were at increased risk for congenital heart disease.

    °Maternal risk factors included a family history of congenital heart disease, maternal diabetes and maternal exposure to a potential teratogen such as lithium or rubella.

    °Specific risk factors identifed during pregnancy included extra cardiac fetal anomaly, intrauterine growth retardation, fetal hydrops, polyhydramnios, fetal cardiac dysrhythmia, or suspected congenital heart disease based on a routine obstetric scannin.

•Elective studies were scheduled at 18 and 24 weeks gestation and other pregnancies were examined as and when they were referred.

•When abnormalities were suspected, pulsed Doppler ultrasound was frequently used to evaluate fetal cardiac hemodynamics.

•Results: 750 fetal echocardiograms were performed on a total of 989 antenatal patients.

    °Cardiac abnormalitles were corrected predicted in 74 cases.

•The largest patient group containing 691 patients was referred for fetal echocardiography because of a **family history of congenital heart disease.**

•Seventy women were referred because a cardiac anomaly had been suspected by the obstetric ultrasonographer.

•A positive diagnosis of congenital heart disease was made when an **extra cardiac anomaly** was the reason in 15 cases of congenital heart disease including three cases of conjoined twins (yield 31%).

•**Fetal hydrops** was the referral reason in 8 cases (yield 18%) whereas fetal dysrhythmia was the referral reason in three cases (yield 5%).

•**Oligohydramnios** and maternal mumps during the first trimester was associated with the two remaining cases.

•Forty-two cases of congenital heart disease were detected before 28 weeks gestation, 15 of which had associated anomalies.

•Cardiac defects were diagnosed after 20 weeks gestation in 32 pregnancies, 14 of which had associated extra cardiac anomalies.

°More than one-third of this group (11 cases), were referred because of non-immune hydrops and atrioventricular septal defect.

•An **atrioventricular septal defect** was found in 18 fetuses.

°In no case the atrioventricular septal defect an isolated anomaly.

°Fourteen fetuses with atrioventricular septal defect also had extra cardiac or chromosomal anomalies.

°Trisomy 21 or Downs syndrome was the most common anomaly, being associated in six cases.

•**Ventricular septal defects** were detected prenatally in 19 fetuses; all defects were moderate or large in size.

°In 14 fetuses the ventricular septal defect was a feature of a complex cardiac anomaly.

°Extracardiac or chromosomal anomalies were found in 11 fetuses.

°The association among trisomy 18, exomphalos, and ventricular septal defects has been described and was found in three more fetuses in this series.

•**Left-sidedcardiac anomalies:** The spectrum of abnormalities in this group includes coarctation of the aorta, aortic atresia, and mitral atresia with intact ventricular septum, which may be described as hypoplastic left heart syndrome.

•**Right-sided cardiac anomalies:** Cardiac anomalies affecting the right side of the heart with intact ventricular septum were diagnosed in nine fetuses.

°All fetuses with anomalies complicated by pulmonary compression died in utero.

°Epstein's anomaly of the tricuspid valve is represented by redundancy and dysplasia of the tricuspid valve with adherence of a variable portion of the septal and often posterior leaflets to the right ventricular wall so that the free portion of the leaflets is displaced downward away from the normal atrioventricular rent.

•Cardiomyopathy or **endocardial fibroelastosis** in the absence of an obstructive cardiac lesion was detected in five fetuses.

°The prognosis is poor.

•False negative diagnoses: A false negative diagnosis of congential heart disease occurred in 17 cases.

•False positive diagnoses: One minor false positive diagnosis made during the period, right ventricular dominance in the fetus examined during the third trimester was considered suspicious and coarctataion of the aorta could not be excluded.

•The prognosis for congential heart disease detected during pregnancy is very poor.

°The survival rate for continuing pregnancies is 17% after one year of follow-up.

°Cardiac abnormalities not detected prenatally were more minor defects which have a better prognosis; the survival rate in the latter group is 81%.

•In total, 46% of congenital cardiac defects diagnosed prenatally had associated extracardiac or choromosomal anomalies.

•A diagnosis of atrioventricular ventricular septal defect should prompt a thorough investigation for additional intercardiac/extracardiac and chromosomal defects.

•A more severe spectrum of congenital heart disease is detected prenatally then that usually encountered by the pediatric cardiologist and postnatal referrals.

•Fetal hydrops associated with a structural cardiac anomaly has a poor prognosis and conservative obstetric management may be appropriate.

•Small ventricular septal defects, secundum atrial septal defects, arterial valve stenoses, and patent ductus arteriosis may be undetectably prenatally.

•Tetrology of Fallot: 1) A cyanotic type of outflow tract lesions of the right heart marked by pulmonic stenosis, 2) interventricular septal defect, 3) overriding dextral position of the aorta and 4) right ventricular hypertrophy.

•Eisenmenger's complex: Cyanotic lesion of outflow tract: 1) Dextoprosition of the aorta, 2) intraventricular septal defect, 3) normal or slightly enlarged pulmonary artery, 4) no right ventricular hypertrophy.]

---

14. What is the minimum predonation hematocrit required of a pregnant patient in anticipation of autologous transfusion at delivery?

    A. 36
    *B.   34
    C. 32
    D. 30
    E. 28

---

p.169   (Herbert W, Owen H, and Collins M. "Autologous blood storage in obstetrics" Obstet Gynecol 1988;72:166)

14. [F & I:•Background: Adverse effects of blood transfusion include transfusion reactions, development of antibodies, and transmission of infection.

•Transfusion of one's own blood minimizes these risks by reducing the need for homologous blood.

•Preoperative collection of autologous blood is safe and effective in decreasing reliance on homologous blood transfusions.

•Patients with placenta previa and previous cesarean section, have a greater incidence of blood transfusion.

•Despite improved blood banking techniques, patients receiving homologous blood are at risk for transmitted infection and blood incompatibility.

°Hepatitis occurs in an estimated 5-10% of blood transfusion recipients; a majority of cases are non A, non B for which there is not specific screening test available.

•Transmission of human immunodeficiency virus via blood in well known but with the current screening of blood for HIV antibody the risk of developing this infection from blood transfusion is estimated to be 1 in 250,000 or less.

•About 1-3% of blood transfusion recipients will develop alloantibodies to red cell antigens.

•Available forms of autologous blood transfusion: preoperative phlebotomy and autotransfusion.

°The latter can be further categorized into red cell salvage and hemodilution.

°In some settings, eg. with ruptured ectopic pregnancies, freshly shed red cells can be collected, processed and reinfused.

•Isovolemic hemodilution is a technique by which whole blood collected after induction of anesthesia and immediately before incision is replaced by crystalloid solution at a volume ratio of 2:1 or 3:1 of crystalloid to whole blood removed.

•Results: 30 patients provided 55 units of blood.

•Inconsequential mild uterine contractions were occasionally noted to before, during or after the phlebotomy procedure.

•Fetal heart rate tracings were normal and changes in mean diastolic blood pressure and mean pulse were minimal.

•Reactions occurred in only two of 51 phlebotomy procedures.

°Both were transient and responded to position change and oral fluid administration.

•Patients with placenta previa who are stable and who do not require delivery soon after admission are prime candidates for this program.

°40% of patients with this complication require delivery within 24 hours after admission and cannot participate.

•The need for transfusion in obstetric patients is quite low and the cost benefit ratio may not justify participation.

•The number of units that should be predepositied is not clear.

•The average transfusion used in patients with placenta previa is 1.8 units and for those with planned cesarean delivery 2.6 units.

•The minimum hematocrit required for predonation may be less than the current recommendation 34% in non-pregnant individuals.]

---

15. The most important element initiating the active management of labor is

    A. parity
    *B.   regular uterine contractions
    C. rupture of the membranes
    D. station of presenting part
    E. the dilation of the cervix

---

p.255   (Akoury HA, Brodie G, Caddick R, McLaughin BD, and Pugh PA, "Active management of labor and operative delivery in nulliparous women," Am J Obstet Gynecol 1988;158:255.)

15. [F & I:•Background:Four diagnostic categories are identified as mainly responsible for the rise in cesarean births: **Dystocia, repeat cesarean section, breech presentation, and fetal distress.**

•Dystocia is usually limited to first labors, and through repeat cesarean section directly or indirectly accounts for about 60% of all cesarean sections.

•Objective: to examine the effect of **active management of labor** on operative delivery rates in nulliparous women.

•**The most important element in active management of labor is to establish the diagnosis of labor followed by early detection and treatment of nonprogressive labor.**

•Diagnosis was made only if subjective elements of pain presented by the patient (at least two painful contractions every 15 minutes) were confirmed by objective findings of the presence of a fully effaced and/or $\geq$ 2 cm dilated cervix.

°Within 1 to 2 hours of the diagnosis of labor, amniotomy was performed.

•The progress of labor was monitored by pelvic examination every 2 hours.

°If the cervix failed to dilate $\geq$ 1 cm/hr, oxytocin augmentation was started.

°The rate was regulated by a pump with one-to-one nursing care.

°The oxytocin rate was titrated against cervical dilatation, with fetal distress or uterine contractions < 2 minutes apart being limited factors.

•In the second stage of labor, progress was measured by descent of the head.

•It was divided into two phases.

°The first phase from full dilatation until the bearing-down reflex and the second phase from the bearing-down reflex to delivery.

•One hour was allowed for each.

•Oxytocin augmentation was used if the first phase lasted >1 hours.

•A trial of forceps and/or cesarean section was performed if the second phase lasted >1 hour.

•Continuous electronic fetal heart rate monitoring was carried out when women were in active labor.

•Conclusion: Active management of labor in nulliparous women reduced the duration of labor, the use of forceps and the rate of cesarean deliveries with no increase in perinatal morbidity and mortality.]

---

16. Which of the following conditions has the greatest effect on accelerating fetal lung maturity?

    A. insulin dependent diabetes mellitus
    B. intrauterine growth retardation
    C. pregnancy-induced hypertension
    *D.   premature rupture of the membranes
    E. second trimester uterine bleeding

---

p.41(Barkai G, Reichman B, Modan M, Goldman B, Serr DM, and Mashiach S,"The influence of abnormal pregnancies on fluorescence polarization of amniotic fluid lipids" Obstet Gynecol 1988;71:39)

---

16. [F & I:•Background:Fluorescence polarization of amniotic fluid lipids is a highly sensitive method of estimating fetal lung maturity.

•The depolarization of lipid material, measured as the fluorescence polarization value, reflects changes in the alveolar surfactant content of amniotic fluid.

•Conditions resulting in fetal stress, such as pregnancy-induced hypertension, intrauterine growth retardation (IUGR), premature rupture of the membranes, class R diabetes, and vaginal bleeding, may influence surfactant production both quantitatively and qualitatively.

•Objectives:

    °to evaluate the change in amniotic fluid fluorescence polarization value as a function of gestational age and

    °to define the influence of abnormal pregnancy states on the fluorescence polarization value, and thus of surfactant production.

•Material and Methods: •The study population consisted of 518 consecutively obtained amniotic fluid samples that met certain study criteria.

•Subjects with pregnancy induced hypertension were further subdivided into mild and severe cases, and those with diabetes into two groups (class A and insulin-dependent).

•Premature contractions were diagnosed as regular contractions effective enough to produce a significant change in cervical consistency, effacement, and dilatation in two consecutive examinations one hour apart.

•Premature rupture of the membranes was diagnosed only when there was a time interval of at least one hour between rupture of the membranes and initiation of uterine contractions.

•Intrauterine growth retardation was diagnosed when the fetal weight, estimated by ultrasound examination, was below the tenth percentile for a given gestational week.

•Gluck and Kulovich first suggested an association between abnormal conditions in pregnancy and fetal lung maturity.

•Results: An increased proportion of mature fluorescence polarization values and lower mean fluorescence polarization values in subjects with premature rupture of the membranes compared with other groups.

•The very high proportion of mature values (84.6%) obtained between 31-36 weeks in this study suggests a positive effect of premature rupture of the membranes upon surfactant content of amniotic fluid.

    °This enhancement of fetal lung surfactant synthesis further questions the use of antenatal steroid therapy for induction of fetal lung maturity in cases of premature rupture of the membranes.

•An influence of pregnancy induced hypertension, either mild, severe, or of premature contractions, vaginal bleeding, or IUGR on either the mean fluorescence polarization value or the proportion of mature values obtained was **not** demonstrated.

•Gluck and Kulovich reported delayed pulmonary maturation in classes A, B, and C diabetes, and an acceleration of maturation in classes D, F, and R diabetes.

•Qualitative analysis of amniotic fluid phospholipids in gestational diabetic subjects did not demonstrate any difference from nondiabetic pregnancies.

°No adverse effect on either class A or insulin-dependent diabetes on the mean fluorescence polarization values or the maturity rate were shown.

•Evaluation of the influence of abnormal conditions in pregnancy on fetal lung maturity is complicated by the marked effect of gestational age.

°The proportion of immature measurements decreased from 85% at 29-30 weeks' gestation of 0% at 39-40 weeks.]

---

17. What is the platelet count (x 10^9/L) at term, above which an epidural anesthetic can safely be administered?

    A. 20
    B. 50
    C. 67
    D. 75
    *E.   100

---

p.920   (Rolbin SH, Abbott D, Musclow E, Papsin F, Lie LM, and Freedman J, "Epidural anesthesia in pregnant patients with low platelet counts" Obstet Gynecol 1988;71:918)

17. [F & I: •Background: Platelet counts may decrease slightly during the third trimester because of hemodilution, placental trapping, or hyperdestruction. But the platelet count in pregnancy should still exceed the lower limit of the normal range for the nonpregnant adult.

•**Thrombocytopenia** influences the choice of regional anesthetic.

•Objective: to evaluate the use of epidural anesthesia during delivery in 61 patients with periparturient thrombocytopenia.

•In clinical practice history and physical examination are necessary to rule out predisposing medical diseases or obstetrical complications.

•Results: Epidural anesthesia can be safely administered if the platelet count is above 100 x 10^9/L.

•**Epidural hematoma**, although infrequent, is a true surgical emergency and must be decompressed within six hours to prevent permanent paralysis.

°Therefore, for epidural anesthesia to be considered safe in a patient with a platelet count of less than 100 x 10^9/L, the anesthetist must be convinced of the following:

°°1) there is no risk that the platelet count has decreased further; and

°°2) there is no associated platelet dysfunction or other coagulation abnormality.

•Conclusion: Epidural anesthesia is not advised for obstetric patients with platelet counts below 100 x 10^9/L.]

18. For which fetal condition would maternal serum alpha-fetoprotein values be the highest?

    A. diaphragmatic hernia
    B. Down syndrome
    *C.   gastroschisis
    D. omphalocele
    E. spina bifida occulta

p.908   (Palomaki GE, Hill LE, Knight GJ, Haddow JE and Carpenter M, "Second-trimester maternal serum alpha-fetoprotein levels in pregnancies associated with gastroschisis and omphalocele" Obstet Gynecol 1988;71:906)

18. [F & I: •Objective: to determine the maternal α-fetoprotein distribution for gastroschisis and omphalocele.

•Material and Methods: **Omphalocele** was defined as a midline defect of the abdominal wall with herniation of abdominal organs through the umbilical ring.

•**Gastroschisis** was defined as a paraumbilical defect, located on the **right** side of the abdominal wall, with herniation of intestine and **no covering**.

•Results: Among 72,782 pregnancies screened, 33 ventral wall defects in singleton pregnancies without associated open neural tube defects or autosomal chromosome anomalies were found (13 omphalocele, 20 gastroschisis).

•Results: The maternal α-fetoprotein log mean for gastroschisis was considerably **higher** than for omphalocele.

•These MSAFP-related distribution characteristics may occur because the exposed viscera associated with gastroschisis are not covered by a membrane, thereby allowing relatively free diffusion of AFP from the fetal circulation.

    °The membrane that covers the viscera in omphalocele cases may occasionally rupture in utero, and this may account for the higher log SD of these values.

•Gastroschisis can be detected at considerably higher rate than omphalocele, and because of this the overall MSAFP screening sensitivity for open ventral wall defects will vary in any given geographic area, depending on the relative proportions of the two types of lesions occurring in the pregnant population.]

19. "Toe jam" refers to abuse of

    A. marijuana
    B. cocaine
    *C.   toluene
    D. glue
    E. PCP

p.716   (Goodwin TM, "Toluene abuse and renal tubular acidosis in pregnancy " Obstet Gynecol 1988;71:715)

19. [F & I:•Objective: to examine cases of **toluene** toxicity occurring during pregnancy secondary to paint sniffing.

•A sock or rag is coated with spray paint (usually clear or gold), then placed over the nose and mouth of inhalation, this is known as **"toe jam"**.

°Alternatively, the paint may be sprayed into an empty "pop top" can and inhaled from there.

°Two cans per day is considered heavy use.

•The diagnosis of toluene abuse usually requires physical evidence of recent use in an intoxicated subject (paint on the body or the odor of toluene on the breath).

•Measurement of serum toluene and its major urinary metabolite, hippuric acid, is not widely available.

°Detectable levels of toluene can be present five days after toxic exposure.

°Hippuric acid declines more rapidly, but may be present 48 hours after toxic exposure.

•The highly lipid-soluble toluene appears to cross the placenta freely.

•Patients had diminished arterial pH and serum bicarbonate, hperchloremia, and a normal anion gap in the presence of an abnormally high urine pH (6.0).

°These criteria are sufficient for a diagnosis of renal tubular acidosis.

•During pregnancy, primary hyperventilation reduces serum bicarbonate and raises chloride, creating an electrolyte picture similar to that seen with mild renal tubular acidosis.

°Arterial blood gas measurement will show the normal gravida to be slightly alkalotic.

•Classic or type I **renal tubular acidosis** was first linked to toluene abuse in 1974.

°The defect in this form of renal tubular acidosis is a failure of the distal tubule to generate a hydrogen ion gradient.

•The mechanism by which toluene impairs the capacity of the distal tubule to handle hydrogen ion and bicarbonate transport is unclear, but may be an alteration in membrane permeability which is reversible.

•Patients with severe acidosis may require **intravenous bicarbonate** according to standard protocols.

°Urinary potassium loss will cease promptly after correction of the acidosis.

•The most striking complication of renal tubular acidosis in pregnancy is **paralysis due to hypokalemia.**

•Chronic maternal acidosis of up to six weeks' duration can result in decreased fetal oxygen saturation, but is generally well tolerated.

•In this series there were three cases of IUGR.

•Cerebellar dysfunction can occur in infants of toluene abusers.

•They may also have microcephaly, central nervous system dysfunction, minor craniofacial and limb anomalies, and variable growth deficiencies.]

20. The drug of choice for treating typhoid fever in pregnancy is

    *A.   ampicillin
    B. chloramphenicol
    C. clindamycin
    D. gentamicin
    E. metronidazole

p.713   (Seoud M, Saade G, Uwaydah M, Azoury R, "Typhoid fever in pregnancy " Obstet Gynecol 1988;71:711)

20. [F & I:•Background: Typhoid fever is a significant threat where sanitation facilities are inadequate.

•Objective: to present experience with 14 cases of typhoid fever in pregnancy.

•Before the antibiotic era, typhoid fever in pregnancy carried a 60-80% risk of abortion and premature labor, as well as a 15% maternal mortality rate.

•Multiple antimicrobial resistance is mediated by an R factor transferred to S *typhi* through conjugation with R-factor-bearing bacteria.

°These resistant strains appear to be sensitive to **ampicillin, which remains the drug of choice for typhoid fever in pregnancy.**

•Pregnancy does not alter the clinical presentation or laboratory findings of patients with typhoid fever.

°Only one patient had a pulse of 80 beats per minute; the rest of the women had rates between 100-140 beats per minute, with a mean of 108.

•Conclusion: The presence of maternal tachycardia should not exclude the suspected diagnosis of typhoid fever in a pregnant patient.

°All patients that received antipyretics had a hypothermic response.

•Among the pregnant patients who were infected after 20 weeks, three newborns had a complicated neonatal course, and one of them died at the age of 25 days.

•Conclusion: Pregnant patients who contracted the disease late in the second trimester or third trimester, the neonatal outcome does not seem to be affected.]

21. Meconium aspiration syndrome can best be prevented by

    A. awaiting spontaneous amniorrhexis.
    B. direct treacheobronchial suctioning via laryngoscope below the levels of the cords.
    C. nasopharyngeal and oropharyngeal suctioning with a DeLee suction catheter before delivery of the chest followed by chest physiotherapy and postural drainage.
    D. nasopharyngeal and oropharyngeal suctioning with a DeLee suction catheter before delivery of the chest followed by direct treacheobronchial suctioning via laryngoscope below the levels of the cords.
    *E.   averting fetal hypoxia.

p.352   (Falciglia HS, "Failure to prevent meconium aspiration syndrome " Obstet Gynecol 1988;71:349)

21. [F & I: •Objectives: to test the following hypotheses:

°1) Suctioning of the nasopharynx and oropharynx by DeLee suction suction catheter before delivery of the chest results in a reduced rate of meconium aspiration compared with suctioning after chest wall delivery.

°2) There has been a historic reduction in the **rate of meconium aspiration** using combined obstetric and pediatric suction for meconium-stained fluid, compared with no systematic suctioning.

°3) There has been an historic reduction in **mortality** from meconium aspiration using a combined approach compared with no systematic suctioning.

•Results: The rate of meconium aspiration (2%) was the same in both the early and late-suctioning groups. The first hypothesis was rejected.

•In 1975 when DeLee tracheal suctioning was not used, the syndrome occurred in 2% (15 of 742) of the infants. This lead to rejection of the second hypothesis.

•Routine DeLee tracheal suctioning reduced the **mortality** rate from meconium aspiration, from 46% in 1975 to 12.5% in 1983, or 5.8% from 1979-1983.

•**Not** routine before 1978:

°Routine delivery room attendance by pediatricians

°hyperventilation therapy for primary pulmonary hypertension

°the use of muscle relaxants

°prophylactic antibiotics

°pulmonary vasodilators.

•The **increased cesarean section rate** for meconium-stained fluid in 1983 compared with 1975 is another factor that could have reduced mortality.

•Prevention of meconium aspiration seems possible only if there is **no meconium beyond the nasopharynx and oropharynx at the time of delivery.**

»It appears that more attention should be paid to events preceding the aspiration of meconium.

•Fetal asphyxia causes passage of meconium, and may cause pulmonary vasoconstriction and reduced pulmonary blood flow.

°In response to asphyxia and acidosis, the fetus makes substantial respiratory efforts "opens the laryngeal sphincter," and aspirates meconium into the trachea.

•With the reduction in the outflow of pulmonary fetal liquid secondary to reduced pulmonary blood flow, the self-cleansing action of the tracheobroncheal tree is lost, and aspirated meconium remains in the trachea.

»**It is unlikely that any postdelivery method of suction can remove meconium that has progressed to the lower tracheobroncheal tree, where it is inaccessible to the endotracheal tube.**

•The presence of significant amounts of meconium below the vocal cords in 37% of meconium-stained infants, whose oropharynx and nasopharynx were suctioned before delivery of the chest, supports this conclusion and may explain failure to prevent meconium aspiration syndrome in 2% of the infants.

°Intact fetal membranes containing meconium amy be another contributing factor to the inability of aspiration to prevent meconium aspiration syndrome

°°Meconium retained inside fetal membranes until delivery prevents recognition of the event and delays obstetric intervention.

•Meconium aspiration was associated with perinatal asphyxia in 60% of the infants in all study periods.

•Conclusion: Meconium aspiration is predominantly an intrauterine event, the occurs shortly after the onset of asphyxia and passage of meconium.

°Gasping respiratory movements may continue to mobilize meconium beyond the carina after delivery of the infant.

°Postnatal DeLee and tracheal suction may reduce the amount of **upper** airways and the severity of meconium aspiration.

•Deaths were more related to **primary pulmonary hypertension** than to mechanical difficulties in ventilation from small-airway obstruction by meconium.

°Suction alone is not prevention enough.

•Conclusion: The prevention of fetal **hypoxia** may be the best approach and prevention of severe meconium aspiration syndrome.]

---

22. Which of the following is the earliest sign of fetal hydrops accompanying severe Rh isoimmunization?

    A. ascites
    B. blunting of fetal heart rate variability
    C. dilation fo the umbilical vein
    *D.   pericardial effusion
    E. sinusoidal fetal heart rate pattern

---

p.1328   (Parer JT, "Severe Rh isoimmunization-Current methods of in utero diagnosis and treatment," Am J Obstet Gynecol 1988;158:1323)

22. [F & I:•Background: Isoimmunization occurs in three groups of pregnant women:

°(1)   those Rh-negative mothers who were sensitized before the availability of Rh immunoglobulin in the late 1960's;

°(2)   those who failed to be appropriately treated either during pregnancy or post partum or who became isoimmunized despite treatment; and

°(3)   mothers who are isoimmunized by antigens other than the D antigen.

•Objective: to outline the current diagnostic steps and to recount some results of treatment since the intensive utilization of ultrasound imaging and fetal surveillance.

•**Diagnosis of isoimmunization.** Titer at which amniocentesis should be carried out must be **greater than 1:16.**

°A titer of 1:8 may rise subsequently so at that level it must be measured monthly.

•In the case of a titer sufficiently elevated to warrant amniocentesis, the timing of the first procedure is dictated by the **magnitude of the titer and the previous history.**

°Amniocentesis has begun as early as 18 weeks' gestation in cases of severe early previous involvement.

°With a previous isoimmunized but term delivery amniocentesis would not begin until approximately 24 to 26 weeks' gestation.

•The timing of repeat amniocentesis is dictated by the history and also the value of the previous optical density measurement.

•The recent introduction of cordocentesis for the rapid and easy determination of fetal hemoglobin level and hematocrit has added a further refinement to the diagnosis of the severity of anemia in the erythroblastotic fetus.

°It is now possible to determine fetal hematocrit before either the initial or subsequent intrauterine blood transfusion.

•The increments of ΔOD_{450} are considered to be of **limited usefulness** in defining the severity of erythroblastosis in **midtrimester**.

°Midtrimester fetuses with a change in $\Delta OD_{450} > 0.3$ should be prepared for an intrauterine transfusion, and those with a value < 0.2 could be followed by repeat amniocentesis.

•The general guide is to transfuse if the affected fetus has a hematocrit **below approximately 30% or a hemoglobin value 10 gm/dl.**

•**Intrauterine Transfusion done under the high-resolution real-time ultrasound.**

•Of 45 patients who have completed their pregnancy, there were 9 fetal deaths, the live birth rate was 80%.

•There were 120 intrauterine transfusions, averaging 2.7 transfusions per patient.

°3 fetal losses were traumatic deaths, giving a traumatic death risk of 2.5% per transfusion.

°°All were due to laceration or compromise of a major fetal vessel.

°°All were at such an immature age that salvage was not considered possible.

•Six deaths occurred in utero in hydropic fetuses who failed to absorb transfused blood.

•Intravascular transfusions are carried out by **cordocentesis** in the presence of hydrops or in babies with hematocrits <20%.

•Intraperitoneal pressure is measured to maximize the volume of blood transfused, which is up to 25% above that calculated by the formula:

Volume of packed cells = (gestational age [weeks] - 20) x 10 ml.

°High intraperitoneal pressures may compromise umbilical venous flow due to compression.

•**Surveillance after intrauterine transfusion**

•**Hydrops develops when the hemoglobin value is ≤ 4 gm/dl.**

°Hydrops can develop at later gestational ages at somewhat higher hemoglobin levels.

°At a hemoglobin level ≤ 4 gm/dl the fetus becomes progressively **acidotic** with **lactic acidosis.**

°°This by-product of anaerobic metabolism is produced in such quantities that it cannot be cleared by the placenta.

°At hemoglobin levels between 4 and 8 gm/dl there tends to be an umbilical arterial lactic acidosis only, which is cleared by the placenta.

•**At hematocrit values below approximately 25% there is a blunting of the fetal heart rate variability.**

°**fetal movement often persists well below this level.**

°°The **biophysical profile** may not be a particularly valuable technique for determining the severity of anemia in such fetuses.

°However, fetuses with severe anemia will often have **late decelerations** with contractions and thus **contraction stress testing may be more important in evaluating difficult cases.**

•**Timing and mode of delivery.**

•Transfusions are now attempted up to 34 weeks.

•Delivery has not been guided by tests of pulmonary maturity; rather, the fetus has been delivered when it was felt that the hematocrit was sufficiently high for it to tolerate labor and when it reached a gestational age at which prematurity would be a minor problem.

•**Graft versus host reactions** are prevented by **irradiation of the donor blood**, which immobilizes the small lymphocytes.

•Fetal innoculation of **cytomegalovirus** is avoided by the use of cytomegalovirus antibody-negative donors.

•Fetal radiation has been eliminated by the availability of high-resolution real-time ultrasound equipment.

•Intensive care has improved survival of premature neonates born <32 weeks' gestation and allowed successful rescue of fetuses in emergency situations encountered at the time of fetal evaluation or during transfusion.

•Pericardial effusion may be an earlier sign of hydrops.

•There is no direct relationship between the fetal hemoglobin value and hydrops.]

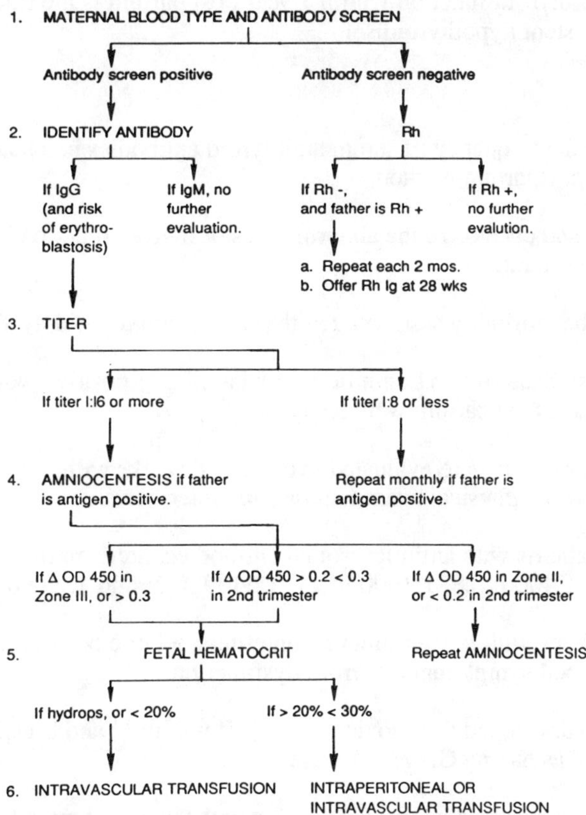

Fig. 1. General guidelines for evaluation and treatment of isoimmunization.

(Reproduced with written permission of the publisher, C.V. Mosby, St Louis, Missouri.)

23. The most common finding in patients who develop post-partum **hypo**thyroidism is

   A.   cold intolerance
   B.   depression
   C.   goiter
  *D.   lack of concentration
   E.   weight gain

p.207   (Hayslip CC, Fein HG, O'Donnell VM, Friedman DS, Klein TA, and Smallridge RC. "The value of serum antimicrosomal antibody testing in screening for symptomatic postpartum thyroid dysfunction," Am J Obstet Gynec 1988; 159:203)

23. [F & I:•Background: Postpartum thyroiditis is a painless, destructive lymphocytic inflammation of the thyroid gland that occurs during the postpartum period and is associated with a high prevalence of serum antithyroid antibodies.

°In the acute phase there is an infiltrative, inflammatory destruction of thyroid parenchyma often manifested by a transient thyrotoxicosis and a nonpainful goiter, generally occurring 6 weeks to 4 months post partum.

°A more prolonged hypothyroid state usually follows, lasting 2 to 6 months or until thyroid follicular epithelial integrity is restored.

°Normalization of thyroid function within 1 year post partum is the rule; however, some patients have persistent hypothyroidism.

•Objectives:

°(1) to determine the frequency of serum antithyroid antibodies in a heterogenous population of American postpartum women,

°(2) to document and categorize the abnormalities of thyroid function in these antibody-positive patients, and

°(3) to evaluate the morbidity associated with post partum thyroid dysfunction.

•Material and Methods: Data from 51 antimicrosomal antibody-positive women evaluated regularly for at least 6 months post partum were analyzed.

•All antibody-positive women were evaluated every 4 to 8 weeks with thyroid function tests, thyroid antibody measurements, physical examinations, and interviews.

°Results: Of the 72 patients with antimicrosomal antibodies, titers on the second postpartum day were 1:100 in 27 patients, 1:400 in 28, 1:1600 in 11, 1:6400 in 5, and 1:25,600 in one patient.

•In contrast to the patients with low antimicrosomal titers, a large percentage of patients with initial titers ≥ 1:400 developed symptomatic thyroid dysfunction.

•Of the 6 patients who developed thyrotoxicosis only, it was mild and transient in four; however, two patients were diagnosed as having Graves' disease.

•Maximal antibody titers occurred between 4 and 6 months post partum, which coincided with peak serum TSH levels.

•The patients with hypothyroidism had three times as many complaints as euthyroid women at 3 to 5 months post partum.

•Approximately 9% of white women tested on the second postpartum day had serum thyroid antimicrosomal antibodies, and 25 or 37 seropositive white patients (64.5%) developed postpartum biochemical thyroid dysfunction.

•In contrast to antimicrosomal antibodies, serum antithyroglobulin antibodies were present in only 0.6% of our patients and were of little value in prediciting postpartum thyroid disease.

•Hispanic women seemed to have an increased frequency and severity of postpartum thyroiditis.

•The necessity of treatment for hypothyroidism also increased as the antibody titer increased.

•An initial antimicrosomal antibody titer of 1:400 was a valuable marker for disease because none of the women with initial titers below this level were treated, whereas women with titers ≥1:400, 30 of 35 (86%) developed biochemical dysfunction, of whom 20 (54%) were treated.

•Although there was a spectrum of disease in women who developed postpartum thyroid dysfunction, a large percentage of our patients required L-thyroxine replacement therapy for hypothyroidism.

•Postpartum symptoms in patients with hypothyroidism were numerous.

°The most worrisome symptoms were the increased frequency of impaired memory and concentration.

°Closer related complaints were increased carelessness and difficulty in completing work.

°Depression was noted in the majority of patients with hypothyroidism.

•The complex symptoms associated with postpartum thyroid dysfunction is a cause for concern because it is probable that women return to work with mental impairments related to postpartum hypothyroidism.

•Serum antimicrosomal antibodies reliably identify women who would benefit from treatment for postpartum thyroid dysfunction.

•Screening for postpartum thyroid disease by clinical parameters alone would not be effective.

•A palpable goiter is **not** a reliable screen for postpartum thyroid disease, because usually it is relatively small and not present before 3 months postpartum.

•Conclusion: The most cost effective method of identifying women with postpartum thyroid disease consists of hospital serum antimicrosomal antibody screening after delivery and follow-up evaluation of antibody-positive patients at 3 months postpartum.

•This method would identify women at highest risk for postpartum thyroid disease requiring treatment as well as a permanent marker to identify those women with underlying autoimmune thyroid disease who may require treatment after a future pregnancy or later in life.]

---

24. At 36 weeks of completed gestation, the chance of a breech presentation spontaneously converting to a vertex presentation is (%)

    *A.   < 20
    B. 33
    C. 50
    D. 67
    E. 75

---

p.1428   (Scaling ST, "External cephalic version without tocolysis," Am J Obstet Gynecol 1987;158:1424)

24. [F & I:Objectives: to report the results of external cephalic version performed in an effort to reduce the incidence of primary cesarean section related to breech presentation and to reduce the incidence of vaginal breech delivery.

•Material and Methods: Sixty six patients underwent 90 attempted external cephalic versions.

•Results: the success rate of external cephalic version at or before 34 weeks was 74.3% and only 45.5% after 34 weeks.

°The overall success rate was 60.6%.

•No fetal or maternal mortality or morbidity occurred.

•One patient with Rh negative blood may have become isoimmunized.

»All patients with breech presentation who were candidates for external version should have an evaluation of the reason for the breech presentation.

•Exclude factors known to be associated with breech presentation.

•There should be an evaluation of fetal well being.

°Forty percent of fetuses undergoing version will exhibit transient bradycardia, tachycardia, or loss of beat-to-beat variability, all indicators of some stress.

•There should be an ultrasound evaluation to assess the **amount of amniotic fluid.**

•The earlier in gestation that the procedure is done, the greater the success.

°The probability of spontaneous conversion to vertex is also higher before 34 weeks gestation.

•There is a rare risk of adverse outcome with fetal distress that may warrant immediate delivery, therefore most authors use a gestational age of $36\frac{1}{2}$ weeks or greater, because the chance of spontaneous version is less than 20% and the pregnancy is essentially at term.

•External cephalic version may protect against premature labor and permit a higher percentage of term deliveries.]

---

25. The most common systemic side effect of the intravaginal application of prostaglandin gel used for the induction of labor is

    A. bronchospasm
    B. diarrhea
    C. headache
    D. hypotension
  *E.   none of the above

---

p.1419 (Rayburn W, Gosen R, Ramadei C, Woods R, and Scott J Jr., "Outpatient cervical ripening with prostaglandin E2 gel in uncomplicated postdate pregnancies," Am J Obstet Gynecol 1987;158:1417)

25. [F & I:•Background: Between 3.5% and 12% of all pregnant women remain undelivered for ≥2 weeks beyond the estimated date of delivery.

°This complication of pregnancy is the most common indication for fetal well-being testing and induction of labor.

•Methods used to prime the "unripe" cervix before labor induction: extraamniotic balloon stretching, the use of *Laminaria*, the application of estradiol gel, and porcine relaxin.

•Clinical trials of prostaglandin E2 gel have shown it can facilitate cervical ripening.

•Objective: to compare the safety and efficacy of PGE2 gel in postdate pregnancies.

•Material and Methods: Singleton pregnancies scheduled for induction of labor for postdate (forty second week) reasons alone and with an unfavorable cervix (Bishop score ≤5) were considered for entry into the study.

•The PGE2 gel was prepared by grinding a whole 20 mg PGE2 suppository and mixing it uniformly with 40 ml methylcellulose gel.

•After a reactive nonstress test, the cervix was swabbed with a rectal swab to remove any discharge.

°A 16-gauge angiocatheter tube was connected to the syringe, and the thawed gel was instilled onto the portio vaginalis of the cervix.

°The patient remained in the semi-Trendelenburg position while uterine contractions and fetal heart rate were monitored intermittently for the next 2 hours by a nurse.

•In the unlikely event of sustained uterine contractions occurring or a worrisome fetal heart rate pattern being noted, precautions were taken to irrigate the upper vagina with normal saline solution and to inject a tocolytic drug (terbutaline 250 µg subcutaneously).

•Duration of labor: the time from the onset of regular (every 3 minutes) or oxytocin induced contractions until delivery.

•A **failed induction** or **failure to progress** during active labor included those women in whom moderately strong and regular uterine contractions did not lead to cervical dilation.

•Results: One hundred and eighteen patients qualified for investigation.

•There were no significant differences in maternal age, race, parity, and pretherapy cervical Bishop scores.

•No systemic side effects were encountered with the gel instillation.

•Labor requiring admission within 8 hours after instillation occurred in 14 (25%) of patients after PGE2 insertion.

•A change in Bishop score ≥3 points was found in almost half of the women who received PGE2.

°Contractions overnight which led to progressive cervical dilatation in the PGE2 group involved 15 women (27%).

•Oxytocin was required for 30 women who received PGE2 and for 59 women who received placebo.

•The time from onset of established labor until vaginal delivery was significantly less for those enrolled in the PGE2 group.

•Infant outcomes were favorable in both groups.]

---

26. Which of the following studies is most sensitive for the detection of amniotic fluid bacterial colonization?

    A. Gram stain
    B. lactic acid dehydrogenase test
    *C.   leukocyte esterase test
    D. limulus amebocyte lysate test
    E. neutrophile count

---

p.122   (Egley CC, Katz VL, and Herbert WNP. "Leukocyte esterase: A simple bedside test for the detection of bacterial colonization of amniotic fluid," Am J Obstet Gynec 1988; 159:120)

26. [F & I]•Background: Neonatal sepsis resulting from chorioamnionitis is secondary only to prematurity as a cause of neonatal morbidity and mortality.

°Chorioamnionitis is a major cause of maternal morbidity.

°Clinical signs and symptoms of chorioamnionitis occur relatively late, making early diagnosis difficult.

•Laboratory tests devised to aid in the early diagnosis of chorioamnionitis include:

°maternal serum C-reactive protein,

°amniotic fluid neutrophils,

°amniotic fluid Gram stain,

°amniotic fluid cultures,

°amniotic fluid lactic dehydrogenase.

•Most of these tests are time consuming and are not particularly sensitive or specific.

•The **leukocyte esterase test** is a rapid, inexpensive test to detect neutrophil activity in urine and other fluids.

•Objective: to examine the relationship between the leukocyte esterase test and the organisms cultured from the amniotic fluid.

•Material and Methods: Fluid was obtained from 44 pregnancy patients at high risk for amnionitis, who had no clinical indication of infection, for example, maternal tachycardia, fetal tachycardia, maternal fever, maternal leukocytosis, or uterine tenderness.

•Each amniotic fluid sample was cultured both aerobically and anaerobically and a Gram stain was performed on an unspun amniotic fluid specimen.

°A positive culture was defined as either moderate of heavy growth.

•In each case one drop of amniotic fluid was tested immediately on its removal for the presence of leukocyte esterase activity by Chemstrip 9 Reagent Strips.

°The leukocyte esterase results were read at 1 minute as negative, trace, +, ++, or +++.

°For the purpose of this study, any reading of trace or greater was called "positive".

•The results of the leukocyte esterase test were not made available to the physicians managing the patients.

°However, the details of the Gram stains and the cultures were available.

•None of the patients were receiving antibiotics at the time of amniotic fluid sampling.

•No patients with meconium staining of the amniotic fluid were included.

•Results: Of the 44 amniotic fluid samples tested, 21 were positive for leukocyte esterase.

•Of the 21 fluid samples positive for leukocyte esterase, all were associated with a positive amniotic fluid culture.

•Of the 23 fluid negative for leukocyte esterase, only 5 (22%) were associated with a positive culture.

°Organisms cultured from the amniotic fluids with **negative** leukocyte esterase tests included *Lactobacillus* species (one), *Staphylococcus epidermidis* (one), *Haemophilus* (two), and *Diptheroids* (one).

°The major organisms cultured from the amniotic fluids with **positive** leukocyte esterase tests included ß-hemolytic streptococcus, *Enterococcus, Peptostreptococcus, Escherichia coli*, and *Bacteroides* species.

•Organisms were found on amniotic fluid Gram stain in 17 samples.

°In 14 (82%) of these the amniotic fluid cultures were positive.

•In samples from the other 27 patients, amniotic fluid Gram stains were negative; organisms were cultured from 12 (44%).

•The sensitivity of leukocyte esterase test in diagnosing chorioamnionitis was 91% and the specificity was 95%.

•Neutrophils contain many destructive enzymes, including the esterases.

°The detection of these enzymes is a marker of white cell activity.

°Ordinary serum or sterile urine without white blood cells will not demonstrate esterase activity.

•Leukocyte esterase was present in all but 2 samples of amniotic fluid from which high virulence organisms were cultured.

•The advantages of leukocyte esterase testing over the Gram stain are that it takes 30 seconds , does not require transportation of samples to a laboratory facility, is inexpensive, and is not subject to subjective interpretation of laboratory personnel.]

---

27. An asymptomatic patient has a unilocular 6 cm ovarian cyst at 16 weeks gestation. The next best step in her management is

    A. biweekly ultrasonogram for cyst growth
    B. culdocentesis for cytological study of peritoneal fluid
    C. laparoscopy with aspiration of cyst
    *D.   ovarian cystectomy
    E. reevaluation in one month

---

p.1033 (Hess LW, Peaceman A, O'Brien WF, Winkel CA, Cruikshank DP, and Morrison JC, "Adnexal mass occurring with intrauterine pregnancy: report of fifty-four patients requiring laparotomy for definitive management," Am J Obstet Gynec 1988; 15:1029)

27. [F & I:•Background: The incidence of adnexal masses occurring in pregnant women is about 1 in 81 to 1 in 2500 live births.

°Approximately half of these masses are <5 cm in diameter, while one-fourth are 5 to 10 cm and 25% are >10 cm in diameter at the time of discovery.

°95% are unilateral, and 65% are asymptomatic at the time of diagnosis.

°94% of those masses <6 cm in diameter that are detected in the first trimester of pregnancy and not surgically removed, resolve spontaneously before the examination 6 weeks post partum, although 75% of those that remain until the second trimester persist until the 6 week examination.

•Approximately 2% to 5% of adnexal masses that are removed during pregnancy are **malignant**, resulting in a malignancy rate of one case per 5000 to 18,000 live births.

•In 1846 Burd reported the surgical removal of an ovarian cyst in a pregnant patient.

•**J. Marion Sims** removed an ovarian tumor from a patient 3 months pregnant who survived an eventually was delivered of a living child at term.

•In 1906 McKerron reported a maternal mortality rate of 21% and a fetal mortality rate of 50% among 720 pregnant women with surgically treated adnexal masses.

•Results: If operation for an adnexal mass occurring in pregnancy is **delayed** until the onset of symptoms, the pregnancy prognosis is **worsened** when compared with that after elective operation.

•**Elective exploration of gravid women having adnexal masses was associated with few adverse pregnancy outcomes and minimal maternal or fetal morbidity.**

•Conclusion: Elective removal of any mass ≥6 cm in diameter that persists until 16 weeks' gestation regardless of its sonographic appearance, unless the mass is suspected to be a uterine leiomyoma, is recommended.

•Sonographic evaluation of the **maternal kidney** if a pelvic kidney or renal cyst is suspected should be undertaken.

•This avoids the risk of emergency, compared with elective operation that can occur when an adnexal mass undergoes acute torsion, acute infarction, or acute hemorrhage.

°This management protocol also avoids the possibility of missing most unsuspected ovarian carcinomas.]

---

28. The underlying pathophysiology of hemorrhagic endovasculitis of the placenta is

    A. diabetes mellitus
    B. graft versus host reaction
  *C.   ischemia
    D. mycoplasma infection
    E. systemic lupus erythematosus

---

p.51   (Shen-Schwartz S, Macpherson T, and Mueller-Heubach E. "The clinical significant of hemorrhagic endovasculitis of the placenta," Am J Obstet Gynec 1988; 159:48)

28. [F & I:•**Hemorrhagic endovasculitis** of the placenta was first described and named in 1980.

°It is important because of its association with perinatal mortality, intrauterine growth retardation (IUGR), and long-term developmental delay.

•Objective: to describe the clinical features of placental hemorrhagic endovasculitis.

•Material and Methods: Criteria for the diagnosis of **placental hemorrhagic endovasculitis** were either one or both of these microscopic features.

°1. Fetal vessel thrombosis associated with vessel wall necrosis, spindle cell proliferation, and red cell entrapment and fragmentation.

°2. Endothelial damage in terminal villi as evidenced by nuclear debris, red cell fragments, stromal hemorrhage, and hypercellularity.

•Up to 52% of infants in cases of hemorrhagic endovasculitis of the placenta were stillborn.

°IUGR, perinatal asphyxia, long-term psychomotor developmental abnormalities, and maternal hypertension or preeclampsia are associated with placental hemorrhagic endovasculitis.

•Placental findings include:

°meconium-stained membranes,

°decreased placental weight,

°umbilical cord abnormalties,

°chronic villitis,

°thrombosis of fetal vessels,

°segmental villous fibrosis, and

°erythroblastosis.

•Viral or mycoplasma-type particles have been seen electron microscopically suggesting that placental hemorrhagic endovasculitis may be an infection that interacts with environmental toxins, altered immune response, changes in prostacyclin levels, and other factors in the maternal-placental-fetal unit.

•Associated features were gestational age of 43 weeks, nuchal cord at delivery, hypertension or preeclampsia, placental fetal vessel thrombosis, infarction, and villitis or unknown cause.

°Nuchal cord was noted in 7 of 13 cases.

•Changes in the umbilical blood flow may be responsible for the vascular changes of placental hemorrhagic endovasculitis.

•Histologic changes of placental hemorrhagic endovasculitis are a result of vascular smooth muscle contraction in fetal vessels that have ischemic and necrotic endothelium.

•Conclusion: Reduced umbilical blood flow may be a link between hemorrhagic endovasculitis of the placenta and its associated maternal and fetal complications.]

---

29. The principle hemodynamic alteration in amniotic fluid embolism is

    A. "shock lung"
    B. acute reflexive adrenal insufficiency
    *C.   impaired left ventricular function
    D. increased pulmonary vascular resistance
    E. splanchnic pooling of effective circulatory volume

---

p.1125   (Clark SL, Cotton DB, Gonik B, Greenspoon J, and Phelan JP, "Central hemodynamic alterations in amniotic fluid embolism" Am J Obstet Gynec   1988; 15:1124)

29. [F & I:•Background: **Amniotic fluid embolism** is characterized by hypoxia, hypotension, cardiovascular collapse with evidence of coagulopathy.

•The principle hemodynamic alteration involved is severe reduction in left ventricular stroke work index indicating impaired left ventricular function.

•Elevations in mean pulmonary artery pressure, paralleled elevations in pulmonary capillary wedge pressure; in all cases pulmonary vascular resistance was within normal limits.]

---

30. The leading infectious cause of congenital deafness in the United States is

    A. Coxackie B virus
    *B.   cytomegalovirus
    C. haemophilus influenzae
    D. mumps
    E. syphilis

p.1189 (Yow Md, Williamson DW, Leeds LJ, Thompson P, Woodward RM, Walmus BF, Lester JW, Six HR, Griffiths PD, "Epidemiologic characteristics of cytomegalovirus infection in mothers and their infants," Am J Obstet Gynec 1988; 15:1189)

30. [F & I:•Background: Approximately 1% of all infants in the United States are congenitally infected by cytomegalovirus.

°Of these, 5% to 10% die or have severe damage (mental retardation, blindness, deafness).

°Of the 95% of infants who are asymptomatic at birth, 15% to 18% will develop problems in infancy or early childhood (deafness, neurological problems, learning difficulties).

°**Cytomegalovirus is the leading infectious cause of mental retardation and congenital deafness in the United States.**

•Objectives: to determine:

°1. the risk factors for the acquisition of cytomegalovirus during pregnancy.

°2. The importance of maternal cytomegalovirus infection as a cause of fetal loss.

°3. The role of maternal antibody in protection of the fetus.

°4. The influence of gestational age at the time of maternal infection on the severity of fetal involvement, and

°5. the immediate and long-term effects of congenital infection in children from birth to 5 years of age.

•Serologically immune status of women when they reach childbearing age is related to their age, socioeconomic group, child-rearing practices, including breast-feeding.

•**Maternal risk factors are: being young and having young children in the home..**

•There was a progressive increase in the seroconversion rate during the second observed pregnancy as compared with the first and during the interval between the two pregnancies.

°This could be the result of the introduction of cytomegalovirus into the family by young children.

•Results: There was an epidemiologic association between fetal death (>20 weeks' gestation) and primary infection in the mother but no association with abortion was found.

•The rate of transmission from mother to living off-spring after primary maternal infection varies from 20% to 50%.

°In mothers who were known to have seroconversion during pregnancy, the rate was 33%.

•The percentage of congenitally infected infants that results from reactivation or reinfection in serologically immune mothers seems to vary depending on the **socioeconomic status of the mother.**

•Primary infection accounts for a greater proportion of infants, than reactivation of latent infection.

•Children with neurological defects have been born to mothers who had infection during all three trimesters.

•Conclusion: Maternal immunity probably protects the infant from disease.]

---

31 In the management of Rh isoimmunization, what is the most accurate method of determining whether a non-hydropic fetus would benefit from a transfusion in utero before 26 weeks gestation?

     A. amniotic fluid ΔOD_{450}
     B. Doppler determination of umbilical artery end diastolic flow
     C. serial maternal antibody titers
     D. ultrasound surveillance of fetus
    *E.   umbilical cord hematocrit

---

p.790   (Berkowitz RL, Chitkara U, Wilkins IA, Lynch L, Plosker H, and Bernstein HH, "Intravascular monitoring and management of erythroblastosis fetalis " Am J Obstet Gynecol 1987;158:783)

31. [F & I:•Background: When transfusion in utero is indicated, the advantages of administering blood intravascularly are

°the antigenic status of the fetal red cells can be confirmed,

°pre and post-transfusion hematocrits can be measured, and

°the transfused cells are not dependent on lymphatic transport from the fetal peritoneal cavity for entry into the circulation.

•The purpose of medicating patients before performing invasive procedures in utero is to minimize patient discomfort, impede fetal movement and reduce the risk of introducing infection.

°Many of the patients are given a combination of meperidine, prochlorperazine, diazepam and cefazolin.

°This combination of drugs heavily sedates some women and lead to exaggerated "sighing" respirations with associated excessive abdominal wall excursions.

•Intravenous ritodrine, 3 mg., is routinely administered before the procedure.

•Intravenous atracirium besylate, which is a short-acting, nondepolarizing neuromuscular blocking agent that is inactivated in the plasma via two nonoxidative pathways was used for fetal sedation.

°Neither the kidneys nor the liver plays a major role in its elimination.

•All of the intravascular transfusions in the first series, and the first 21 in the second series, were straight transfusions.

°The significant overexpansion of a neonate's intravascular space will result in cardiac decompensation, however, the placenta has the extraordinary capacity to function as a low-resistance "sink."

°A straight transfusion can be associated with a **ruptured spleen.**

•While amniotic fluid ΔOD_{450} is usually a reliable indicator of the status of isoimmunized fetuses during the third trimester, they correlate very poorly with actual hematocrit values in the **second** trimester.

°Other modalities of fetal assessment, such as serial maternal antibody titers and early ultrasonic evidence of hydrops, have also proved to be very **unreliable** for detecting hemolytic disease requiring therapy when the anemia is early in its evolution.

°The only truly accurate way to determine whether a non-hydropic fetus would benefit from a transfusion in utero before 26 weeks' gestation is to directly measure its hematocrit.]

---

32. At 27 weeks an ultrasound examination made because of polyhydramnios shows a distended stomach but no other abnormality. What karyotype is most commonly associated with this condition?

A. 45, XO
B. 46, XX, p5-
C. 46, XX
*D.   47, XX, 21+
E. 47, XYY

---

p.558   (Miro J and Bard H, "Congenital atresia and stenosis of the duodenum: The impact of a prenatal diagnosis " Am J Obstet Gynecol 1988;158:555)

32. [F & I:•Background: Atresia and stenosis of the small intestine in neonates form a group of congenital malformations that have a global incidence in the order of 0.5/10,000.

°The prognosis depends on the presence of associated malformations, the level of prematurity of the infant, and how soon the diagnosis is made after birth.

•A prenatal diagnosis of bowel obstruction should diminish the morbidity related to delay in diagnosis, especially in cases of duodenal obstruction where the poorly feeding newborn infant may not exhibit a distended abdomen or vomit bile.

°This is in sharp contrast to the infant with a more distal obstruction who presents symptoms of abdominal distension and bile-stained vomitus.

•Objective: to compare the outcome of infants with small bowel obstruction diagnosed prenatally with that of those diagnosed with obstruction after birth.

•An obstruction distal to the ligament of Treitz is more difficult to diagnose because its echographic image is less characteristic, and the image may be confused with a transient dilatation of the normal intestine.

•Results: In 13 cases of obstruction diagnosed prenatally, 12 were located in the duodenum.

•Until recently it was believed that a prenatal diagnosis of duodenal atresia was impossible before 24 weeks of gestation.

•There is a statistically significant association between polyhydramnios and a prenatal diagnosis of duodenal obstruction.

°**The closer the intestinal lesion is to the stomach, the more likely polyhydramnios and stomach dilatation are present.**

•The benefits of prenatal diagnosis in duodenal atresia are a decrease in the delay before operating and the morbidity from metabolic complications.

•The **fetal anomalies** associated with duodenal obstruction are numerous.

°Despite the fact that a diagnosis is usually made too late for any choice about the outcome of the pregnancy, the parents should be prepared for the possibility of multiple malformations in the infant and the possibility of the chromosomal anomaly **trisomy 21.**]

---

33. What is the most common X-linked **lethal** disease in man?

    A. agammaglobulinemia
    *B.   Duchenne muscular dystrophy
    C. glucose-6-PD deficiency
    D. hemophilia
    E. vitamin D resistant rickets

p.548   (Katayama S, Montano M, Slotnick RN, Lebo RV and Golbus MS, "Prenatal diagnosis and carrier detection of Duchenne muscular dystrophy by restriction fragment length polymorphism analysis with pERT 87 deoxyribonucleic acid probes " Am J Obstet Gynecol 1988;158:548)

33. [F & I:•Background: Newer methods of antenatal diagnosis are based on the findings that the deoxyribonucleic acid (DNA) complement in every cell of an individual is identical, and that a hereditary defect detectable at this level is recognizable in any nucleated cell type, including amniocytes and chorionic villi cells.

°This technology utilizes restriction endonucleases, enzymes that cleave DNA at specific nucleotide base sequence recognition sites.

°Direct identification of DNA mutations is possible by virtue of the specificity of these enzymes.

°A single nucleotide change in an enzyme's recognition site is detectable because the enzyme no longer recognizes and cuts the nucleotide sequence or because a recognizable sequence is generated.

•**Duchenne muscular dystrophy is the most common X-linked lethal disease in man, with an incidence of approximately one in 4000 male live births.**

•A boy affected with Duchenne muscular dystrophy usually exhibits signs before the age of 6 years, is confined to a wheelchair by age 12, and dies by age 20.

•**Serum creatine phosphokinase activity** has been depended on to indicate Duchenne muscular dystrophy carrier status.

°creatine phosphokinase activity is elevated in only 70% obligate carriers and is of limited utility.

°**Fetal serum creatine phosphokinase activity cannot be used as a diagnostic indicator of Duchenne muscular dystrophy, because not all affected fetuses will manifest the disease with an elevated creatine phosphokinase activity by 21 menstrual weeks, such that creatine phosphokinase values of normal and affected fetuses overlap.**

°Several reports of Duchenne muscular dystrophy in girls with balanced X autosome translocations are consistent with the Duchenne muscular dystrophy locus on the **short arm of the X chromosome.**

°The normal X chromosome is inactivated in all cells, leaving the gene loci on the translocated X chromosome to be expressed.

°Because the translocation breakpoint is within the Duchenne muscular dystrophy locus, the phenotype is expressed in these girls.

°A series of single copy DNA sequences from the short arm of the X chromosome have been isolated.

•Objective: to report experience with the restriction fragment length polymorphism analysis with the use of pERT 87 probes for carrier detection and prenatal diagnosis in families of individuals with Duchenne muscular dystrophy.

•The reliability of these probes requires that there be minimal meiotic crossover between the actual Duchenne muscular dystrophy gene mutation and the DNA used as a probe.

°The diagnoses are 92% to 96% reliable, and the patients should be so counseled.

•Restriction fragment length polymorphism analysis may differentiate Duchenne muscular dystrophy caused by a spontaneous mutation from that caused by an inherited mutation.

°Because one third of Duchenne muscular dystrophy is caused by spontaneous mutation, its recognition greatly reduces the concerns of the at-risk-family to the small likelihood of uncertainty that can result from meiotic recombination.]

---

34. The overall accuracy of the L/S ratio and phosphatidylglycerol level in predicting respiratory difficulty is (%)

    A. 75
    B. 80
    C. 85
    *D.   90
    E. 98

---

p.534   (Hallman M, Arjomaa P, Mizumoto M, Akino T, "Surfactant proteins in the diagnosis of fetal lung maturity. I. Predictive accuracy of the 35 kD protein, the lecithin/sphingomyelin ratio, and phosphatidylglycerol " Am J Obstet Gynecol 1988;158:531)

34. [F & I:•Background: The sensitivity and specificity of the L/S ratio are increased when phosphatidyglycerol is also determined.

•The major human surfactant-associated protein is an oligomer with a unit molecular weight of 35 kD.

•Objective: to assess the value of the 35 kD protein assay for the clinician managing high-risk pregnancies.

•Results: The 35 kD surfactant protein defined a population of fetuses that developed RDS if they were born within 48 hours after the amniotic fluid specimen was taken.

°These fetuses include 59% of all cases of RDS.

•The lung profile (L/S ratio and phosphatidylglycerol) and the 35 kD protein complement each other in improving the predictive accuracy, sensitivity, and specificity.

•The predictive accuracy of the 35 kD protein analyses was not affected by contaminants in the amniotic fluid.

°Changes in amniotic fluid volume and in the centrifugal force used to sediment cellular debris did affect the values obtained for the 35 kD protein concentration.

°In contrast the predictive accuracy of the L/S ratio and phosphatidylglycerol/total phospholipid should not be affected by changes in amniotic fluid volume.

°Phospholipid rich contaminants do disturb these indices, although less than the biophysical indices of lung maturity.]

---

35. Which factor is most predictive of therapeutic failure in the treatment of post-cesarean endomyometritis?

    A. parity
    B. infant weight
    *C.wound infection
    D. type of uterine incision
    E. type of anesthesia

---

p.428   (Alvarez RD, Kilgore LC, and Huddleston JF, "A comparison of mezlocillin versus clindamycin/gentamicin for the treatment of postcesarean endomyometritis," Am J Obstet Gynecol 1988;158:425.)

35. [F & I:•Background: Endomyometritis is the most common infectious complication of cesarean delivery.

•**Mezlocillin** is effective in the treatment of postpartum endomyometritis.

•The combination of **clindamycin and gentamicin** results in cure rates > 90% in patients with postcesarean endomyometritis.

•Objective: to elucidate factors significant for predicting therapeutic outcome and associated factors of increased febrile morbidity.

•Material and Methods:

°Criteria for inclusion were a diagnosis of **endomyometritis** based on a single oral temperature measurement of > 100.4°F at least 24 hours from the time of cesarean section, uterine or parametrial tenderness on bimanual examination, and informed consent.

°All study patients had received a **prophylactic** gram of cefazolin during their cesarean section after the umbilical cord was clamped.

°Eligible patients were then prospectively randomized to receive either:

    °°(1)   mezlocillin, 3.0 gm intravenously every 4 hours, or

    °°(2)   clindamycin phosphate, 600 mg. intravenously every 6 hours, and gentamicin sulfate, initially 1.5 mg/kg body weight, then 1.0 mg/kg body weight intravenously every 8 hours.

•A **therapeutic cure:** resolution of fever and uterine or parametrial tenderness within 72 hours after the start of therapy.

•therapeutic failure: no resolution of the above signs and symptoms within this period.

°A **"side effect failure"** adverse reactions led to cessation of therapy.

•When there was a cure, the regimen was continued until the patient remained afebrile with resolution of signs and symptoms for 48 hours.

°Oral antibiotics were **not** administered upon discontinuation of intravenous medications.

•When there was a therapeutic failure, the patient was reevaluated.

°In therapeutic failures on mezlocillin, therapy was empirically changed to clindamycin and gentamicin and either ampicillin or cefazolin.

°In therapeutic failures on clindamycin and gentamicin, ampicillin or cefazolin therapy was added.

•When there was an adverse reaction, patients taking mezlocillin were treated with gentamicin and clindamycin, and mezlocillin was discontinued.

°Therapy for those patients taking gentamicin and clindamycin was changed to gentamicin and metronidazole when there was an adverse reaction to clindamycin, and to cefoxitin when there was a side effect to gentamicin.

•Ninety-six post-cesarean section patients with endomyometritis were enrolled; 47 received mezlocillin and 49 received clindamycin and gentamicin.

•Results: The mezlocillin and clindamycin/gentamicin groups had success rates of 74.5% and 85.7%

•**The most significant factor in predicting the therapeutic result was the presence or absence of a wound infection.**

•Mezlocillin belongs to the class of penicillin antimicrobials known as ureidopenicillins.

°Its range of activity includes those pathogens commonly isolated in postcesarean endomyometritis, such as *Escherichia coli, Klebsiella pneumoniae, Proteus* sp., *Bacteroides* sp., groups B and D streptococci, *Peptococci,* and *Peptostreptococci.*

•Conclusion: Mezlocillin was as effective and comparable to clindamycin and gentamicin in the treatment of postcesarean endomyometritis.

•In the analysis of factors prognostic for therapeutic outcome positive blood or urine culture results were **not** helpful.

°This adds to the controversy of the need for routine blood and urine cultures in the evaluation of patients with endomyometritis.

°Wound infections were delineated as the most significant factor for predicting therapeutic outcome.

•The number of vaginal examinations in patients diagnosed with cephalopelvic disproportion was associated with febrile morbidity.]

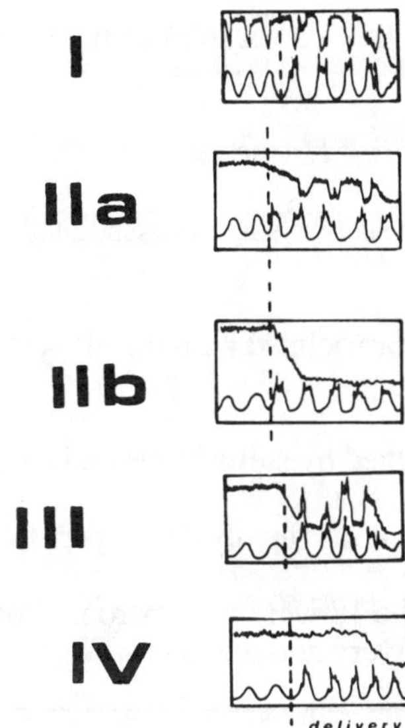

(Reproduced with written permission of the The American College of Obstetricians and Gynecologists.)

36. Which of the these tracings in the second stage of labor most likely reflects fetal acidosis?

    A. Type I
    B. Type IIa
    *C.   Type IIb
    D. Type III
    E. Type IV

p.750   (Piquard F, Haiung R, Mettauer M, Schaefer A, Haberey P and Dellenbach P, "The validity of fetal heart rate monitoring during the second stage of labor" Obstet Gynecol 1988;72:746)

36. [F & I:•Objective: to assess the value of fetal heart rate monitoring during the end of the second stage of labor.

   •This revised classification was therefore adopted and six types of FHR pattern were obtained, corresponding to the following definitions:

    °type 0-stable heart rate;

    °type 1- decelerations at each contraction and maintenance of a normal baseline between the contractions;

°type 2a-decreased baseline between 90-120 beats per minute, with decelerations often occurring during the contractions;

°type 2b-decreased baseline under 90 beats per minute, with frequent decreased variablity;

°type 3-severe fall of the baseline associated with marked accelerations during the contractions; and

°type 4-fall of the baseline under 90 beats per minute, but occurring much later, practically at the extreme end of labor.

•The second stage of labor is a time of risk for the fetus.

°Although a longer duration of the second stage is associated with an increase in preinatal morbidity and mortality.

•Type 0 and type 1 FHR patterns were associated with the highest Apgar scores, and type 3 with the lowest.

°The degree of fetal hypoxia is judged by shifts in pH and lactate increased from type 0 to 3.

°In type 3, a clear-cut metabolic acidosis rapidly developed.

•Results: This group of whom 15 of the 18 were primiparous showed the longest duration for the final stage, the highest rate of operative delivery and the lowest Apgar scores.]

---

37. Which of the following symptoms of cardiorespiratory distress in a heart transplant recipient is LEAST likely to be manifested during pregnancy?

    A. palpitations
    B. orthopnea
    C. edema
    D. dyspepsia
    *E.   chest pain

---

p.492   (Kossoy LR, Herbert CM, Wentz AC, "Management of heart transplant recipients: Guidelines for the obstetrician-gynecologist," Am J Obstet Gynec 1988; 159:490)

37. [F & I:•Survival rates after heart transplantation average approximately 80% at 1 year, 65% at 2 years and 60% at 5 years.

•After heart-lung transplantation a 1 year survival of approximately 70% can be expected.

•For women most heart and heart-lung transplantation centers recommend tubal ligation if the patient has not been sterilized; the patients health usually dictates that the procedure be done after the transplantation.

•The effectivness of the intrauterine contraceptive device may decrease in association with immunosuppressive therapy.

°Also, the increased risk of infection, ranging from endometritis to pelvic inflammatory disease, that is inherent with intrauterine contraceptive device use makes it unacceptable in an immunosuppressed population.

•Barrier methods such as condoms, sponges, foams, and diaphragms, are safe choices when reproductive capacity is to be preserved.

•The conscientious use of barrier methods can be quite effective, has essentially no risk, and offers some protection against infection and cervical dysplasia.

•The metabolic effects of oral contraceptives, which can predispose to complications including stroke, thromboembolic disease, myocardial infarction, and hypertension, must be balanced against the noncontraceptive benefits of pill use, including decreased menorrhagia and intermenstrual bleeding, predictable and usually scant bleeding, potential long-term protection against benign breast disease, ovarian cysts, ectopic pregnancy, endometrial and ovarian cancer, and pelvic inflammatory disease.

•The effect on lipoproteins is different for estrogens and progestins: estrogen even in low doses increases high-density lipoprotein cholesterol levels and decreases low-density lipoprotein cholesterol levels; the progesting which do not all have identical effects, in general do the opposite.

    °**Norethindrone** has the least metabolic impact among those progestins available in the United States.

•At low dose, pills can cause or aggravate hypertension or further increase the incidence of thromboembolism.

    °It would be undesirable for the patient undergoing heart or heart-lung transplantation who already has hypertension because of azathioprine and prednisone.

    °Coronary artery disease in the allograft, a known complication of the transplant procedure, is present in 40% of transplant recipients by 2 to 5 years after transplantation; whether the oral contraceptive would exacerbate or prevent this occurrence is unknown.

•Several formulations of oral contraceptives (monophasic levonorgestrel, triphasic levonorgestrel, monophasic cypoterone acetate, triphasic gestodene, biphasic desogestrel) may not have any effect on lipid or glucose metabolism.

•**Risk for the Mother:**

•Cardiorespiratory changes. Easy fatigability, chest discomfort, dyspnea, orthopnea, palpitations, and peripheral edema occur during normal pregnancy and are related to changes in blood volume and hemodynamics.

    °**Chest pain, a sign typical of myocardial ischemia, will not be present in the heart transplant recipient because of the lack of afferent reinnervation of the graft.**

    °Maternal blood volume rises by an average of 40% above nonpregnant levels.

    °Almost all of the increment is achieved by midpregnancy, the rise beginning in the first trimester with a plateau after week 30 of gestation.

•Hemodynamically the most significant changes is an increase in cardiac output (the product of heart rate and stroke volume).

    °The early increment in cardiac output associated with pregnancy is due largely to an increase in stroke volume.

    °As pregnancy proceeds, heart rate increases, but cardiac output remains unchanged or declines due to a progressive fall in stroke volume.

    °The mothers oxygen consumption (which includes that of the fetus) increases progressively both at rest and at exercise.

°In normal pregnancy, the maximum cardiac output is reached at lower levels of exercise, because the pregnant woman starts from a higher level or cardiac output than when she is not pregnant.

°Because the graft remains denervated, function at rest and during exercise depends on intrinsic cardiac mechanisms and their response to catecholamines released during activity.

°A rise in central venous pressure and volume will result in an increase in stroke volume by means of the Starling mechanism still active in the heart transplant recipient.

°The circulating catecholamine levels rise, increased heart rate and contractility permit a further increase in cardiac output.

•Rejection. Immunosuppressive drug therapy must be continued and prepregnancy levels of these drugs in plasma will be maintained unless manifestations of toxicity or acute rejection mandate alterations.

•Gastrointestinal Disorders: Gastroesophageal reflux occurs more commonly during gestation and may add to the esophagitis and dyspepsia that afflict any transplan recipient.

°The ulcerogenic effect of corticosteroids is also well known and "stress ulceration" must be considered

°Antacid therapy is useful and agents such as calcium hydroxide are being used.

•Infection: Bacterial, viral, and fungal infections are more common in individuals with immunosuppression and are of particular concern during pregnancy, because they represent a potential hazard to both mother and fetus.

°Uncommon organisms are frequently associated with immunosuppression and cultures should always be performed when infection is suspected.

°Antibiotics are indicated for any forceps operation other than a simple outlet procedure and certainly with the earliest signs of infection.

°Prophylactic antibiotics are indicated for cesarean section regardless of the presence of labor or ruptured membranes.

°After primary infection with cytomegalovirus, the virus remains dormant, capable of being reactivated.

°°The most notable of these influences are **immunosuppression**, allograft rejection, and the hormonal changes of pregnancy.

°80% to 90% of those who develop primary cytomegalovirus infection after transplantation receive their infection via the renal allograft itself.

°Antilymphocyte preparations, when given in addition to azathioprine and prednisone, appear to have the greatest potentiating effect on cytomegalovirus infections.

•**Risk to the Infant:**

•Immunosuppressive regimens use three agents: cylosporine A, azathiopirne, and prednisone.

•Cyclosporine: Cylosporin has the ability to suppress the immune response without significant myelotoxicity.

°The effectiveness of cyclosporine is reduced by its nephrotoxicity.

°Untoward effects include hypertrophy of the gum, impairment of hepatic function, gastrointestinal intolerance, hirsutism, benign tumors of the breast, and tremor.

°Cyclosporin crosses the placental barrier, and is present in the fetal circulation during gestation at concentrations similar to those in the mother.

•Azathioprine: Azathioprine is an imidazole derivative of 6-mercaptopurine.

°The side effects of azathioprine are predominately dose dependent and **marrow suppression is the most common toxic effect.**

°There is an increase in infections caused by ordinary microbial pathogens and by unusual bacteria and viruses.

°°Other side effects: cutaneous rashes, gastrointestinal upset, and hypersensitivity hepatitis.

°Azathioprine in pregnancy is relatively safe because the great majority of pregnancies in kidney transplant recipients have successful outcomes.

•Prednisone: Prednisone and prednisolone are corticosteroid agents with less mineralocorticoid activity than cortisol and an intermediate-duration half-life.

°The long-term administration of corticosteroids is not teratogenic in human pregnancies.

•Infections. About 1% of infants born in the United States have congenital cytomegalovirus infection, an incidence that equates to about 36,000 new cases each year; fortunately there are no adverse sequelae in most infected newborns.

°Only 5% to 10% of those infected have the more virulent form, associated with fatal illness or moderate hepatosplenomegaly, jaundice, and petechiae.

°Late complications develop almost invariably among survivors in this group.

°Another 10% of infants with subclinical congenital infection will have degrees of perceptual neurologic, psychomotor, or behavioral complications during their preschool years.

•In the event of maternal infection with the **rubella** virus in the first trimester, approximately 20% of infants will have abnormalities detectable at birth, and in another 10% to 15% hearing loss and other defects will become apparent later.

°There is a smaller risk when maternal infection occurs during the second trimester (up to week 20 of pregnancy).

°The most frequent combination seen at birth includes a cardiac lesion, cataracts, and low birth weight.

°Characteristic lesions include petechial rash, hepatosplenomegaly, jaundice, characteristic transient long bone lesions, microphthalmia, glaucoma, and meningoencephalitis.

°The use of gammaglobulin in pregnant women who have been exposed to rubella may modify the infection.

•Risk for the neonate: Sixty to 70% of the infants born to mothers with a renal transplant have an uncomplicated neonatal course.

•Eight percent to 45% of the babies delivered of patients taking immunosuppressive drugs are **small for gestational age.**

•Breast feeding: Women taking immunosuppressive drugs have the same milk concentration of IgA as do women taking no medications.

•The general practice has been to advise mothers who are taking immunosuppresive drugs **not** to breast feed to avoid any potential risk to the neonate.

•**Gynecologic problems of the heart transplation recipient.**

•**Gynecologic cancer:** Immunodeficiencies predispose to the development of de novo cancers.

•Gynecologic cancer occurs in 8.6% of patients who develop de novo neoplasm after transplantation and is the third most frequent type of cancer in these patients.

•**Bone loss.** Glucocorticoid agents decrease bone formation by inhibiting osteoblastic activity and increasing bone resorption.

°Corticosteroids also induce hypercalciuria and inhibit internal calcium absorption, leading to **secondary hyperparathyroidism.**

•Correction of estrogen deficiency should be combined with the use of progestin in a woman with an intact uterus to reduce the risk of endometrial cancer.

°Of the alternatives to estrogen, calcitonin prevents postmenopausal bone loss; sodium fluoride increases trabecular bone volume.

°The combination of those agents, and **hydroclorothiazide** if hypercalciuria is present, is a rational approach to prevent glucocorticoid-induced osteoporosis.

°**Because most of the bone loss in corticosteroid-treated patients occurs in the axial skeleton, the spine is the appropriate site for monitoring such loss.**

•The use of corticosteroid agents may also predispose patients to the development of aseptic necrosis of the femoral head.]

---

38. Which of the following antibiotics given in the usual intravenous doses for intrapartum sepsis would be LEAST concentrated in the fetal membranes?

   *A.   ampicillin
   B.   cefoxitin
   C.   clindamycin
   D.   gentamicin
   E.   mezlocillin

---

p.124 (Gilstrap LC III, Bawdon RE and Burris J, "Antibiotic concentration in maternal blood, cord blood, and placental membranes in chorioamnionitis" Obstet Gynecol 1988;71:124)

38 [F & I:•Background: Acute chorioamnionitis results in maternal and neonatal morbidity, and occurs in up to 3% of all pregnancies.

•Objective: to ascertain the concentrations of various antibiotics in maternal blood, cord blood, and placental membranes obtained from women with chorioamnionitis.

•Material and Methods: 25 women with clinical diagnosis of acute chorioamnionitis who received antibiotics while in labor.

•Clindamycin, cefoxitin, ampicillin, and mezlocillin were studied.

•Results: **Ampicillin** had the highest cord blood to maternal blood ratio, but one of the lowest placental membrane to maternal blood ratios.

°Ampicillin levels in the placental membranes was about one-fourth that in maternal blood, whereas the gentamicin level in membranes was approximately four times that in the maternal blood.

•Ampicillin and gentamicin in combination are frequently used to treat chorioamnionitis, but this regimen fails to provide coverage against many of the anaerobes common to female pelvic infections.

•For broader coverage either the addition of clindamycin to this regimen or broader-spectrum antibiotics such as cefoxitin or mezlocillin would be used.]

---

39. Which of the following would be the LEAST helpful in managing abnormalities of the active phase of labor?

    A. ambulation
    B. expectant observation
    C. maternal sedation
    D. oxytocin stimulation
    *E.   x-ray pelvimetry

---

p.1171 (Thurnau GR, and Morgan MA, "Efficacy of the fetal-pelvic index as a predictor of fetal-pelvic disproportion in women with abnormal labor patterns that require labor augmentations," Am J Obstet Gynec 1988; 159:1168)

39. [Facts and Issues:•Background: To avoid prolonged unsuccessful labor trials and difficult operative vaginal deliveries associated with abnormal labor patterns, an accurate means of prospectively identifying the presence or absence of fetal-pelvic disproportion is needed.

•The **fetal-pelvic index** was devised to prospectively identify fetal-pelvic disproportion.

°The fetal-pelvic index accurately predicted the presence or absence of fetal-pelvic disproportion in 32 of 34 women delivered of neonates who weighed $\geq$4000 gm.

•Objectives:

°to evaluate the accuracy of the fetal-pelvic index (the ability to identify the presence or absence of fetal-pelvic disproportion) in women with abnormal labor patterns that require labor augmentation and

°to compare it with the Colcher-Sussman x-ray pelvimetry and ultrasonographically derived estimated fetal weight $\geq$4000 gm.

•Material and Methods: An adequate trial of labor was defined as:

°1) uterine contraction $\geq$ 40 mm Hg in intensity and 60 seconds in duration,

°2) a frequency of at least three contractions in 10 minutes, and

°3) cervical dilatation of $\geq$ 5 cm for a minimum of two hours.

•Individually measured anteroposterior diameter (APD) and transverse diameter (TD) of the fetal cranium, fetal abdomen, maternal pelvic inlet, and maternal midpelvis were used to compute respective circumferences (C) of the fetal head (HC), fetal abdomen (AC), maternal pelvic inlet (IC), and maternal midpelvis (MC) by the following equations:

$$C = (TD + APD) \times \tfrac{1}{2}\,\pi.$$

°According to the four circumference differences between the fetus and the maternal pelvis (HC - IC, HC - MC, AC - IC, AC - MC), a fetal-pelvic index number was derived from the sum of the two greatest positive circumference values.

°A **positive** fetal-pelvic index indicates the presence of **fetal-pelvic disproportion**, and a negative fetal-pelvic index value indicates the absence of fetal-pelvic disproportion.

•When abnormalities of the active phase of labor encountered the five management options are:

°1) maternal sedation or analgesics,

°2) ambulation,

°3) expectant observation,

°4) oxytocin stimulation of myometrial contractions, and

°5) cesarean section.

•With regard to the accurate recognition of the type of abnormal labor pattern, two major approaches that have emerged are the cervicographic analysis of labor, and the manometric analysis of labor abnormalities.

°Cervicographic analysis evaluates labor progress by means of graphic illustration of the rate of cervical dilation.

°Three types of abnormal labor pattern are described:

°°1)primary dysfunctional labor (**protraction** pattern),

°°2) secondary arrest of cervical dilation (**arrest** pattern), and

°°3) a combination of the protraction and arrest disorders of active phase dilation (**combined** pattern).

•Malposition (occipitoposterior, brow, face, asynclitism, and compound presentation), breech presentation, heavy maternal sedation, and premature rupture of the membrances are considered the major causitive factors associated with the **protraction** pattern.

•In contrast, fetal-pelvic dispropotion is present in approximately 50% of the patients with **arrest** disorders; however, excessive maternal sedation and fetal malposition are other primary considerations.

•With regard to the **combined** pattern, fetal-pelvic disproportion is present in the majority of patients.

°Other common factors include malposition and excessive maternal sedation.

•The basis of manometric analysis is the measured electromechanical activity of the uterus.

°Disorders of the active phase of labor are divided into the two categories

°°hypotonic dysfunction (insufficient contractions) and

°°hypertonic dysfunction (inefficient contractility).

•Treatment of uterine activity disorders depends on their cause.

•Before administration of an intravenous oxytocin labor augmentation to a patient with hypotonic dysfunction, fetal-pelvic disproportion and an abnormal fetal lie must be ruled out.because of the risk of a difficult operative vaginal delivery and the subsequent increased perinatal morbidity and mortality.

•Results: Evaluated in 46 patients with abnormal labor patterns that required augmentation assessing fetal-pelvic disproportion by x-ray and ultrasonography.

°When used independently neither x-ray pelvimetry nor ultrasonography derived estimated fetal weights ≥4000 gm accurately identified the presence or absence of fetal-pelvic disproportion.

°In contrast the fetal pelvic index had a sensitivity of 71% and a specificity of 95% and an overall predictability of of 83% and a positive predictability of 94%.

•Persistent occipitoposterior presentation may be a special category.

°Of the seven patients with false-negative fetal-pelvic disproportion values, 6 had fetuses that persisted in an occitioposterior presentation that led to operative intervention when the patients failed to progress.

•The concept of fetal-pelvic index is to compare the fetal head and abdominal circumference with respect of maternal inlet in midpelvis circumference.

°With this approach, each pregnancy can be individualized with regard to the measurements of the fetus (passenger) and respective maternal pelvis (passage) when the observed uterine contraction pattern (power) is coupled with these data, the "three P's" can be accurately evaluated before implementation of appropriate therapy.]

---

40. Clinically useful in the treatment of septic shock during pregnancy, all of the following EXCEPT

    *A.   dexamethasone
    B. dobutamine
    C. dopamine
    D. norepinephrine
    E. phenylephrine

---

p.414   (Lee W, Clark SL, Cotton DB, Gonik B, Phelan J, Faro S, Giebel R, "Septic shock during pregnancy," Am J Obstet Gynec 1988; 159:410)

40. [F & I:•Background: Septic shock can have a mortality rate as high as 80% in nonpregnant patients.

•Objective: to identify the clinical and hemodynamic factors associated with septic shock in pregnancy.

•There is a wide variety of aerobic and anaerobic pathogens in the pelvis.

°*E. coli, Klebsiella-Enterobacter, Proteus mirabilis*, and *Pseudomonas aeruginosa* and anaerobic streptococci and bacteroides.

°About 20% of postpartum patients exhibit transient bacteremia after cesarean section; the low incidence of obstetric septic shock reflects the generally good health of the reproductive age population.

•Results: **Prolonged rupture of the membranes with development of chorioamnionitis or postpartum endometritis is the major risk factor commonly preceding the development of obstetric septic shock.**

°The diagnosis of septic shock should be suspected in febrile and hypotensive patients with a prior history of a recent surgical procedure such as cervical conization, laparotomy, or uterine dilatation and curettage–especially when there are retained products of conception.

•The risk of maternal mortality increases as associated complications become superimposed on the septic hypotension.

°These complications may include pulmonary edema, adult respiratory distress syndrome, disseminated intravascular coagulation, and thromboemboli.

•Maternal septic shock was characterized by decreased peripheral vascular resistance with depressed left ventricular function; there is a normal to increased cardiac output with a decrease in systemic vascular resistance in the early stages of septic shock.

°Despite normal to elevated cardiac output, echocardiographic evidence of myocardial depression was found in 55% of 20 nongravid patients who were serially studied by invasive hemodynamic and imaging evaluations.

°Myocardial depression has an important role in the pathogenesis of septic shock.

•**Early stages of septic shock** involve low systemic vascular resistance and high cardiac output with a relative decrease in intravascular volume.

•**Late or cold shock** subsequently involves the superimposition of an endogenous myocardial depressant factor and results in decreased cardiac output and continued low systemic vascular resistance in the absence of pressor agents.

•Some invasive hemodynamic parameters may be predictive of clinical outcome.

°The two nonsurviving patients appeared to have a lower initial mean arterial pressure, stroke volume index, cardiac index, and left ventricular stroke work index when compared with survivors.

°The smallest increases in systemic vascular resistance indices after therapy occurred in nonsurviving patients.

•**Left ventricular stroke work index** appeared to be a good indicator of cardiac performance after drug or fluid therapy, because this parameter significantly improved before removal of the pulmonary artery catheter in survivors.

•Obstetric patients with septic shock tend to have depressed myocardial function and often require inotropic therapy.

°Ventricular function curves provide a useful index of cardiac performance and allow a more rational choice of therapy when inotropic and vasoactive agents are used.

°The overall goal of such therapy should be to obtain the best left venticular work at the lowest filling pressure.

•Generally supportive measures for septic shock during pregnancy should include antibiotic regimens that will provide preliminary **broad-spectrum coverage** for organisms such as *E. coli*, enterococcus, and anaerobic bacteria until culture results are available.

°Aminoglycoside maintenance dosages should be titrated in relation to serum peak and trough levels.

°There must be a careful search for infected or necrotic foci that can result in persistent bacteremia, as evident in three women whose septic conditions were related to retained products of conception after uterine dilatation and curettage.

•Supportive care should include control of maternal fever with **antipyretics or hypothermic cooling blankets.**

°In the antepartum patient, correction of maternal acidosis, hypoxemia, and systemic hypotension will usually improve any associated fetal heart decelerations.

•Aggressive therapy of obstetric septic shock must achieve a rapid and effective reversal of organ hypoperfusion, improvement of oxygen delivery, and correction of acidosis.

°Priority should be given to cardiopulmonary support, with the additional understanding that other major organ systems can also be severely affected.

•Patients condition should be stabilized with **volume repletion, inotropic therapy, and peripheral vasoconstrictor drugs.**

°The total amount of crystalloid administered should be guided by the presence or absence of maternal hypoxemia secondary to pulmonary edema and left ventricular filling pressures as best estimated by the pulmonary capillary wedge pressure.

°Myocardial performance will be optimized according to the Frank-Starling mechanism at pulmonary capillary wedge pressures of 14 to 16 mm Hg.

°Preload optimization is mandatory before the initiation of inotropic therapy.

•**Blood component therapy** can also be an important adjunct if the patient has experienced significant hemorrhage or has developed an associated coagulopathy.

•Efforts should be directed toward improving myocardial performance and vascular tone of the shock state persists despite volume replacement and adequate hemostasis.

°Inatropic agents such as dopamine, dobutamine, or isoproterenol are excellent choices for improving myocardial contracitility.

°**Dopamine** is the first-line drug of choice for treating septic hypotension when inotropic therapy is indicated.

°°Dopamine is a chemical precursor of norepinephrine that has α-, β-, and dopaminergic recptor-stimulating actions.

°°At low doses (0.5 to 2.0 μg/kg/min), this sympathomimetric amine acts primarily on the dopaminergic receptors, leading to vasodilation and improved perfusion of the renal and mesenteric vascular beds.

°°Higher dopamine dosages (2.0 to 10.0 μg/kg/min) are associated with predominant effects on the β_1-receptors of the heart.

°The ß-adrenergic effects are responsible for improved myocardial contractility, stroke volume, and cardiac output.

°Much higher dopamine dosages (greater than 15 to 20 µg/kg/min) will elicit an α-adrenergic effect, similar to a norepinephrine infusion, and result in generalized vasoconstriction.

°This can be detrimental to organ perfusion.

°A systemic cardiac index >3 L/min/m² should be maintained.

•If satisfactory ventricular function is not achieved with dopamine, a second inotropic agent such as **dobutamine** (2 to 10 µg/kg) should be added to the dopamine regimen.

°This drug is a direct myocardial ß$_1$-receptor stimulant that increases cardiac output with only minimal tachycardia.

•**Isoproterenol** should be considered a third-line agent that can be titrated at 1 to 20 µg/min.

°This drug acts primarily on ß-adrenergic receptors to increase contractility and heart rate, however, potential side effects may include ventricular ectopy, excessive tachycardia, and undesired vasodilatation.

•**Digoxin** is a commonly used cardiac glycoside that may be added to the above regimen to improve the force and velocity of contractility of myocardial contraction.

°Intravenous digoxin should be given under continuous electrocardiographic monitoring with special attemtion of serum potassium levels.

•A peripheral vasoconstrictor may be administered if there is reduced systemic vascular resistance index accompanied by a systolic blood pressure <80mm Hg despite inotropic therapy.

°Maintenance of afterload appeared to be a major hemodynamic determinant associated with maternal survival.

°**Phenylephrine** (1 to 5 µg/kg/min) is the initial drug of choice for this purpose due to its pure α-adrenergic activity, which increases systemic vascular resistance.

°**Norepinephrine** is only indicated for patients with septic shock and decreased afterload who do not respond to volume loading, inotropic therapy, and phenylephrine.

°°This drug is a mixed adrenergic agonist with a primary effect on the α-receptors, leading to gereralized vasoconstriction and increased systemic vascular resistance..

•The potential benefit of short-term **steroid** therapy for septic shock is controversial, but much of the available evidence does not support is usefulness under these circumstances.]

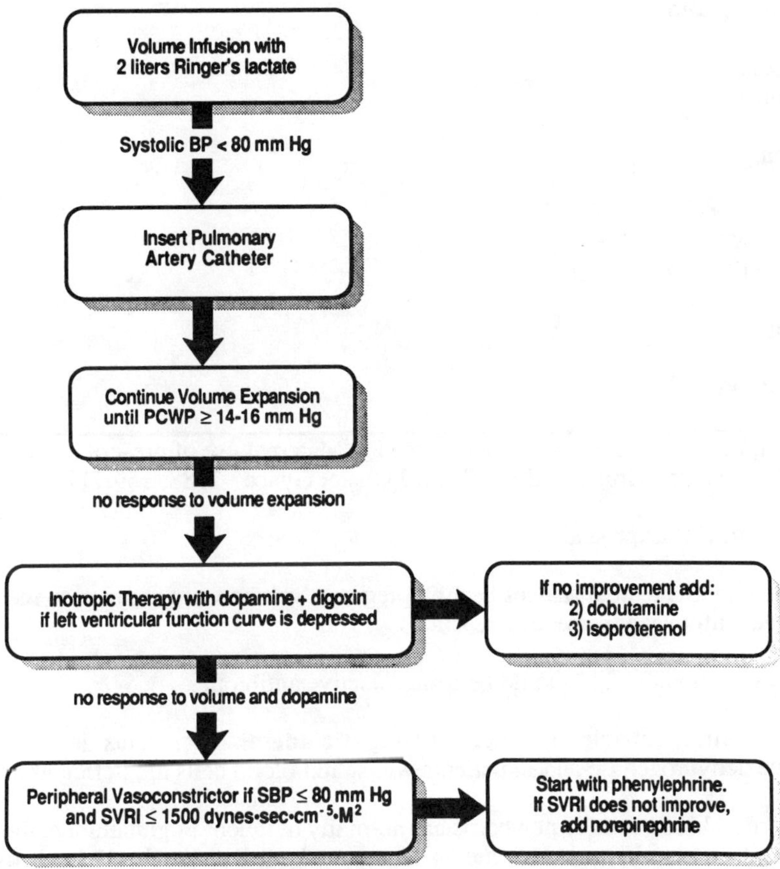

Fig. 2. Hemodynamic algorithm for obstetric septic shock. *BP,* Blood pressure; *PCWP,* pulmonary catheter wedge pressure; *SBP,* systolic blood pressure; *SVRI,* systemic vascular resistance index.

(Reproduced with written permission of the publisher, C.V. Mosby, St.Louis, Missouri.)

Directions: Each group of numbered words or phrases is preceded by a list of lettered items. MATCH the lettered item most closely associated with the numbered word or phrase. Each item may be used once, more than once, or not at all.

For each drug listed below, MATCH the most likely fetal effect.

    A. lithium
    B. nitrofurantoin
    C. propanolol
    D. thiazide
    E. valproate

41. hypoglycemia   Ans: C

42. anemia   Ans: B

43. CNS malformation   Ans: E

44. thrombocytopenia   Ans: D

45. cardiac malformation   Ans: A

p.1174   (Piper JM, Baum C, Kennedy DL, and Price P, "Maternal use of prescribed drugs associated with recognized fetal adverse drug reactions ," Am J Obstet Gynec   1988; 159:1173)

41-45. [Facts and Issues:•Background:

•Objective: to quantitate the instances healthy pregnant women were exposed to medications generally associated with fetal adverse drug reactions.

•Urinary tract infection therapy should be from selective antibiotics.

°Nitrofurantoin is capable of inducing **hemolytic anemia** in patients deficient in glucose-6-phosphate dehydrogenase and in patients whose red blood cells are deficient in **gluthathione**.

°Red blood cells of newborns are normally deficient in glutathione, the use of nitrofurantoin could become hazardous to the fetus after the 37th week of gestation and care should be exercised in prescribing late in pregnancy.

°Oral sulfonamides late in pregnancy should be avoided on similiar grounds.

°Sulfonamides compete with the bilirubin for binding to plasma albumin.

•The best drug therapy for the management of hypertension in pregnancy has not been identified.

°Propranolol and thiazide diuretics may be useful in the management of pregnant long-term hypertensive patients if used judciciously.

•Anticonvulsant therapy should be prescribed in the lowest possible dosage.

•The decision regarding how best to treat a pregnant patient should favor drug avoidance when the drug in question carries a risk and the benefit is slight or maybe obtained from another drug.

°From this prospective, the use of thiazide diuretics for the treatment of physiologic edema of pregnancy or the use of phenobarbital as a hypnotic sedative is difficult to justify.]

Obstetrical ultrasound findings:

    A.   aortic root dilatation
    B.   hypoplasia of the middle phalanx of the 5th digit
    C.   periventriuclar hemorrhage
    D.   pseudohydrocephalus
    E.   ventriculomegaly

46. microcephaly   Ans: C

p.23   (Stoddard R, Clark S, and Minton S., "In utero ischemic injury: Sonographic diagnosis and medicolegal implications," Am J Obstet Gynec   1988; 159:23)

46. [F & I:•Background: The diagnosis of cerebral vascular hemorrhage in utero and congenital hydrocephalus secondary to unexplained fetal intraventricular hemorrhage can be made by means of improved ultrasound technology.

   •Cerebral hemorrhage in the preterm infant is a well known occurrence.

   °Most neonatal hemorrhage occurs in the first 72 hours of life, with 50% of the cases occurring in the first 24 hours.

   °The pathogenesis of such hemorrhage relates to the fragility of the premature germinal matrix and possible peripartum physiologic stress.]

47. tetralogy of Fallot   Ans: A

p.129   (Devore GR, Siassi B, and Platt LD. "Fetal echocardiography. VIII. Aortic root dilatation--A marker for tetralogy of Fallot," Am J Obstet Gynec   1988; 159:127)

47 [F & I]•Background: Tetralogy of Fallot, which occurs in 7% to 10% of children with congenital heart disease, has increased in incidence during the past decade.

   •The fetal cardiovascular screening evaluation to be performed in all fetuses undergoing ultrasound examination has been suggested.

   °The image that has been suggested is the four-chamber inflow tract view.

   °The high ventricular septal defect and underdeveloped pulmonic outflow tract seen with tertralogy of Fallot are subtle and more difficult to detect.

   °A dilated aortic root, commonly seen in the newborn with tetralogy of Fallot, could be observed during the "screening examination" of the fetal heart by imaging of the aortic outflow tract.

   •Objective: to determine whether aortic root dilatation occurs during the second and third trimesters of pregnancy in fetuses with tetralogy of Fallot and

   °to examine the clinical presentation to ascertain associated factors that could affect perinatal management.

   •Penicillin has been suggested as a cardiovascular teratogen.

   •A four chamber view for each fetus undergoing ultrasound examination was suggested.

•Results: In this study 7 cases of tetralogy of Fallot were identified in utero and all demonstrated dilatation of the aortic root when compared with cardiovascular (biventricular outer dimension) and noncardiovascular (biparietal diameter, head circumference, abdominal circumference, femur length) organ systems.

•The clinical management of the fetus with tetralogy of Fallot is dependent of the gestational age at the time of diagnosis.

°Of the four fetuses diagnosed in the second trimester, three had noncardiovascular malformations and one did not.

•Two of the three fetuses diagnosed in the third trimester had structural defects of noncardiovascular organ systems as well as trisomy 18.]

---

48. osteogenesis imperfecta   Ans: D

p.176   (Brons JTJ, van der Harten HJ, Wladimiroff JW, van Geijn HP, Dijkstra PF, Exalto N, Reuss A, Niermeijer MF, Meijer CJLM, and Th NF."Prenatal ultrasonographic diagnosis of osteogenesis imperfecta," Am J Obstet Gynec   1988; 159:176)

48. [F & I:•Background: Osteogenesis imperfecta is a clinically and genetically diverse disorder of connective tissue, characterized by fragile, brittle, and osteoporotic bones, blue sclerae, impaired hearing, defective dentition, and hyperlaxibility of the joints.

•Objective: to describe experience with prenatal ultrasound diagnosis of osteogenesis imperfecta in seven cases with radiologic and pathologic follow-up.

•Prenatal diagnosis of osteogenesis imperfecta was based on ultrasound findings of abnormal length and aspect of the fetal limbs, for example, shortening, bowing, fractures, differences in length and shape between left and right, hypoechogeneity, and diminished or absent acoustic shadowing.

°In addition other abnormalities of other parts of the fetal skeleton (e.g., rib fractures, hypoechogeneity of the skull and spine), deformation of the membranous fetal skull touching the uterine wall; clear visibility of the cerebral structures, giving the cerebral ventricles almost the appearance of hydrocephalus (i.e., pseudohydrocephalus); and narrow chest.

•Material and Methods: 7 cases were studied. Indications for ultrasonography included polyhydramnios, and a previous child born with osteogenesis imperfecta.

•Results: The biparietal diameter was normal in all seven fetuses; the abdominal circumference was normal or small for gestational age.

°In most cases the chest was narrow compared with the abdomen; the heart completely filled the chest.

•Osteogenesis imperfecta is classified into four groups based on clinical and genetic criteria.

•Osteogenesis imperfecta type I, IIA, and IV are thought to be autosomal dominant. Type IIB, IIC, and III are thought to be autosomal recessive but possibly new dominant mutations.

•Most studies indicate that properly classified cases of osteogenesis imperfecta are homogenous within families.

•Results: Osteogenesis imperfecta type IIA could be diagnosed as early as 15 weeks gestation, and osteogenesis imperfecta types IIB and III at 23 and 19 weeks, respectively.

°Prenatal diagnosis of osteogenesis imperfecta IIB, IIC, and III requires a longer observation period because of a later onset.

•In the cases of limb shortening and underossification of the skeleton, there are two possiblities other than osteogenesis imperfecta: congenital hypophosphatasia and achondrogenesis type I.

°These three skeletal dysplasias, however, are almost equally severe and usually are fatal during the neonatal period, with the exception of the regressive form of osteogenesis imperfecta (types I and IV).]

---

49. trisomy 21   Ans: B

---

p.181   (Benacerraf BR, Osathanondh R, and Frigoletto FD. "Sonographic demonstration of hypoplasia of the middle phalanx of the fifth digit: A finding associated with Down syndrome," Am J Obstet Gynec   1988; 159:181)

49. [F & I:•Background: Sonographic evidence of Down syndrome (trisomy 21) is a thickened skin roll at the back of the occiput that correlates well with the diagnosis in the second trimester.

°This abnormality is present in 40% of second trimester fetuses with Down syndrome, 60% of the affected fetuses are not detected by this imaging method.

•Hypoplasia of the middle phalanx of the fifth digit is a well-established radiographic sign of Down syndrome and is present in 60% of affected individuals.

•Objective: to examine specifically the middle phalanx of the fifth digit in five fetuses between 17 and 20 weeks' gestation known or suspected to have Down syndrome.

•Results: An abnormal appearance of the middle phalanx of the fifth digit with radial curving of that finger could be used as another sonographic sign, in addition to the excess skin roll at the back of the occiput, for the antenatal detection of Down syndrome during ultrasound examinations.]

---

50. agenesis of corpus callosum   Ans: E

---

p.184   (Lockwood CH, Ghidini A, Aggarwal R, and Hobbins JC. "Antenatal diagnosis of partial agenesis of the corpus callosum: A benign cause of ventriculomegaly," Am J Obstet Gynec   1988; 159:184)

50. [F & I:•Background: Agenesis of the corpus callosum represents a **benign** cause of ventriculomegaly.

•The callosal structions form in a rostral to caudal fashion, completing their development by approximately 17 weeks' gestation.

°When partial agenesis occurs, it usually involves the posterior-caudal segment; the splenium is absent, but the anterior callosal structures (rostrum and genu) are preserved.

•Diagnosis of complete agenesis of corpus callosum is made on transverse scan by the findings of superior displacement and enlargement of the third ventricle, lateral displacement of the frontal horns with a concave appearance to their medical border and a dilation of the posterior horns of the lateral ventricles.

°Views in the coronal and sagittal planes demonstrate an absence of the characteristic echo-spared structure delineated superiorly by the echogenic pericallosal cistern and inferiorly by the cavum septi pellucidi, cavum vergae, and the third ventricle.

•The significance of agenesis of the corpus callosum is poorly understood.

•Partial or complete agenesis of the corpus callosum is frequently associated with other central nervous system abnormalities in psychologic and autopsy series.

°Specific associated defects include interhemispheric cysts, Dandy-Walker malformations, Arnold-Chiari type II malformations, encephaloceles, and neurofibromas.

°In addition, agenesis of corpus callosum can be found in a number of well-defined syndromes, including trisomies 13 and 18, Shapiro syndrome, Rubenstein-Taybi syndrome,acrocallosal syndrome, Aicardi syndrome, and Andermann syndrome.

•Posterior ventriculomegaly, the most prominent finding of this condition, must be differentiated from early hydrocephalus.

°Early hydrocephalus is usually associated with involution of the choroid plexuses and a worsening of ventricular dilation over time.

°Persistant posterior ventriculomegaly should also be differentiated from bilateral porencephalic cysts.]

A.   laminin
B.   plasma cholinesterase
C.   plasma urokinase-type plasminogen activator antigen
D.   serum 5-nucleotidase
E.   sulpiride

---

51. abruptio placentae   Ans: B

---

p.147   (Cherukuri R, Minkoff H, Feldman J, Parekh A, and Glass L. "A cohort study of alkaloidal cocaine ("Crack") in pregnancy" Obstet Gynecol 1988;72:147)

51. [F & I:The growing popularity of alkaloidal cocaine ("crack") as a drug of abuse has led to widespread use during pregnancy.

•Crack is almost pure cocaine and is not destroyed by moderate heating.

°When it is smoked, large quantities are delivered to the pulmonary vascular bed, producing an effect similar to that occurring with intravenous injection.

•Among the perinatal events reported in association with cocaine use are abruptio placentae, spontaneous abortion, prematurity, and congenital malformations.

•In laboratory animals intravenously administered cocaine can alter fetal oxygenation by reducing uterine blood flow and impairing oxygen transfer.

•Objective: to describe the association of crack with pregnancy outcome.

•Results: Cocaine, when used in its alkaloidal form (crack) during pregnancy in a group of women with inadequate or not prenatal care, has a deleterious effect on perinatal outcome.

•Cocaine blocks the presynaptic reuptake of the neurotransmitters norepinephrine and dopamine, resulting in tachycardia, vasoconstriction and a sudden but transient rise in blood pressure.

°The activity of **plasma cholinesterase**, which metabolizes cocaine, is lower in pregnant women, fetuses, and neonates, enhancing the above effects.

•Neonates exposed to both crack and cocaine had a higher incidence of low birth weight and a significant increase in the rate of congenital anomalies compared with a non-drug-exposed group.

•The increased incidence of intrauterine growth retardation observed may be partially a consequence of chronic hypoxia and that the shortened gestational period may be related to an altered catecholamine response, because large doses of epinephrine can enhance myometrial contractility.

•Conclusion: Many of the adverse outcomes noted among crack users may be related to life styles rather than pharmacologic effects.]

---

52. intrahepatic cholestasis   Ans: D

---

p.171   (Alvi M, Amer N, and Sumerin I. "Serum 5-nucleotidase and serum sialic acid in pregnancy" Obstet Gynecol 1988;72:171)

52. [F & I:•Background: The enzyme 5-nucleotidase is one of the alkaline phosphatases with increased activity in diseases of the liver and biliary tract.

•Alkaline phosphatases activity in serum increases not only in diseases of the liver and biliary tract but also in diseases of the bone in childhood, adolescence, and pregnancy because of the contributions of alkaline phosphatase from different tissues.

•Determination of **serum 5-nucleotidase** is used to differentiate between liver disease and nonliver conditions in the presence of an elevated serum alkaline phosphatase activity.

•Serum 5-nucleotidase and serum sialic acid concentration are used as tumor markers.

•Drugs affecting liver function which produce a cholestatic effect are androgens, estrogens, and anabolic drugs.

°Very high levels of progesterone and estrogens in the later stages of pregnancy predispose to cholestasis of pregnancy and the consequent increase in both serum alkaline phosphatase and 5 nucleotidase.

•The pathogenesis of intrahepatic cholestasis of pregnancy is still unknown, although the disease probably represents a genetically predisposed abnormal reaction of maternal liver to estrogen hormones.

•The sialic acids are a group of acylated neuraminic acids found in glycoproteins of plasma membranes and other cellular constituents, such as glycoprotein hormones and enzymes.

•Objective: to study the level of serum 5-nucleotidase and serum sialic acid in pregnancy.

•Material and Methods: Two hundred and nineteen consecutive patients.

•**Cholestasis of pregnancy was defined as itching without a known cause in a pregnancy women with or without laboratory evidence of the liver dysfunction.**

•Results: No consistent increase in 5-nucleotidase mean group values with the progress of pregnancy.

•Sialic acids are carbohydrate components of plasma membranes, and their turnover increases in rapidly growing tissues whether cancerous or otherwise.

°The increase in sialic acid in pregnancy is not unexpected.

•Serum sialic acid level can be a useful indicator of tumor or its growth, even in the presence of pregnancy.]

Directions: Each set of lettered headings below is followed by a list of numbered words or phrases. For each numbered word or phrase select:

     A.   if the item is associated with (A) only
     B.   if the item is associated with (B) only
     C.   if the item is associated with both (A) and (B)
     D.   if the item is associated with neither (A) nor (B)

In a patient post-operative day 2 following cesarean section:

     A.   cecal volvulus
     B.   pseudoobstruction of colon
     C.   both
     D.   neither

53. abdominal pain, tenderness, hyperactive bowel sounds   Ans: C

54. mechanical obstruction   Ans: A

55. colonoscopic decompression   Ans: B

p.1202   (Fanning JO and Cross CB, "Post-cesarean cecal volvulus," Am J Obstet Gynec   1988; 15:1200)

53-55. [F & I:•Background: Two prerequisites for the development of cecal volvulus are: Cecal hypermobility and a fixed point around which rotation can occur.

•Predisposing causes after cesarean section include postoperative ileus, physical dislocation of the cecum, and, possibly, partial rectosigmoid obstruction by the postpartum uterus.

    °**Signs and symptoms** include crampy abdominal pain and tenderness, nausea, vomiting constipation, cystic mass in the mid or upper abdomen, and high pitched bowel sounds.

•Leukocytosis and elevated temperature are **not** consistent findings.

•**The main diagnostic aid is abdominal x-ray.**

    °Features consistent with **cecal volvuli** are dilated cecum in an ectopic position, single cecal fluid level, and distended loops of small bowel often located to the right of the cecum.

•**Early** operative treatment is imperative to prevent **cecal perforation.**

•The main **differential diagnoses** in post-cesarean section large intestinal distention include cecal and sigmoid volvuli and pseudo-obstruction of the colon.

    °**Sigmoid volvuli** may be differentiated by the absence of distended loops of small bowel on abdominal x-ray examination and the characteristic findings on barium enema and sigmoidoscopy.

    °**Pseudo-obstruction of the colon** is characterized by marked dilation of the transverse colon and cecum in the absence of mechanical obstruction.

•Abdominal x-ray differentiation from cecal volvuli includes continuous gaseous distention with minimal fluid and normal fecal content, preserved regular haustration, thin and well-defined septa, and smooth intercolonic contour.

°Colonic pseudo-obstruction, with no evidence of perforation or ischemia, can be treated by colonoscopic decompression, and if successful obviates laparotomy.]

    A.   symmetrical growth retardation
    B.   asymmetrical growth retardation
    C.   both
    D.   neither

56. impaired uteroplacental blood flow   Ans: B

57. intrinsic fetal abnormalities   Ans: A

58. predicted by sonographic estimation of fetal weight   Ans: C

---

p.1152 (Berkowitz GS, Chitkara U, Rosenberg J, Cogswell C, Walker B, Lahman EA, Mehalek KE, and Berkowitz RL, "Sonographic estimation of fetal weight and Doppler analysis of umbilical artery velocimetry in the prediction of intrauterine growth retardation: A prospective study," Am J Obstet Gynec 1988; 15:1149)

56-58. [F & I:•Background: The cause of IUGR is multifactorial but impaired uteroplacental blood flow is a major etiological factor.

•During the third trimester of pregnancy, an elevated systolic to diastolic ratio is indicative of increased vascular resistance and is predictive of a small for gestational age infant.

•Objective: to examine whether Doppler velocity waveform studies of the umbilical artery give a better or an earlier prediction of IUGR than estimation of fetal weight by sonographic biometry.

•Material and Methods: Continuous-wave Doppler ultrasound studies with a 4 MHz transducer and an Angioscan spectrum analyzer were used to identify and obtain the velocity wave-forms in 168 patients.

•Results: While the sonographic estimation of fetal weight is a more sensitive predictor of IUGR than is the systolic to diastolic ratio of the umbilical artery, umbilical artery studies have a higher specificity and predictive value of a positive test.

•The substantially higher sensitivity rates for the umbilical artery studies in asymmetric as opposed to symmetric growth retardation would be expected since asymmetric growth retardation is frequently associated with impaired uteroplacental blood flow, whereas a symmetrically small infant more commonly results from intrinsic fetal abnormalities.

•Conclusion: Velocimetry studies of the umbilical artery may be of value in the early detection of IUGR, but this finding needs to be confirmed in a larger series.]

At 16 weeks gestation

    A. elevated maternal serum alpha-fetoprotein
    B. decreased maternal serum alpha-fetoprotein
    C. both
    D. neither

59. karyotyping from amniotic fluid indicated   Ans: C

60. increased incidence of congenital anomalies   Ans: A

61. increased incidence of fetal loss   Ans: C

---

p.712   (Burton BK, "Outcome of pregnancy in patients with unexplained elevated or low levels of maternal serum alpha-fetoprotein" Obstet Gynecol 1988;72:709)

59-61. [F & I:•Background: In second trimester the finding of an elevated MSAFP value may lead to the detection of underestimated gestational age, multiple gestation, fetal death, oligohydramnios, or other open fetal defects such as omphalocele and gastroschisis.

•Unusually low MSAFP levels in the second trimester may be found on further testing to be associated with overestimated gestational age, missed abortion, non-pregnancy, molar pregnancy or field chromosomal abnormalities.

°Often no explanation for the elevated or low MSAFP levels are found at ultrasonography or amniocentesis.

•Objective: to explore the relationship between unexplained elevated or low MSAFP levels and adverse pregnancy outcomes.

•Results: Patients with unexplained MSAFP elevations exhibited a significantly increased incidence of fetal loss beyond 20 weeks gestation, low birth weight, neonatal death, fetal congenital anomalies.

•Congential anomalies were observed in 21 of 338 chromosomally normal fetuses or infants who were evaluated adequately.

°Of these 21 cases, congenital malformations were detected in six cases in the second trimester by ultrasonography performed to evaluate the significance of the elevated MSAFP level.

°The six cases included, five of hydrocephalus and one of severe osteogenesis imperfecta.

°Excluding these cases, the 14 fetal losses and five known chromosomal anomalies, 16 of 325 women with live birth delivered an infant with at least one malformation.

•All 361 patients with unexplained MSAFP elevations had fetal karyotypes performed on cultured amniotic fluid cells.

°Five chromosomal abnormalities were identified: two cases of triploidy, two 47,XXX and one 46,XX,1q- karyotype.

•676 patients had low MSAFP levels.

•113 women had low MSAFP levels, not explained by ultrasonography.

°26 of these 113 women who had an amniocentesis had normal fetal karyotypes.

•Most of the malformations in fetuses with elevated MSAFPs originated during the period of organogenesis at least several months before MSAFP determinations.

•Women with unexplained MSAFP elevations are at increased risks for fetal chromosomal abnormality.

•Although the value of fetal karyotyping may be debatable when the amniotic fluid AFP is normal, it is clearly important when the amniotic fluid AFP is elevated.

°A significant percentage of infants with trisomy 18 or 13 have open fetal defects such as spina bifida or omphalocele, that will lead to amniotic fluid AFP elevation.

°The patient's decision regarding pregnancy termination may depend on whether the fetus has a major chromosomal abnormality.

•Patients with unexplained low levels of MSAFP did not exhibit an increased incidence of low birth weight, neonatal death, or fetal congenital malformations.

°They did experience a significantly increase of fetal loss.]

Considering the preterm (<1701 g) of the mother with

    A. toxemia
    B. hypertension without toxemia
    C. both
    D. neither

62. increased incidence of pneumothorax   Ans: B

63. increased incidence of coagulopathy   Ans: B

64. increased incidence of germinal matrix hemorrhage   Ans: B

---

p.573   (Leviton A, Kuban KCK, Pagano M, Brown ER, Krishnamoorthy KS, and Allred EN, "Maternal toxemia and neonatal germinal matrix hemorrhage in intubated infants less than 1751 g " Obstet Gynecol 1988;72:571)

62-64. [F & I:•Background: Infants born to toxemic women are at reduced risk of respiratory distress syndrome and retinopathy of prematurity.

•Material and Methods: 272 intubated infnats who weighed less than 1751 g were enrolled in a clinical trial of phenobarbitral prophylaxis of postnatal germinal matrix hemorrhage.

•To be included each infant had to satisfy the following criteria:

°1) birth weight less than 1751 g,

°2) endotracheal intubation before the 12h hour after delivery,

°3) absence of an obvious major congenital anomaly,

°4) cranial ultrasonogram obtained during the first 12 hours showing no evidence of intracranial hemorrhage,

°5) a blood phenobarbital level of less than 5 µg/mL, and

°6) parental consent that the infant could be randomized to receive either phenobarbital or placebo.

•Most postnatal intracranial hemorrhage occurs between the 12th-36th hour of life.

•An echodensity in the area over the caudate nucleus was essential for the diagnosis of germinal matrix hemorrhage.

•Results: Infants born to toxemic mothers had one tenth the risk of germinal matrix hemorrhage than infants born to mothers that did not have toxemia.

•Infants born to women who are hypertensive or toxemic are at lower risk of respiratory distress than those born to women without either of these entities.

°Infants with respiratory distress are at increased risk of intracranial hemorrhage.

°An explanation for the reduced risk of germinal matrix hemorrhage in infants born to toxemic women is that these infants are at reduced risk of respiratory distress.

•Infants with a coagulopathy appear to be at increased risk of germinal matrix hemorrhage, and infants who receive fresh frozen plasma are at reduced risk of hemorrhage into the lateral cerebral ventricles.

°Preterm infants born to toxemic mothers are less likely than their peers to have a coagulopathy.

°Toxemia might reduce the risk of germinal matrix hemorrhage via a reduction in the risk of neonatal coagulopathy.

°Coagulopathy was defined by a platelet count of less than 75,000, or a prothrombin time or a partial thromboplastin time prolonged by five seconds.

•Toxemic women are $3\frac{1}{2}$ times more likely than women without toxemia to receive barbiturates in the days just before delivery.

°No infant born to the 8 toxemic women who received barbiturates had a germinal matrix hemorrhage.

°This is comparable to the germinal hemorrhage rate of 4.1% among infants born to toxemic women who did not receive barbiturates.

•None of the infants born to the 12 toxemic women who received dexamethasone developed germinal matrix hemorrhage, as compared with only 5% (one of 20) of those born to toxemic women who did not receive dexamethasone postnatally.

•Infants born to women with late toxemia have passed the gestational ages for the high risk of germinal matrix hemorrhage.

•Conclusion: The reduced risk of neonatal germinal matrix hemorrhage associated with maternal toxemia is as prominant in infants who received phenobarbital as in infants who received placebo.

•**The window of vulnerability to germinal matrix hemorrhage is relatively confined to the first days after delivery between the 28th-32nd weeks of gestation.**

°The two other disorders that have their onset at this time are RDS and the retinopathy of prematurity.

°Both occur less frequently than expected in infants born to toxemic women.

•Infants who developed pneumothorax have relative odds of germinal matrix hemorrhage of 2.

•The risk of germinal matrix hemorrhage may be influenced by intracranial maturation processes.

•Conclusion: Infants born to toxemic women, but not those born to hypertensive nontoxemic women, are at reduced risk of pulmonary problems and of germinal matrix hemorrhage.

»"Protective" effects of maternal hypertension are conveyed not by phenomena common to maternal hypertension, but by physiologic effects relatively unique to toxemia.]

Directions: For each of the questions or incomplete statements below, ONE or MORE of the answers or completions given is correct. In each case select:

A.	if only 1, 2 and 3 are correct
B.	if only 1 and 3 are correct
C.	if only 2 and 4 are correct
D.	if only 4 is correct
E.	if all are correct

---

65. Effects of prolonged neonatal phototherapy include

1. decreased unconjugated bilirubin
2. hyperthermia
3. increased insensible water loss
4. retinopathy

---

p.1492   Ans: E   (Rayburn W, Donn S, Piehl E, Compton A, "Antenatal phenobarbital and bilirubin metabolism in the very low birth weight infant" Am J Obstet Gynecol 1988;159:1491)

65. [F&I:•Background: Serum bilirubin concentrations are greater in premature than full-term infants, which reflects an immaturity of hepatic microsomal enzyme activity.

•Neurologic damages attributed to relatively low levels of bilirubin occurs despite the absence of classic findings of kernicterus.

•Phenobarbital lowers serum bilirubin concentrations by the induction of hepatic-conjugating enzymes, notably glucuronyl transerase.

•Objective: to determine whether phenobarbital may have a stimulating effect on the immature fetal hepatocytes, thereby diminishing the severity of hyperbilirubinemia in the premature infant.

•The in-utero exposure to phenobarbital results in higher postnatal serum levels of conugated bilirubin at birth.

°This phenomenon may be indicative of microsomal enzyme induction, presumable hepatic glucuronyl transferase.

•Prolonged phototherapy in the very low birth weight infant is associated with increased insensible water loss, hyperthermia and retinopathy.

•Conclusion: Antenatal barbiturate therapy can increase fetal/neonatal bilirubin conjugation.

°The issue of whether antenatal phenobarbital for the prevention of neonatal intraventricular hemorrhage is effective, remains unsolved.]

---

66. Clinically useful in identifying patients at risk for pregnancy-induced hypertension

1. rollover test
2. isometric handgrip exercise
3. calcium/creatinine ratio and microalbuminuria
4. angiotensin II pressor response

---

p.1452   Ans: E   (Rodriguez MH, Masaki DI, Mestman J, Kumar D, and Rude R, "Calcium/creatinine ratio and microalbuminuria in the prediction of preeclampsia" Am J Obstet Gynecol 1988;159:1452)

---

66. [F&I:•Background: Methods of identifying pregnant women at risk for preeclampsia include angiotensin II pressor response test, the rollover test, the isometric handgrip exercise test, and the mean arterial pressure test.

°These tests have limitations as screening tools in the clinical setting because of either they're complexity, the high incidence of false-positive results, or the subjective nature of result interpretation.

•Objective: to determine whether the presence of microalbuminuria or hypocalciuria or both in the pregnant women who are free of symptoms can predict the subsequent development of preeclampsia.

•Patients and methods: Normal pregnant women between 24 and 34 weeks of gestation where invited to participate.

°Women were excluded from the study if they had a history of chronic hypertension, diabetes, renal disease if at the time of entry into the study they had a blood pressure that was ≥140/90 mm Hg or if they had any evidence of proteinuria by the dip stick method.

°Once the patients were entered into the study, a first morning fasting urine specimen was analyzed for microalbuminuria, and calcium and creatitnine levels.

°No dietary alterations were recommended.

•The calcium concentration (in milligrams per deciliter) was divided by the creatinine concentration (in milligrams per deciliter) to derive the calcium/creatinine ratio.

•Slightly increased excretion of albumin is predictive of the development of clinical nephropathy in insulin-dependent diabetic patients.

°Because proteinuria is one of the classic signs of preeclampsia it was hypothesized that the presence of microalbuminuria or hypocalciuria might be predictive of preeclampsia.

•Classically preeclampsia is a disease of primigravid patients with at least $\frac{2}{3}$ rds of the cases occurring in this group.

°Only 40% of patients in whom preeclampsia developed were primigravid.

•Results: The presence of microalbuminuria and a low calcium/creatinine level may be a screening tool between 24 to 34 weeks gestation for predicting the development of preeclampsia in patients who are free of symptoms.

°When used as a single test, the urinary calcium/creatinine ratio is a better predictor of preeclampsia than the urinary microalbumin concentration, and it is easily and inexpensively available.]

---

67. The human yolk sac is the embryonic source of

1. blood cells
2. epithelia of the respiratory and digestive tracts
3. primitive germ cells
4. yolk

---

p.1191   Ans: A   (Reece EA, Scioscia AL, Pinter E, Hobbins JC, Green J, Mahoney MJ, and Naftolin F, "Prognostic significance of the human yolk sac assessed by ultrasonography ," Am J Obstet Gynec 1988; 159:1191)

---

67. [Facts and Issues:Background: **The human yolk sac contains no yolk material.**

•It is the embryonic source of blood cells and blood vessels, primitive germ cells, and epithelia of the respiratory and digestive tracts, and it may account for the transfer of nutrients to the embryo at early stages in it development.

•A portion of the early yolk sac becomes incoporated into the embyronic mid-gut and contributes to the aformentioned cells and tissues and maybe described as the provisceral yolk sac.

•Objectives:

°to establish normative secondary yolk sac dimensions between 6 and 12 weeks gestation and

°to compare the secondary yolk sac diameter in patients with aneuploidy or spontaneous abortions with the diameter in patients with euploidy and normal pregnancy outcome.

•Results: The secondary yolk sac can be consistently seen by sonography between 6 and 12 weeks'.

•Although there is a slight increase in yolk sac growth between 6 and 12 weeks gestation, the yolk sac diameter did not vary significantly in abnormal conditions such as aneuploidy or spontanous abortion.

•The primary yolk sac develops from the inner cell mass, opposite the amniotic cavity.

•As the amniotic cavity enlarges, it divides the yolk sac.

•The provisceral yolk sac forms the ventral side of the embryo while the remainder of the primary yolk sac is extruded to lie on the surface of the placenta between the amniotic and chorionic membranes.

•Before the provisceral yolk sac becomes incorporated into the fetus to form part of the primitive gut, the endodermal cells actively proliferate, even after the liver assumes its hematopoietic function.

•These endodermal yolk sac cells contain abundant rough endoplasmic reticulum, glycogen, golgi bodies, and lysosomes, and presumably have the capacity for active biosynthesis.

•The yolk sac is the source of several embryonic proteins including alpha-fetoprotein, transferrin, prealbumin, albumin, alpha-1 antitrypsin, and apolipoproteins.

•Because the amnion does not come in contact with chorion leave until about the third month of gestation, transfer of nutrients to the fetus may occur via the yolk sac as an expansion or satellite of the fetal gut.

•The size of the extruded portion of the secondary yolk sac was found to be an insensitive predictor of the embryonic status and its potential outcome.]

---

68. In considering vaginal delivery after cesarean section, conditions predisposing to uterine dehiscence include

1. use of prostaglandin E suppositories to ripen unfavorable cervix
2. use of oxytocin
3. unknown scar
4. single layer closure

p.809   Ans: D   (Pruett KM, Kirshon B, and Cotton DB, "Unknown uterine scar and trial of labor " Am J Obstet Gynecol 1988;159:807)

68. [F & I:•Background: Success rates for vaginal birth after cesarean section range from 66% to 82%.

•A single-layer uterine closure technique that does not include imbrication could effect outcome of a vaginal birth after cesarean section.

•Objective: to demonstrate that prior **unknown** uterine incision in patients undergoing trial of labor does not place the mother or fetus at a greater risk than that which occurs in patients with a known incision type.

•Results: The success rate of vaginal birth after cesarean section in patients in this study was 59%.

•**There was no significant difference between the different types of uterine scars and the incidence of uterine dehiscence.**

•The incidence of uterine dehiscence is not statistically increased with an unknown scar over that seen in patients with a prior low cervical transverse incision.

•The use of oxytocin in patients undergoing trial of labor remains a controversial issue.

°Data from this study is consistent with the finding that oxytocin augmentation is not related to a significantly increased incidence of uterine dehiscence.

•The incidence of uterine dehiscence ranges from 0.7% to 6% in patients undergoing a trial of labor.

•Results: The incidence of uterine dehiscence in patients having a **single-layer uterine closure** was 5.2%.

°The overall incidence of uterine dehiscence was 2.8%.

°The incidence of uterine dehiscence is slightly **greater** with the single-layer closure; however, the risk of catastrophic rupture does not appear to be increased.

•Conclusion: Allowing a trial of labor in a patient with an unknown uterine scar does **not** place the mother or fetus at greater risk than the risk for a patient with a known low cervical transverse incision.

•Oxytocin use does **not** increase the incidence of uterine dehiscence and may be used judiciously in the laboring patient with a prior uterine incision.

•Although the risk of uterine dehiscence may be slightly increased with single-layer closure compared with that of double-layer closure, the overall rate of dehiscence is comparable to that of prior reports on trial of labor after previous cesarean section.]

---

69. Factors which decrease insulin sensitivity during pregnancy include

    1.   hPL
    2.   hCG
    3.   hPRL
    4.   glucagon

---

p.620   Ans: A (Langer O, Anyaegbunam A, Brustman L, Guidetti D, Levy J, and Mazze R, "Pregestational diabetes: Insulin requirements throughout pregnancy " Am J Obstet Gynecol 1988;159:616)

69. [F & I:•Background: Management of **pregestational** diabetes (existence of diabetes prior to conception) may be require tight metabolic control to reduce maternal and perinatal morbidity and mortality.

°**Type I diabetes** is a disorder characterized by insulin **deficiency;**

°**Type II** diabetes is characterized by insulin **resistance.**

•Objective: to determine the nature of insulin requirements throughout the pregnancies of women with **pregestational** diabetes.

•Methods: At entry the initial insulin dosage was changed for both type I and type II patients on the basis of a fixed protocol.

°Independent of a previous regimen all patients were placed on multiple injections (AM: regular and NPH; predinner: regular; bedtime: NPH when needed; regular at lunch).

°The total dosage of insulin was calculated according to actual body weight (0.7 unit/kg).

°For all patients dietary assessment consisted of a 24-hour recall diet plus history (including sociocultural factors).

°Dietary management consisted of an overall caloric intake based on prepregnancy body mass index (obese, 25 cal/kg; nonobese, 30 cal/kg; underweight, 35 cal/kg) divided into three meals and four snacks synchronized to the insulin administration.

•Results: Overall insulin requirements 2 weeks after initiation of treatment **increased** by 26% for subjects with type I diabetes and by 34% for subjects with type II diabetes to reach normal glucose levels.

•For Type I diabetes, total insulin requirements remained stable during the first trimester with a significant **increase** occurring between the eighth and twelvth gestational weeks.

•For Type II diabetes initial total insulin requirements remained relatively **stable**, increasing by 15% between entry and the thirtieth gestational week.

•The subjects with type II diabetes consistently required more insulin to reach target levels than the subjects with type I diabetes.

•The triphasic pattern of insulin requirement appears to mimic the changing endocrinopathic needs in pregnancy.

°Levels of counterregulatory hormones, prolactin, human chorionic gonadotropin, and human placental lactogen increase throughout pregnancy, and may contribute to the decrease in insulin sensitivity and the consequential increase in insulin resistance.

°The contribution of body mass to this observation may be due to the heightened insulin resistance among obese pregnant women.

°The combination of increased homonal production with greater body mass may produce a synergistic effect resulting in the triphasic insulin increase observed in both type I and type II diabetes.]

---

70. Criteria for diagnosing endomyometritis post-partum include

1. oral T elevated >100.4° at least 6 hr apart
2. uterine or parametrial tenderness
3. negative urinalysis
4. negative chest x-ray

---

p.405   Ans: E   (Stovall TG, Ambrose SE, Ling FW, Anderson GD, "Short-course antibiotic therapy for the treatment of chorioamnionitis and postpartum endomyometritis," Am J Obstet Gynec 1988; 159:404)

70. [F & I:•Background: Chorioamnionitis develops in 0.5% to 2.0% of all term pregnancies, but increases to 25% when rupture of the membranes exceeds 24 hours.

•Cesarean section increases the postpartum infection rate up to 20-fold over that of patients who have a vaginal birth.

•Objective: to evaluate the effectiveness of a short course of parenteral antibiotics without the addition of oral antibiotics in a high-risk obstetric population being treated for chorioamnionitis or endomyometritis.

•Material and Methods: One hundred six consecutive women with chorioamnionitis or endomyometritis were enrolled.

°All patients undergoing cesarean section were treated with intravenous prophylactic cefazolin, either as a single 2 gm dose or as three 1 gm doses after the umbilical cord was clamped.

°Patients who delivered vaginally were not given prophylactic antibiotics.

•The diagnosis of chorioamnionitis was defined as the presence of documented ruptured membranes, maternal fever >100.4 F, uterine tenderness, and maternal or fetal tachycardia.

•As soon as the diagnosis was made, patients with chorioamnionitis were treated with inravenous ampicillin (1 gm every 6 hours) and gentamicin (100 mg loading dose followed by 80 mg every 8 hours).

•**The diagnosis of endomyometritis was defined as the presence of febrile morbidity (two oral temperature readings >100.4° F taken at least 6 hour⁁ apart, excluding the first 24 hours post partum), uterine or parametrial tenderneṣṣ, and no evidence of pulmonary tract, urinary tract, or wound infection as documented by a negative urinalysis with a negative follow up culture and physical examination.**

°Therapy for this group consisted of intravenous clindamycin (900 mg every 8 hours) premixed with gentamicin (100 mg loading dose, followed by 80 mg every 8 hours).

•In all patients the serum creatinine level was determined before the start of treatment, and gentamicin peak and trough levels were measured at the time of the third dose.

•Antibiotics were continued in all patients until the oral temperature was <99.5° F for 12 to 24 hours and until there was no evidence of pelvic abscess or uterine tenderness.

°Antibiotics were then discontinued and the patients were discharged.

°The patient was instructed to record her temperature at home twice a day and to report any temperature >100.0° F.

°No oral antibiotics were given as continuation of inpatient treatment.

•A retrospective review of charts from 40 consecutive patients with a diagnosis at discharge of chorioamnionitis and 40 consecutive patients with endomyometritis before the start of this study was used as a control group.

°This control group of patients was treated with an additional 5 to 7 days of dosing with a broad-spectrum oral antibiotics.

•Results: Of the 106 patients only 2 were readmitted, both as a result of superficial wound separation.

°No patient had an infectious complication.

•Conclusion: A shorter course of parenteral antibiotics without the addition of an oral antibiotic has results comparable to the standard extended treatment regimines.]

71. Pregnant women with essential hypertension have an increased risk of developing

    1.   acute renal failure
    2.   coagulation disturbances
    3.   pregnancy-induced hypertension
    4.   increased peripheral insulin resistance

p.446　　Ans: E　(Bauman WA, Maimen M, Langer O, "An association between hyperinsulinemia and hypertension during the third trimester of pregnancy," Am J Obstet Gynec　1988; 159:446)

71. [F & I:•Background: Pregnant women with hypertension are at increased risk for superimposed preeclampsia or eclampsia, abruptio placenta, acute renal failure, stroke, and coagulation disturbances.

    •During pregnancy there is a cumulative retention of about 700 mgEq of sodium, distributed between the maternal excellular volume and the products of conception.

        •**Insulin** has several physiologic effects that may affect sodium and water balance, vascular resistance and cardiac contractility and could potentiate sodium retention during pregnancy.

    •Objective: to measure serum glucose and plasma insulin response to an oral glucose load in normotensive and hypertensive women **without** diabetes during the third trimester of pregnancy.

    •Results: There is a sub-group of women who developed hypertension and hyperinsulinemia during the third trimester of pregnancy.

    •Insulin responses to a 50 g oral glucose were greater in 19 subjects with severe hypertension who had normal glucose tolerance compared with aged matched normotensive controls.

    •Hypertension during pregnancy increases the risk for intrauterine growth retardation.

    •**Human placental lactogen** is a major factor responsible for the insulin resistance of later pregnancy.

    •There were **no** significant placental lactogen differences noted among any of the groups.

    »Because glucose tolerance was similiar in all groups, peripheral insulin resistance must have been markedly increased in the subgroup with hyperinsulinemia and hypertension.]

72. Useful in the management of a prolapsed cord at 26 weeks gestation when vaginal delivery is not imminent

    1.   bladder distention
    2.   elevation of presenting part out of pelvis
    3.   ritodrine
    4.   epidural anesthesia

p.279　　Ans:　　A　(Katz Z, Shoham (Schwartz) Z, Lancet M, Blickstein I, Mogilner BM, and Zalel Y. "Management of labor with umbilical cord prolapse: A 5-year study" Obstet Gynecol 1988;72:278)

72. [F & I:•Background: Methods of alleviating cord compression include manual or positional elevation of the presenting part to a level above the pelvic brim if delivery is not imminent and the fetus is still alive, and preparations for urgent cesarean section are made.

    •Objective: to review the perinatal outcome of cases or cord prolapse managed by filling the bladder with 500-700 mL of sterile saline and by intravenous ritodrine.

•Material and Methods. 51 cases of umbilical cord prolapse in which delivery was not imminent (eg, full dilatation and crowning presenting part), the gestational age was more than 26 weeks (by menstrual history and first trimester ultrasonography), and the fetus was still alive.

•Immediately after the diagnosis of cord prolapse, 500-700 mL of sterile 0.9% saline was rapidly introduced into the bladder through a Foley catheter.

•Concomitantly, an intravenous infusion of ritodrine was started.

°The rate of infusion was adjusted and titrated to arrest the uterine contractions, with careful monitoring of maternal pulse and blood pressure.

°If the cord protruded from the vagina, it was gently returned and the introitus closed with a wet, warm gauze tampon.

•In 41 cases, the contractions were completely arrested 5-10 minutes after starting the ritodrine infusion.

°Most of the side effects from ritodrine, such as cardiac failure, pulmonary edema, severe hypotension, or vomiting were noted.

°After abdominal delivery of the fetus 10 U of IV oxytocin was administered.

°No cases of postpartum atony or hemorrhage were seen.

•**Signs of fetal distress were seen in 33 cases before ritodrine was started, compared with only eight cases, mainly variable decelerations, during ritodrine infusion.**

•Most of the infants had 5-minute Apgar scores of 7 or more.

•There was not statistical difference between small and large infants with regard to fetal heart rate decelerations or Apgar scores.

•The mean prolapse to delivery interval was 36 minutes.

•**Prompt cesarean section after 26 weeks' gestation is the treatment of choice when cord prolapse is diagnosed, when the fetus is still alive, and when delivery is not imminent.**

•There were 4 perinatal deaths among all 73 cases of prolapsed cord.

•All surviving infants were discharged in good condition.]

---

73. True statements about premature rupture of the membranes with a cerclage in place include

1. The risk of infection is not increased compared to patients who do not have a cerclage in place.
2. Delivery will take place within 2 to 3 days.
3. The risk of prematurity exceeds the risk of infection for the neonate.
4. If the cerclage is left in place the pregnancy will be prolonged.

p.110   Ans: A (Yeast JD, Garite TR, "The role of cervical cerclage in the management of preterm premature rupture of the membranes" Am J Obstet Gynecol 1988;158: 106)

73. [F &I:•The fetus is at immediate risk for two significant problems after premature rupture of membranes, 1) preterm delivery and 2) infection.

°Infection is a less significant risk to the fetus than are the risks of prematurity but it potentiates the problems associated with prematurity.

°Maternal risks associated with infection may prolong hospitalization and require multiple antibiotic therapy.

•Objective: to evaluate the role of cervical cerclage in place at the time of premature rupture of the membranes and its impact on subsequent outcome.

•Material and Methods: Only patients with an estimated gestational age of 23 to 36 completed weeks were included.

•Membrane rupture was confirmed by sterile speculum examination and the presence of vaginal pooled fluid, ferning, and a positive Nitrazine test result.

•Patients were monitored from a minimum of 30 minutes with electronic fetal monitors to rule out antepartum fetal distress.

•An ultrasound examination was then made to confirm gestational age, rule out anomalies, and localize a pocket a pocket of fluid for amniocentesis.

°If amniocentesis could be preformed, fluid was submitted for Gram stain, culture, and fetal maturity studies.

°All patients with a positive Gram stain, positive culture, or mature fetal pulmonary studies were excluded from study.

•Patients referred with a cervical cerclage and premature rupture of the membranes had the cerclage removed before or immediately after admission.

•Management was expectant until the onset of labor, evidence of fetal distress, amnionitis, or documentations of fetal maturity.

•Antibiotics were only used in patients with a diagnosis of chorioamnionitis or endometritis.

•No corticosteroids were used to enhance fetal pulmonary maturity.

•All neonates delivered began receiving prophylactic antibiotic therapy.

•The diagnosis of respiratory distress syndrome was made on the basis of clinical signs, radiologic findings, and oxygen requirements for a minimum of 24 hours.

•Thirty-two patients were studied.

•Slightly more than 27% of the patients were unable to enter the expectant management arm.

•Conclusion: The presence of a cervical cerclage at the time of membrane rupture does not appear to have any immediate impact on the subsequent qualification for expectant management.

•More than 65% from both the cervical cerclage group as well as the control group were delivered in <48 hours after membrane rupture.

•The latency data from premature rupture of the membranes until delivery reveals that only two patients in the study group exceeded 7 days of latency.

°Four patients in the control group had pregnancy extended 7 days beyond premature rupture of the membranes.

•50% of the babies born in the study group qualified for the diagnosis of respiratory distress syndrome, and more than 34% of the babies in the control group were similarly affected.

°The incidence of neonatal infections was quite low in both groups.

•Delivery to prevent sepsis does not seem warranted in either group.

•Conclusion: The management of preterm premature rupture of the membranes complicated by the presence of a cervical cerclage is not affected by the presence of the cerclage if it is removed soon after premature rupture of the membranes.]

---

74. Clinically useful for establishing fetal karyotype in midtrimester

    1.   amniocentesis
    2.   cordocentesis
    3.   transabdominal chorionic villus sampling
    4.   transcervical chorionic villus sampling

---

p.345   Ans: A   (Hogdall CK, Doran TA, Shime J, Wilson S, and Teshima I, "Transabdominal chorionic villus sampling in the second trimester," Am J Obstet Gynecol 1988;158:345)

74. [F & I:•Background: Transabdominal chorionic villus sampling is an alternative to transcervical chorionic villus sampling in the first trimester.

°The use of transabdominal approach may reduce the risk of intrauterine infection after the procedure and early pregnancy loss associated with the transcervical route.

•Objective: to report a second-trimester transabdominal chorionic villus sampling experience.

•When the placenta was anterior or fundal in location, transabdominal chorionic villus sampling could be accomplished relatively easily.

°The procedure was not performed when the placenta was posterior and low lying.

•Increase in serum α-fetoprotein was comparable to the increase seen after chorionic villus sampling in the first trimester.

•Chromosome results were obtained in all samples > 5 mg.

•The mitotic index of the chorionic villus cells did not decrease.

•A rapid karyotype result is important when patients who are at increased risk for fetal chromosome disorders present for prenatal diagnosis near 20 weeks' gestation.

•Amniocentesis is not usually possible with significant oligohydramnios.

•Sampling of fetal cord blood by fetoscopy or ultrasound-guided percutaneous puncture has been used to establish a lymphocyte culture for obtaining a rapid cytogenetic diagnosis.

•Midtrimester transabdominal chorionic villus sampling should be considered in patients who need to have karyotypes done near 20 weeks.

°Another potential benefit for transabdominal chorionic villus sampling is the possibility of performing deoxyribonucleic acid studies on villi in the second trimester.]

---

75. Which of the following variables increase as term approaches in a normal pregnancy?

    1. fetal tone
    2. fetal breathing
    3. fetal movement
    4. fetal heart rate accelerations

p.334   Ans: C (Baskett TF, "Gestational age and fetal biophysical assessment," Am J Obstet Gynecol 1988;158:332.)

75. [F & I:•Background: Maternal perception of fetal movement was not affected by gestational age.

°With advancing gestational age, the number of fetal heart accelerations rises progressively.

°As gestational age increased, so did the amount of time the fetus spent making breathing movements.

•Objective: to report the results of fetal biophysical tests with regard to gestational age between 26 and 44 weeks.

•Results: The NST and fetal breathing movements were more likely to be falsely abnormal in the early third trimester in pregnancies destined to have a normal perinatal outcome.

•The NST fetal breathing movements, fetal tone, and amniotic fluid volume were more often abnormal in prolonged pregnancies compared with term pregnancies, this may not mean the same thing since these patients were induced and delivered if the biophysical profile score was equivocal or if the amniotic fluid volume was abnormal.]

76. A fetus is noted to have a heart rate of 200 bpm at 30 weeks gestation. Further evaluation of the pregnancy should include

    1. amniotic fluid L/S ratio
    2. fetal cardiac assessment
    3. fetal karyotype
    4. assessment of maternal thyroid function

p.289   Ans: E (Cameron A, Nicholson S, Nimrod C, Harder J, Davies D, and Fritzler M, "Evaluation of fetal cardiac dysrhythmias with two-dimensional, M-mode, and pulsed Doppler ultrasonography," Am J Obstet Gynecol 1988;158:286.)

76. [F & I:•Background: Approximately 2% of pregnancies exhibit a fetal cardiac dysrhythmia.

•Objective: to review the diagnosis and management of fetuses with a cardiac dysrhythmia and construct an algorithm to assist the clinician in the assessment and appropriate referral to a tertiary center.

•In 1969 the first case of supraventricular tachycardia causing fetal hydrops was diagnosed in utero.

•Fetal dysrhythmias are difficult to detect because of the wide variation in normal heart rate.

•The normal heart rate gradually decreases from 140 bpm at 20 weeks to 130 bpm at term, with a range of ± 20 bpm.

°Short episodes of slowing or acceleration are common, and occasional extrasystoles are considered a normal variation and a function of immaturity.

•Methods: Episodes of dysrhythmia lasting longer than 10 seconds were considered abnormal.

•Only an **electro**cardiogram can properly characterize fetal dysrhythmias.

°Insulating effects of the vernix limit the current use of a fetal electrocardiogram between 28 and 34 weeks.

•Two-dimensional and M-mode **echo**cardiography aid in the diagnosis and evaluation of fetal dysrhythmias.

•Results: All 26 patients with irregular fetal heart rate had a good outcome, and none of the patients converted to a tachycardia or bradycardia.

°Since extrasystoles are not associated with fetal hypoxia, distress, or an adverse perinatal outcome, such cases could be managed in the office with auscultation or nonstress testing after an initial fetal cardiac structural ultrasound examination.

•5–10% of all tachycardias may be associated with a structural abnormality.

•Traditionally the fetus whose lungs are mature is delivered immediately and in utero drug therapy is used for treatment of an immature fetus.

•When there is ultrasonic evidence of severe cardiac failure,.antiarrhythmic treatment may be less effective and prompt medical intervention is imperative.

•In this series one of the fetuses with hydrops and atrial flutter responded to a combination of digoxin and verapamil, but the ascites persisted until the later addition of maternal furosemide treatment.

•The response to medical therapy is often gradual, and in the absence of fetal deterioration and fetal lung immaturity, urgent delivery should be avoided, but intense fetal surveillance is mandatory.

•Of all the fetal dysrhythmias, **fetal bradycardias have the worst prognosis.**

°Accurate diagnosis of fetal bradycardias is essential, since this arrhythmia may be misinterpreted as fetal distress and a cesarean section may be performed unnecessarily.

•The presence of **complete heart block** should alert the echocardiographer to the possibility of serious structural heart disease or connective tissue disease, and a complete fetal cardiac examination should be performed.

°Four of the five patients with complete heart block had anti-RO(SSA) antibodies detected in maternal serum.

•The type of cardiac anomaly and the presence of other congenital abnormalities are important, since these may be one manifestation of a lethal cardiac or chromosomal condition and knowledge of which might alter management.

°Fetal karyotyping either by amniocentesis or fetal blood sampling may be indicated.

•After the fetal bradycardia is fully evaluated, monitoring, specifically for ultrasonic evidence of cardiac failure, is required.

°With cardiac failure, evidence of fetal distress, a poor biophysical profile or decreased fetal movements, delivery is necessary.

•The degree of heart block can be determined by examination of the fetal aortic and inferior vena cava waveforms and using pulse Doppler ultrasonography.

°This technique is also useful in the follow-up of fetal bradycardias, since any progression in the degree of block can be detected.

•The other main role of pulsed Doppler ultrasonography is in the estimation of aortic volume flow in both tachycardias and bradycardias.

•Aortic volume blood flow is maintained within the normal range only until the heart rate drops to approximately 50 bpm or exceeds 230 bpm.

°Outside of this range the blood flow diminishes.

»The patient should be instructed regarding daily fetal movement counting and have weekly biophysical profile testing and fetal cardiac ultrasound evaluation, and if maternal antiarrhythmic drug therapy is given, regular drug levels should be checked.]

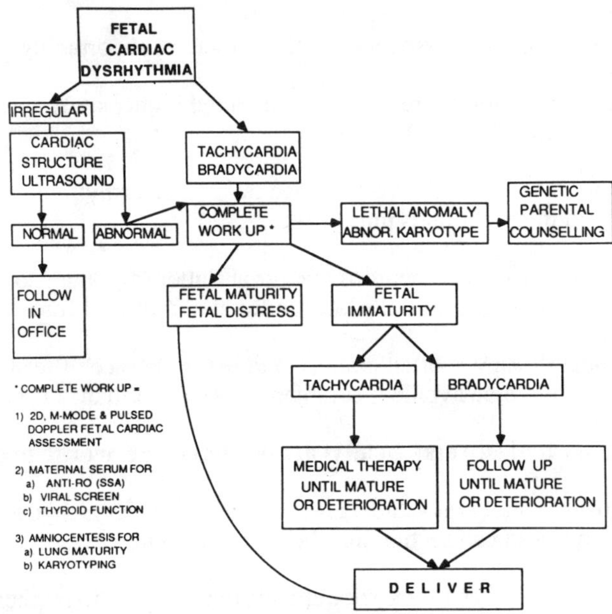

Fig. 1. An algorithm for the management of fetal cardiac dysrhythmia.

(Reproduced with written permission of the publisher, C.V. Mosby, St.Louis, Missouri.)

---

77. Mothers carrying hepatitis B surface antigen can be expected to have

    1. more stillbirths.
    2. more infants with congenital anomalies.
    3. infants with lower birth weight.
    4. infants who have a 90% risk of contracting hepatitis.

p.488 Ans: D   (Pastorek II JG, Miller JM and Summers PR, "The effect of hepatitis B antigenemia on pregnancy outcome " Am J Obstet Gynecol 1988;158:486)

77. [F & I:•Background: Neonates born to mothers testing positive for hepatitis B surface antigen are at risk for vertical receipt of the virus, with subsequent development of antigenemia, hepatitis, cirrhosis, and even hepatocellular carcinoma.

   °In areas of high prevalence such as the Orient, as many as 40% of hepatitis B cases may be the result of perinatal vertical transmission of the virus, which makes perinatal vertical transmission of the disease one of the most important modes of transmission of the disease worldwide.

•The fact that perinatal transmission of hepatitis B may be interrupted by immunotherapy at the time of delivery has prompted recommendations for screening high-risk pregnant women for hepatitis B surface antigenemia.

•High risk groups, however, may include only half of women with positive antigen tests for hepatitis B who are at risk for transmitting the hepatitis B virus vertically.

   °**Therefore, it may be necessary to screen all pregnant women in order to identify infants needing vaccination.**

•To ascertain the affect of hepatitis B on pregnancy and its outcome.

•In mothers carrying the hepatitis B surface antigen, roughly 10% of their infants will develop hepatitis B infection in utero, presumably via transplacental viral passage.

   °**The remaining 90% of neonates, who are not infected at birth, run the risk of contracting hepatitis B of up to 90%, especially in cases where the mother has positive tests for hepatitis B e antigen as well.**

•If hepatitis B antigenemia in the mother were to predict a poor pregnancy outcome independently of postnatal hepatic compromise (i.e., if there were indications of a high stillbirth rate or perhaps a high incidence of fetal anomalies attributable to the infection), then substantial financial and human commitment to such screenings may not be warranted.

•Results: This was a retrospective study of 60 pregnant women who tested positive for hepatitis B antigen and an equal number of controls with negative tests to the virus, in a population whose prevalence of antigenemia during pregnancy is 0.88%.

   °Both pregnancy course and pregnancy outcome are unaffected by the antigenemia.

•Also maternal factors including weight gain, hemoglobin level, and morbidity and fetal outcome parameters such as gestational age at birth, birth weight, Apgar scores, and neonatal morbidity were all found to be equivalent between the two groups.

•The only significance exhibited noted between the two groups was an increase in birth weight of an average of 381 gm in Oriental patients, in the group with hepatitis B.

   °This may be explained by a significantly longer gestation in the Oriental patients with hepatitis].

---

78. Common central hemodynamic findings in severe preeclampsia include

   1.   Hyperdynamic ventricular function
   2.   Low central venous pressure
   3.   Low colloid osmotic pressure
   4.   No pulmonary hypertension

---

p.454   Ans: E   (Clark SL, Cotton DB, "Clinical indications for pulmonary artery catheterization in the patient with severe preeclampsia " Am J Obstet Gynecol 1988;158:453)

---

78. [F & I:•**Central hemodynamics of severe preeclampsia:**

•**(1)Preload:** Central venous pressure is a measure of preload of the right side of the heart.

°It is less important than assessment of preload of the **left** side of the heart, reflected in the **pulmonary capillary wedge pressure.**

°When central venous pressure is used clinically, the assumption is that preload of the right and left sides of the heart (end-diastolic pressure or volume) are roughly equivalent.

°This assumption is valid only in the absence of right or left ventricular dysfunction and the presence of normal cardiac values.

•Patients with severe preeclampsia act as if they were severely hypovolemic and have pulmonary capillary wedge pressures in the low to normal range.

°A typical example is the patient in whom a minimal dose of hydralazine results in an abrupt and profound drop in blood pressure.

°This reduction in preload is manifested by the tendency of patients with severe preeclampsia to develop hypotension in response to minimal blood loss.

•Effective circulating intravascular volume in severe preeclampsia is usually **low.**

•Central venous pressure and pulmonary capillary wedge pressure often do not correlate in severe preeclampsia.

°**Central venous pressure is a clinically unacceptable measurement of preload in the patient with severe preeclampsia.**

•Conclusion: Pressure should be managed clinically or a pulmonary artery catheter should be placed in order to obtain a valid assessment of left ventricular preload.

•**(2)Afterload:**

•Afterload reflects the impedance to the ejection of blood from the ventricles.

°Afterload cannot be measured directly but rather is a calculated parameter derived from clinical assessment of mean pulmonary capillary wedge pressure and cardiac output.

°Afterload of the **right** side of the heart is reflected in **pulmonary vascular resistance** while afterload of the **left** side of the heart is reflected in **systemic vascular resistance.**

•There is a variably elevated systemic vascular resistance in patients with severe preeclampsia.

•Cardiac output will vary inversely with systemic vascular resistance.

•Marked elevation in systemic vascular resistance may have a detrimental effect on cardiac output, leading to pulmonary edema.

•Blood pressure is as dependent upon cardiac output as it is upon systemic vascular resistance:

$$\text{Mean arterial pressure} = CO \; x \; SVR \; x \; k,$$

where CO is cardiac output and SVR is systemic vascular resistance.

•A patient with elevated blood pressure may be hypertensive on the basis of either elevated systemic vascular resistance or elevated cardiac output.

•Systemic vascular resistance may be lower in pregnancy than in nonpregnant patients.

•Oliguric patients may experience renal arterial spasm quite out of proportion to the generalized increase in systemic vascular resistance.

°Systemic vasospasm in severe preeclampsia may affect various arterial beds differently .

•**Contractility.**

•Contractility describes an inherent property of the myocardium and is reflected in the ability of the ventricles to pump blood independent of preload-dependent Starling forces.

•Most patients with severe preeclampsia have **hyperdynamic left ventricular function.**

•**(2) Clinical applications:**

•**Control of hypertension.**

•**Hydralazine** hydrochloride remains the mainstay of intrapartum antihypertensive therapy for severe preeclampsia.

°A diastolic pressure of 110 mm Hg is the level above which acute antihypertensive therapy is mandatory.

°When administered intravenously in boluses of 5 to 10 mg hydralazine promptly lowers blood pressure to acceptable levels.

°If systemic vascular resistance is elevated and cardiac output is depressed to a point where the cardiac output is not meeting the patient's physiologic needs, reduction of systemic vascular resistance with arterial dilators such as hydralazine will result initially in improved cardiac output and no net change in blood pressure, while the peripheral blood pressure may remain unchanged, such therapy may in fact be beneficial in terms of perfusion of maternal organs, including the uteroplacental bed.

°Only after initial reductions in systemic vascular resistance have allowed cardiac output to normalize will further reductions in systemic vascular resistance be reliably reflected in a fall in blood pressure.

•Patients with acute hypertension and are unresponsive to standard doses of arterial dilators including hydralazine and trimethaphan may have increased cardiac output.

•With **normal** systemic vascular resistance, arterial dilators could not be effective.

°Cautious control of cardiac output is a more physiologically appropriate method of controlling hypertension.

°This may be done either by altering Starling forces by decreasing preload with the use of venous dilators such as **nitroglycerin** or by a direct effect on myocardial contractility with ß-**adrenergic receptor blockers.**

•Patients in whom hypertension fails to respond to conventional doses of hydralazine are candidates for pulmonary artery catheterization to guide further hemodynamic manipulation.

(3)Pulmonary edema.

•In any patient pulmonary edema may occur by one of three mechanisms.

°(1) pulmonary edema may be **cardiogenic**, implying either an absolute increase in preload (as in iatrogenic volume overload) or

°(2) a relative increase in preload (as in left ventricular failure).

°(3) **Decreases in colloid osmotic pressure** and **alterations in pulmonary capillary** integrity may contribute to clinical pulmonary edema.

•Placement of a pulmonary artery catheter in a patient with severe preeclampsia and pulmonary edema allows precise assessment of the type of pulmonary edema present (cardiogenic versus non-cardiogenic), thus allowing the physician to specifically tailor therapy to the underlying physiologic aberration.

•**Hemodynamic manipulation in noncardiogenic pulmonary edema consists of lowering the wedge pressure with diuresis to the lowest level compatible with acceptable cardiac output and peripheral perfusion.**

•**Oliguria.**

•Oliguria is an infrequently encountered complication of severe preeclampsia.

•Most young women with healthy kidneys can tolerate oliguria for a considerable length of time without developing acute tubular necrosis.

•Three subsets of patients with severe preeclampsia and severe oliguria unresponsive to a single fluid challenge have been described.

°Most patients were found to have **low** wedge pressures, mild to moderate elevations of systemic vascular resistance, and normal cardiac output.

°°In these patients oliguria was associated with inadequate preload and responded rapidly to **further crystalloid infusion.**

°A second group of patients were oliguric on the basis of **severe systemic vasospasm and inadequate cardiac output.**

°°Oliguria in these patients responded to aggressive **afterload reduction.**

°The final group of patients appeared to be hypertensive principally on the basis of **elevated cardiac output.**

°°These patients exhibited high cardiac output, hyperdynamic ventricular function, normal or mildly increased systemic vascular resistance, and adequate preload, yet they were oliguric with urinary specific gravities exceeding 1.030.

°°Analysis of the above hemodynamic parameters implies the presence of selective renal arteriospasm out of proportion to systemic vasospasm.

°In the oliguric patient with severe preeclampsia in whom delivery is anticipated within an hour or two, withholding any therapy in anticipation of spontaneous reversal after delivery may be justified.

•**(3)Anesthesia:**

•Patients with severe preeclampsia have an increased risk of serious hypotension associated with the administration of epidural anesthetics.

•**When cautiously administered, an epidural anesthetic is not associated with an increase in maternal hypotension or fetal distress and may actually improve intervillous blood flow in patients with severe preeclampsia.**

•Induction of **general anesthesia**, on the other hand, is often associated with **blood pressure elevations** that may be especially hazardous for the patient who is already hypertensive.

•**Safety:**

•Rare complications including lethal arrhythmias, cardiac or great vessel trauma, and pulmonary infarction have all been reported.

°Such complications are usually the result of poor insertion or maintenance technique.

•More frequent complications such as pneumothorax are largely complications of obtaining central venous access rather than being specific to the pulmonary artery catheter itself.]

---

79. Microbes associated with endotoxin production

      1.   fusobacterium
      2.   mycoplasma
      3.   E. coli
      4.   Candida albicans

---

p.1048   Ans: B   (Romero R, Roslansky P, Oyarzun E, Wan M, Emamian M, Novitsky TJ, Gould MJ, and Hobbins JC, "Labor and infection. II. Bacterial endotoxin in amniotic fluid and its relationship to the onset of preterm labor," Am J Obstet Gynec   1988; 15:1044)

79. [F & I:•Background: **Endotoxin** or lipopolysaccharide is a component of the cell wall of gram-negative bacteria.

•Endotoxin can be detected in the amniotic fluid of patients with gram-negative intraamniotic infections with the **Limulus amebocyte lysate assay.**

°Lipopolysaccharide may play a role in the onset of labor.

•Lipopolysaccharide ican induce prostaglandin production by macrophages directly or through the release of monokines such as interleukin-1 and tumor necrosis factor.

•The mechanisms responsible for the onset of labor in cases of gram-negative intraamniotic infection may involve lipopolysaccharide.

•Objective: to examine the relationship between endotoxin concentration in amniotic fluid and the presence or absence of labor in women with premature rupture of membranes.

•Results: Normal amniotic fluid enhances the reaction of lipopolysaccharide and Limulus amebocyte lysate.

•Of all patients with premature rupture of the membranes and endotoxin in their amniotic fluid, those in active labor had **higher** concentrations of endotoxin than those without labor.

°The standard use in the assay was E. *coli* lipopolysaccharide, which has a midrange activity in comparison to that of other bacterial endotoxins.

•Endotoxin was able to demonstrated in five patients without demonstrable gram-negative infections.

°In these women only mycoplasma species, gram-positive bacteria, or *Candida albicans* grew.

•Endotoxin is not known to occur in mycoplasma species.

•Because there is a great overlap between patients with and without infection it is unlikely that endotoxin is the only factor responsible for the onset of labor in cases of intraamniotic infection.

•Because of the limited success of antibiotic therapy in endotoxin septicemia, a new therapeutic modality with an antiendotoxin antibody is being developed.

---

80. Types of human papilloma virus associated with squamous papillomas of the larynx and respiratory tract seen in infants delivered through a contaminated birth passage include

    1. 35
    2. 11
    3. 18
    4. 6

---

p.1412   Ans: C   (Schwartz DB, Greenberg MD, Daoud Y. and Reid R., "Genital condylomas in pregnancy: Use of trichloroacetic acid and laser therapy.," Am J Obstet Gynecol 1987;158:1407)

80. [F & I:•Background: Although **respiratory papillomatosis** is infrequent, this complication can be catastrophic, producing mortality or significant long-term morbidity in affected children.

•**Podophyllin** is contraindicated in pregnancy because absorption into the general circulation can result in severe side effects for both mother and fetus, including maternal flaccid paralysis, hypokalemia, coma, and death.

°Teratogenicity has been demonstrated in laboratory animals.

•**5-fluorouracil** is absorbed after topical administration.

°Because of cytotoxic and antimitotic actions, this drug is also contraindicated in pregnancy.

•Objective: to determine the efficacy of therapy, and maternal and perinatal morbidity with the use of trichloroacetic acid and carbon dioxide laser surgery during pregnancy.

•This retrospective case control study was designed to evaluate

°(1) whether prenatal treatment of exophytic condylomas with trichloroacetic acid and carbon dioxide laser surgery would successfully remove overt lesions at the time of delivery and thereby avoid the problem of having to allow vaginal delivery through a field of genital condylomas, and

°(2) whether laser photovaporization during pregnancy produced a detectable increase in perinatal or maternal morbidity.

•Material and Methods: •**Technique of trichloroacetic acid application.**

°Trichloroacetic acid is a caustic and astringent agent that acts by precipitating proteins at the site of local application.

°**85%** trichloroacetic acid was used.

°°trichloroacetic acid therapy does not cause inflammation (in contrast to podophyllin), but produces a white slough that peels off in a few days.

°The cure rate from a single application is limited to approximately 20% to 30%.

°A treatment may need to be repeated every 7 to 10 days.

•**Technique of carbon dioxide laser surgery.**

•Surgical control is relatively easy obtained through the manipulation of two physical parameters, average power density and beam geometry.

°Power density was kept within the 1000 to 2000 W/cm^2 range by making incremental variations in spot diameter such that energy intensity suited the speed of hand movements comfortable to the individual surgeon.

°Power density was always maintained above 750 W/cm^2.

•The beam geometry was "flattened" by partial **defocusing**, to produce a round (rather than drill-like) impact crater.

•Treatment margins were set with the colposcope, after acetic acid soaking, such that destruction encompassed both condylomatous lesions and all areas of subclinical papillomaviral infection.

•Results: At the time of delivery, condylomas had been successfully eradicated by a combination of laser surgery and 85% trichloroacetic acid application in 31 (97%) of the 32 women treated.

•Twenty-nine patients had no lesion recurrence after laser surgery.

°3 women had recurrences which occurred within 2 to 8 weeks after laser ablation.

•The only immediate postoperative complication was acute pylonephritis.

•Two patients were treated with tocolysis to suppress uterine activity.

•One patient required cesarean section for extensive recurrent disease.

•No laryngeal papillomas in offspring was found.

•Condyloma lesions may enlarge and cover the perineum, the vagina, and cervix to the point of causing extreme discomfort and impeding urination of defecation.

°With such large lesions the potential for dystocia and the risk of severe **hemorrhage** preclude vaginal delivery.

•Large perineal condylomas are prone to secondary **infection** by vaginal and rectal bacteria, thereby predisposing to intrapartum fetal infections.

•Most anogenital condylomas result from sexually transmitted HPV types 6 and 11.

°HPV types 6 and 11 cause squamous papilloma of the larynx and respiratory tract.

•Respiratory papillomatosis exists in a juvenile and an adult form.

°The larynx is the most common primary site, but the papillomas may spread to the trachea and throughout the respiratory tract.

°Respiratory obstruction is the most serious consequence.

°There is no consistently curative treatment, and recurrence is the rule, leading to repeated treatments and lifelong morbidity.

•The latent period may be very long,and clinical expression may not occur for many years.

•Maternal condylomas occur in 55% to 65% of infants with respiratory papillomas, and the lifetime risk of developing laryngeal papilloma for children born to mothers with condylomas is estimated to be 1 in 30.

•A single laser treatment effectively eradicated all clinically apparent disease in 29 of 32 patients.

•Whether to proceed to cesarean section or to allow vaginal delivery depends on the size, location, and number of lesions.

•Conclusion: Extensive or recurrent condylomas are best treated with carbon dioxide laser ablation, using a high rate of energy delivery, and "flattened" beam profile, and a power density in the range of 1000 to 2000 W/cm^2.]

---

81. A pregnant patient complained of pain over the right portion of her lower back . Examination revealed a normal hip joint and no tenderness or contracture over the adductor muscles on the right. Findings corroborative of sacroiliac joint dysfunction include pain upon

    1.   manually pressing the pelvis apart
    2.   manually pressing the pelvis together
    3.   placing the left heel on the right knee and rotating the leg outward
    4.   palpation of the right sacrospinous ligament

---

p.72   Ans: A   (Berg G, Hammar M, Moller-Nielsen J, Lindén U, Thorblad J, "Low back pain during pregnancy," Obstet Gynecol 71:71,1988)

81. [F & I: •Background: The hormonal effect of pregnancy increases biomechanical strain on ligaments, muscles, and the skeleton.

•Objectives:

°to ascertain prospectively the incidence, time of onset, and severity of low back pain in pregnancy, and

°to identify causes for severe low back pain among those women either unable to continue work outside the home or unable to take care of domestic tasks without assistance.

•Materials & Methods: The orthoneurologic examination was performed with the woman standing, walking, and lying.

•The presence and degree of scoliosis and tilting of the pelvis were noted, as was asymmetry of movements in the spine during rotation, flexion, and extension.

•Postural asymmetry of the pelvis was tested in the absence or presence of a lateral pelvic tilt, where a torsion of one ilium in relation to the other may have occurred.

°The iliolumbar, sacrospinal, and sacrotuberal ligaments were examined for tenderness and strain.

°Contractures and tenderness in the muscles of the pelvis, hip, and thigh were noted.

•The diagnosis of **symphysiolysis** was made in those women who were complaining of pain and/or tenderness over the symphysis.

°This pain was usually worsened by exercise, straining, and walking on stairs.

°The pain and tenderness was reproduced by pressure over the symphysis.

•When Patrick's test, Derbolowski's test, and the sacroiliac joint fixation test were **positive**, the sacroiliac joint of one or both sides was considered to be engaged.

°The diagnosis of **sacroiliac joint dysfunction** was also made if either of the provocation tests was positive.

•**No** diagnoses of sacroiliac joint dysfunction based on asymmetries of the pelvis alone was made; there had to be pain at provocation testing and/or a disturbed motion of the sacroiliac joint.

•**Treatment** included

°the **trochanteric belt,** made from rigid cloth and strapped around the pelvis to hold it together and minimize the movements in the sacroiliac joint and the symphysis; and

°immobilization, performed by the two participating orthopedic surgeons using a technique described by Maitland and Corrigan.

•Dysfunction of the sacroiliac joint was found in two-thirds of the women with severe back pain, results that agree with earlier opinions.

•Symphysiolysis was significantly more common among women with dysfunction of the sacroiliac joints than among pregnant women without backache, supporting earlier suggestions that hormonal effects are an important cause of instability in the pelvis.

•Most women treated with the trochanteric belt reported good results.]

---

82. Cystic fibrosis

    1.   is an autosomal recessive disorder
    2.   has a gene locus on chromosome 7
    3.   carriers of the gene are asymptomatic
    4.   cannot be detected in first trimester pregnancies

---

p.213   Ans: A (Nugent CD, Gravius T, Green P, Larsen JW Jr, MacMillin MD, Donis-Keller H, "Prenatal diagnosis of cystic fibrosis by chorionic villus sampling using 12 polymorphic deoxyribonucleic acid markers. " Obstet Gynecol 1988;71: 213)

82. [F & I: •Background: Cystic fibrosis is a common **autosomal recessive** disorder in whites, with a carrier frequency of one in 22 and an incidence of one in 2000 newborns.

°Carrier parents for cystic fibrosis gene have a one in four chance of having a cystic fibrosis-affected child in each pregnancy.

•There is a genetic linkage of a DNA marker to cystic fibrosis gene, its chromosomal origin on **chromosome 7**, as well as additional markers.

•DNA markers , or restriction fragment length polymorphisms, detect sequence variation among individuals: they can often be used to follow the inheritance of cystic fibrosis in families with at least one affected individual, provided each parent is heterozygous for at least one marker locus.

•Cystic fibrosis had been diagnosed by measuring enzyme activity of alkaline phosphatase isoenzymes or disaccharidases in amniotic fluid.

°The sensitivity of these methods is 90% with a false positive rate of 5%.

°These tests are not applicable to first trimester diagnosis by chorionic villus sampling.

•A case of prenatal diagnosis of cystic fibrosis using 12 polymorphic DNA markers that flank the cystic fibrosis locus on chromosome 7 was presented.

•The usefulness of **linkage markers** in presymptomatic diagnostic tests depends on their genetic distance from the disease gene and on their informativeness.

°For cystic fibrosis there is a set of restriction fragment length polymorphism DNA probes that detect polymorphism within a few centimorgans of the cystic fibrosis gene.

•The ultimate goal in presymptomatic diagnostic testing for cystic fibrosis is the direct detection of mutations that lead to cystic fibrosis, so that carrier testing can be done for any individual in the population.

•This advance awaits the cloning of the gene and characterization of all mutations that lead to cystic fibrosis.]

---

83. A gravida 2, para 1 is diagnosed as having a complete placenta previa, confirmed by ultrasound, at 24 weeks gestation after an episode of uterine bleeding requiring hospitalization. After 24 hours bleeding stops. Further management to prolong the pregnancy includes

    1.   tocolysis
    2.   bed rest at home
    3.   cerclage
    4.   alpha-hydroxyprogesterone

p.545   Ans: A (Arias F, "Cervical cerclage for the temporary treatment of patients with placenta previa " Obstet Gynecol 1988;71:545)

83. [F & I: Background: Between 40% and 75% of patients with placenta previa who have their first bleeding episode between 12-28 weeks gestation, deliver by 30 and 34 weeks, respectively.

•Perinatal mortality is 8.1% for previa overall and 37% for those patients delivering infants with a birth weight under 1500 grams.

°Patients with previa who start bleeding **early** in gestation have lower hematocrits, require a larger number of transfusions, and have more bleeding episodes than other patients with placenta previa.

•Objective: to limit the frequency and severity of complications with placenta previa by using a **cervical cerclage** for the temporary treatment of this problem.

•Materials and Methods: 25 Patients between 24-30 weeks gestation, of whom 20 had complete placenta previa and 5 had partial placenta previa, demonstrated by ultrasound examination.

•Control patients were treated with bedrest in the hospital until delivery, terbutaline (2.5 mg. orally every four to six hours) to prevent preterm contractions, and glucocorticoid treatment (betamethasone, 12 mg. intramuscularly in two consecutive doses 24 hours apart) to accelerate fetal lung maturity when they reached 28 weeks of gestation.

•The cervical cerclage was placed after the cessation of all bleeding.

•The procedure was performed under general anesthesia using a 5 mm **Mersilene** band, which was attached to the cervix in a purse-string fashion, as described by McDonald.

•**Indomethacin** (initial dosage, one 50-mg rectal suppository one hour before surgery, followed by 25 mg orally every six hours for eight doses) was given to prevent uterine contractions during the perioperative period.

•Patients in both the study and control groups had ultrasound examinations every three weeks to reconfirm the placental localization and follow fetal growth.

•The management of placenta previa by means of cerclage was proposed in 1959.

•Since the most likely mechanisms for bleeding in placenta previa was partial detachment of the placenta brought about by progressive formation of the lower uterine segment, cervical cerclage was thought to act by halting placental separation.

•This study was limited to patients who were less than 30 weeks gestation because they bleed early and have a worse prognosis and the advantage of the cerclage procedure could be more clearly delineated.

•Results: Gestational age at delivery, prolongation of pregnancy and birth weights were greater in patients treated with cerclage than in those who received conventional, expectant treatment.

•The number of units of **blood** transfused between randomization and deliver was significantly higher for patients in the control group than for those in the cerclage group.

•There was no significant difference in the number of units of blood transfused at the time of delivery reflecting a similar magnitude of intrapartum blood loss for patients in both groups.

•A number of **cesarean hysterectomies** performed was high because the number of patients (11 of 25) who had previous cesarean sections.

°The risk of placenta previa and **accreta** increases almost linearly with the number of previous cesarean sections.

•Problems exist concerning the use of cerclage in the treatment of placenta previa:

°First, the possibility of using cerclage in patients who were **misdiagnosed** for placenta previa.

°97% of all asymptomatic patients with second-trimester echographic evidence of placenta previa will **not** have a previa term.

°Second potential problem is that there is a **false sense of security** given to the patient by initial results.

°Third, the possibility of concealed bleeding after the cerclage.

°°All patients were specifically instructed to report any lower abdominal pain and were followed by periodic ultrasound, paying special attention to the search for **retroplacental clots**.

•Conclusion: The use of cervical cerclage in patients with symptomatic placenta previa early in gestation has real advantages without increasing maternal morbidity.]

84. Indications for transabdominal cerclage for recurrent pregnancy loss include patients with

    1. congenitally short cervix
    2. T-shaped uterine cavity from DES exposure in utero
    3. penetrating forniceal lacerations
    4. subseptate uterus

p.865   Ans: B (Herron MA and Parer JT, "Transabdominal cerclage for fetal wastage due to cervical incompetence" Obstet Gynecol 1988;71:865)

84. [F & I:•Background: For some women with cervical incompetence the transvaginal approach for cervical cerclage is **not** effective.

•Women with the following conditions may benefit from the transabdominal procedure.

°1. Congenitally short or extensively amputated cervix.

°2. Marked scarring of the cervix, as after unsuccessful transvaginal cerclage.

°3. Deeply notched multiple cervical defects.

°4. Penetrating forniceal lacerations.

°5. Subacute cervicitis.

°6. Wide or extensive cervical conization.

°7. Cervicovaginal fistulas after abortion.

°8. A previously failed vaginal approach to cervical cerclage.

•Objective: to evaluate the transabdominal cervicoisthmic approach to cerclage in a rigidly selected group of women.

•8 patients were selected for the procedure based on one or more of the above criteria, excluding subacute cervicitis.

•The operation was carried out between 13 and 18 weeks; the mean age of placement was 14.5 weeks.

°General anesthesia was used, with midline vertical abdominal incisions.

°The suture (5 mm mersilene band) was placed as close as possible to the junction between the firm cervix and the soft uterine isthmus.

°The knot was buried beneath the bladder flap.

•Results: There was one intraoperative failure, in a woman with a surgically absent cervix.

•The eight patients had 11 successful pregnancies out of a total of 13; thus the pregnancy salvage rate post-cerclage was 85%.

•All of the fetuses were delivered in the third trimester.

•All patients had ancillary bed rest during their pregnancies, and some almost complete bed rest; half also had **tocolytics**.

•**The most common complication was blood loss.**

°Three women required blood transfusion.]

---

85. A patient who is 16 weeks pregnant is found to have a breast mass which on needle aspiration is diagnosed as carcinoma. Indicated in her further management

    1.   chemotherapy
    2.   mammography
    3.   mastectomy
    4.   radiation therapy

---

p.863   Ans: B (Parente JT, Amsel M, Lerner R, and Frank Chinea, "Breast cancer associated with pregnancy" Obstet Gynecol 1988;71:861)

85. [F & I:•Background: Breast cancer is the most frequent cause of cancer death in women in the United States.

•Breast cancer during pregnancy represents 2-5% of all breast cancers.

•Palpable masses are difficult to diagnose during pregnancy because of breast engorgement resulting from hormonal changes.

•Mammography or xeroradiography is an indicated diagnostic tool even in pregnancy, particularly for high risk patients or those with suspicious palpable lesions.

°The amount of radiation exposure to the patient is less than 0.1 rad; with proper shielding, the exposure to the fetus is negligible.

•Recurrence can be confirmed by fine-needle biopsy.

•Abortion did not appear to improve the prognosis in one patient.

•Radiation therapy is contraindicated during pregnancy.

°In most cases in which radiotherapy is considered the treatment of choice, the pregnancy is either terminated before treatment starts or, if the diagnosis is made in the later stages and the medical condition permits, pregnancy is allowed to continue until viability, at which time labor is induced or cesarean section is performed.

•Chemotherapy as an adjuvant treatment may be administered after organogenesis-embryogenesis is complete.

•Permanent sterilization should be considered, as oral contraceptive pills or other estrogen therapy are contraindicated after breast cancer.

•Pregnancy after treatment for breast cancer is permissible, but consideration must be given to such factors as age, parity, and stage of disease.

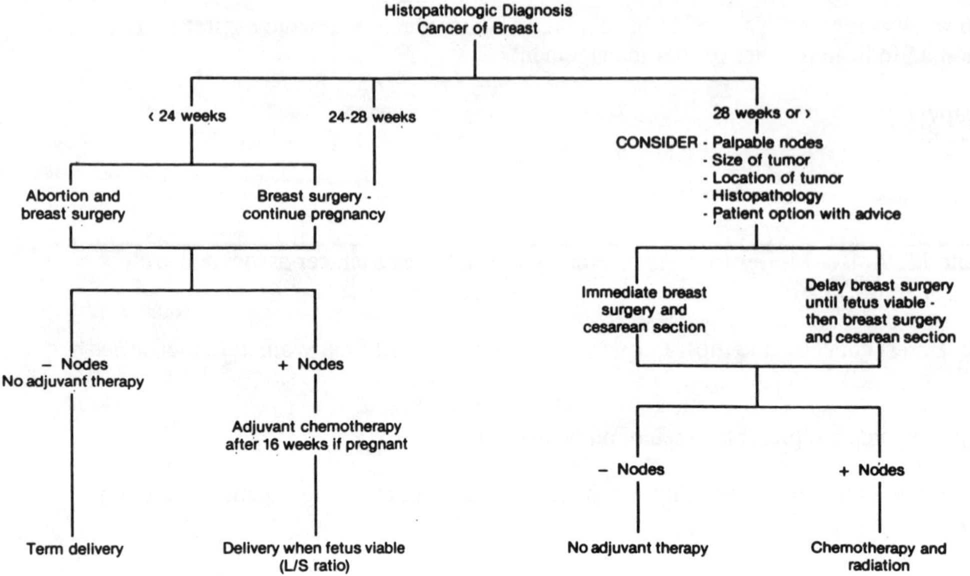

Figure 1. Suggested management of breast cancer in pregnancy.

(Reproduced with written permission of the The American College of Obstetricians and Gynecologists.)

---

86. Hypothyroidsim during pregnancy is associated with an increased risk for

1.   abruptio placentae
2.   anemia
3.   postpartum hemorrhage
4.   preeclampsia

---

p.111   Ans: E   (Davis LE, Leveno KJ, Cunningham FG,"Hypothyroidism complicating pregnancy" Obstet Gynecol 1988;71:108)

86. [F & I:•Background: Fewer than 60 cases of untreated hypothyroidism complicating pregnancy have been described in the English literature since 1897.

•Material and Methods: 25 hypothyroid women were followed through 28 pregnancies.

•Patients were considered in two groups.

°In the first group, 14 women had 16 pregnancies during which they were clinically hypothyroid and/or had chemical hypothyroxinemia.

°The second group included 12 pregnancies in women with histories of hypothyroidism but with subclinical hypothyroidism, which was defined as abnormally high serum TSH levels despite normal serum thyroxine (T4).

•The causes of hypothyroidism in the study subjects were as follows.

°Subtotal thyroidectomy in 10 women.

°Surgery was for Graves' thyrotoxicosis in six, Hashimoto's thyroiditis in two, papillary carcinoma in one, and an unknown indication in one.

•7 women had radioiodine for thyrotoxicosis

•In another 7, primary hypothyroidism was diagnosed a mean of 8.6 years before pregnancy.

•The remaining woman had hypothyroidism that followed septic cavernous sinus thrombosis at age five.

•Nearly 20% had no clinical findings, despite markedly abnormal chemical tests.

•Preeclampsia, abruptio placentae, stillbirths, anemia, postpartum hemorrhage, and cardiac dysfunction were frequent, especially with overt hypothyroidism.

°proteinuric hypertension complicated 32% of the 28 pregnancies and was identified in 7 women (44%) with overt hypothyroidism.

°°5 of these 25 women had underlying chronic hypertension.

•The hematocrit was < 26% initially during 5 of 16 pregnancies in overt hypothyroidism.

•Postpartum hemorrhage from uterine atony complicated 5.

•Perinatal losses were common and related to preeclampsia and placental abruption.

•Results: 7 of 16 pregnancies (44%) in overtly hypothyroid women were complicated by preeclampsia; two of these women also had placental abruption and two had heart failure.

•hypertension is common in nonpregnant hypothyroid patients, and improves after long-term T4 replacement.

•**Anemia**, a common finding with hypothyroidism, has been attributed to erythropoietin deficiency, pernicious anemia, decreased iron absorption, and bone marrow suppression.

°Nonpregnant hypothyroid women are prone to **excessive surgical blood loss** and, although the etiology is unclear, platelet dysfunction and factor VIII deficiency may normalize after T4 replacement.

•2 women had ventricular dysfunction , one of whom was subsequently hypothyroid.

•Myocardial dysfunction results from decreased alpha- and beta-receptors in the myocardium and down regulated myosin adenosine triphosphatase activity.

•One fourth of infants weighed less than 2000 g.

°Low birth weight was usually associated with preeclampsia or placental abruption and not idiopathic preterm labor.]

87. Pregnancies in which there is elevated maternal serum alpha-fetoprotein and oligohydramnios are associated with

    1. deformations
    2. intrauterine growth retardation
    3. pulmonary hypoplasia
    4. renal agenesis

p.338   Ans: E (Richards DS, Seeds, JW, Katz VL, Lingley LH, Albright SG, and Cefalo RC, "Elevated maternal serum alpha-fetoprotein with oligohydramnios: Ultrasound evaluation and outcome " Obstet Gynecol 1988;71:337)

87. [F & I:•Background: An elevation of maternal serum alpha-fetoprotein unexplained by structural fetal anomalies visible on ultrasound may be associated with adverse pregnancy outcome.

    °The combination of unexplained elevations of MSAFP and second-trimester oligohydramnios has been associated with an exceptionally poor prognosis.

•Material and Methods: Screened patients were referred for further evaluation when two MSAFP levels were greater than 2.25 multiples of the median, or if a single level was 3.0 multiples of the median or greater.

•A detailed ultrasound examination was then performed to confirm gestational age, exclude multiple gestation, search for fetal malformations, and assesss the amniotic fluid volume.

•The term "severely decreased" generally indicated **less than a 2 cm** pocket of fluid in at least two dimensions, and "moderately decreased" meant little or no fluid behind the back, with a 2-4 cm pocket in the region of the fetal small parts.

•Patient were given the following options:

    °1) attempted amniocentesis for cytogenetic studies and amniotic fluid AFP determinations,

    °2) pregnancy termination, or

    °3) expectant management with serial ultrasound examinations to confirm the persistence of oligohydramnios and the presence of any suspected fetal anomalies, with the option of elective pregnancy termination up to 21 weeks.

•During the study period 19 pregnancies were evaluated with MSAFP values and oligohydramnios.

    °The mean fetal age at the time of initial sonographic evaluation was 18.4 weeks.

    °The mean initial MSAFP elevation was 4.1 multiples of the median.

•Elevated MSAFP is associated with poor pregnancy outcome, regardless of the amniotic fluid volume.

    °Complications reported include low birth weight, pregnancy induced hypertension, fetal distress, and perinatal death.

•There have been a limited number of cases reported in which elevated MSAFP levels and second timester oligohydramnios coexist.

    °Outcomes have been very poor, with only three of 33 pregnancies producing suriving infants.

•In this series there was a lower incidence of fetal death at less than 24 weeks and a much lower incidence of fetal/neonatal deaths at greater than 24 weeks.

•When malformations are present in association with oligohydramnios, the prognosis for the fetus is extremely poor.

•For those cases with elevated MSAFP and oligohydramnios, the published series offer little hope for a good outcome, even if no anomalies are seen on ultrasound.

°Serial ultrasound examinations seem to be helpful in determining which patients are likely to have good outcomes.

°When the amniotic fluid was found to be only moderately decreased or normal on a subsequent examination, four of five infants survived.

•All six fetuses with severely decreased fluid on subsequent examinations had abnormal outcomes.

°Of the two pregnancies that were continued, one spontaneously aborted at 20 weeks; the other infant delivered prematurely at 24 weeks with postural deformities and pulmonary hypoplasia, and died.

°The other four pregnancies were electively terminated, and all four fetuses had compression deformities.

°It seems likely that with oligohydramnios of sufficient severity and duration to cause postural deformities, pulmonary hypoplasia would have been inevitable.

•Mechanisms by which these two findings are related can only be speculated.

°Lack of fetal renal clearance of AFP with primary kidney disease could result in higher fetal serum levels and increased transplacental passage.

°Possibly there is fetal excretion of AFP across pulmonary membranes, which is altered by primary oligohydramnios.

°Placental disease could allow fetomaternal hemorrhage, with fetal hypotension and subsequently decrease urine output.]

---

88. Twin zygosity can be determined prenatally by

1. blood group antigens
2. HLA typing
3. oligonucleotide probes
4. ultrasound

---

p.956   Ans: E (Kovacs B, Shahbahrami B, Platt LD, and Comings DE, "Molecular genetic prenatal determination of twin zygosity," Obstet Gynec 1988; 72:954)

88. [Facts and Issues:•Background: Protein markers such as histocompatibility antigens (HLA) and blood group antigens exhibiting heritable polymorphisms can resolve questions of paternity, zygosity, and identity.

°Heritable polymorphisms detected in DNA after digestion with restriction endonucleases and Southern blot hybridazation have been found.

°Termed "restriction fragment length polymorphisms," they are genetic markers for the identification of genes responsible for heritable disorders and in the prenatal diagnosis of fetuses with affective genetic diseases.

°The most polymorphic are located in regions of the human genome that consist of short stretches of of repetitive sequences.

°Polymorphisims in these regions (termed minisatellites or hypervariable regions) are due to variations in the number of small repeat sequences that make up the regions.

°Many hypervariable regions are disbursed throughout the human genome and DNA probes complimentary to them have been used to determine identity.

•Synthetic oligonucleotide probes that detect hypervariable regions in the genome of humans have been discovered.

°The probes identify a highly individual specific DNA patterns even in closely related persons and have used to detect chimerism after bone marrow transplantation in HLA-matched siblings.

•Identification of chromosomal heteromorphisms or protein polymorphisms (blood group antigens etc.) may help; but infrequent polymorphism of these markers results in a failed test.

•Synthesized probes have been used to determine at the molecular level the zygosity of twins prenatally.

°The advantages of this technique are accuracy, reliability and simplicity.

°The probability that two individuals may share all fragments detected by a single proble is related to the mean population frequency of alleles detected by the probe.

°The probability of any two unrelated persons having identical patterns is one in 300 billion.

°For siblings, this number is reduced to one in 300,000.

°The false positive probability of using both probes is 5.6×10^{-10} for siblings.

°This results in a false positive rate for prediction of monozygosity significantly less than with any other method.

•Monozygositic twins suffer greater morbidity and mortality than do dzygotic twins.]

---

89. Intrapartum treatment of intraamniotic infection results in

    1.   lower incidence of neonatal sepsis
    2.   increased incidence of late neonatal sepsis
    3.   shorter maternal hospital stay
    4.   increased incidence of nosocomial infection

---

p.827   Ans: B (Gibbs RS, Dinsmoor MJ, Newton ER, and Ramamurphy RS, "A randomized trial of intrapartum versus immediate postpartum treatment of women with intra-amniotic infection," Obstet Gynec 1988; 72:823)

89 [Facts and Issues: •Objective: to report the results of a prospective randomized trial of intra- versus immediate postpartum treatment of intraamniotic infection.

•Material and Methods: Intraamniotic fever is based on maternal fever of 100° F or higher and rupture of the membranes plus two or more of the following:

°maternal tachycardia (more than 100 beats per minute),

°uterine tenderness,

°purulent or foul amniotic fluid,

°fetal tachycardia (more than 160 beats per minute), or

°maternal leukocytosis.

•Results: Neonatal sepsis was reduced significantly by beginning therapy during labor rather than immediately after birth.

°This study was limited to cases where gestational age >34 weeks because of concern for the the high mortality accompanying neonatal sepsis in infants who weigh less than 2000 grams.

°This study was also arbitrarily limited to women with cervical dilatation 4 cm or more in view of the potential adverse effects that defer treatment for too long.

•Improved maternal outcome was demonstrated by three measures: shorter hospital stay, fewer febrile days, and a lower maximum postpartum temperature.

•Conclusion: Benefits to the neonate were demonstrated in that there was less neonatal sepsis and a significantly hospital stay without any cases of late sepsis.]

---

90. At 41 weeks, a patient has a non-reactive non-stress test after 40 minutes, adequate amniotic fluid, and satisfactory intrauterine physical assessment by ultrasound. The Bishop score is 9. Appropriate further management options include

   1.   repeat NST in 2 hours
   2.   medical induction of labor
   3.   contraction stress test
   4.   amniocentesis

---

p.553   Ans: A   (Bochner CJ, Williams J III, Castry L, Medearis A, Hobel CJ, and Wade M, "The efficacy of starting postterm antenatal testing at 41 weeks as compared with 42 weeks of gestational age " Am J Obstet Gynecol 1988;159:550)

90. [F & I:•Background: Perinatal morbidity, including fetal asphyxia, intrapartum distress, meconium aspiration, and postmaturity, increases significantly each week from 40 weeks on.

•Objective: to compare the neonatal outcomes of patients with antenatal fetal testing starting at 41 weeks of gestation with

°(1) patients who delivered between 41 and 42 weeks without having had testing and

°(2) patients who started testing at 42 weeks.

•Methods: The **contraction stress tests** were performed and results were classified according to the standard protocol and criteria of Freeman et al.

•The **amniotic fluid volume** was considered adequate if at least one pocket measured 3 cm vertically, and decreased if the larges vertical pocket was < 3 cm.

•The twice-weekly antepartum testing protocol included amniotic fluid assessment, nonstress tests and, when necessary, contraction stress tests.

•The **nonstress tests** were performed for up to 40 minutes, with abdominal stimulation if the test was not reactive after 20 minutes, followed by amniotic fluid assessment.

°A nonreactive nonstress test was repeated 2 hours later, if the amniotic fluid was determined to be adequate and the cervix was unfavorable for induction.

°A contraction stress test was done if the nonstress test was again nonreactive.

°°If the contraction stress test was negative, patients were retested in 3 to 4 days.

•Abnormal testing, leading to labor induction, included

°(1) decreased amniotic fluid,

°(2) bradycardias or repetitive variable or late decelerations during the nonstress test or contraction stress test, or

°(3) a nonreactive nonstress test in a patient subsequently noted to have an inducible cervix.

•Patients with normal test results were seen twice weekly until they went into labor or had labor induced at the discretion of their personal physicians.

•All patients were managed with continuous electronic fetal heart rate monitoring throughout labor.

°**Fetal distress in labor** was defined clinically as

°°(1) repetitive late decelerations,

°°(2) repetitive moderate or severe variable decelerations with either $pH < 7.20$ or decreased variability, or

°°(3) prolonged bradycardia.

•Patients were divided into those who did and those who did not receive antenatal testing starting at 41 completed weeks.

•The number of elective inductions, as well as the individual parameters of adverse perinatal outcome (including intrapartum fetal distress, low Apgar scores, meconium aspiration, stillbirths, and major perinatal morbidity and death) **were not significantly different between the groups.**

°**The incidence of cesarean sections due to fetal distress was higher in the group without testing; this difference approached but did not reach significance.**

°The tested group did not have any perinatal deaths or major morbidity, whereas the **untested group had three stillbirths, three cases of meconium aspiration, and seven instances of major neonatal morbidity, including four infants with seizures.**

°°Combined, the total number of averse outcomes in the untested group resulted in a significantly increased incidence of neonatal morbidity compared with the group with testing ($p < 0.5$).

•In this study, patients who were at risk were identified and delivered before 41 weeks.

°°Therefore, the study patients were at low risk for an adverse outcome, even without the use of antenatal testing.

°Conversely, the incidence of intrapartum fetal distress in the untested group was **almost** significantly greater, and when the total number of adverse perinatal outcomes was combined in this group, the incidence of morbidity was significantly increased compared with the tested group.

•Conclusion: Postterm testing starting at 41 weeks may decrease postterm perinatal mortality as well as intrapartum fetal distress.]

---

91. Advantages of transvaginal ultrasound diagnosis of placenta previa include

    1.   better visualization of a posterior placenta
    2.   full bladder not necessary for the study
    3.   increased image resolution
    4.   more accurate in obese patients

---

p.567   Ans: E   (Farine D, Fox HE, Jakobson S, and Timor-Tritsch IE, "Vaginal ultrasound for diagnosis of placenta previa " Am J Obstet Gynecol 1988;159:566)

J-9-566 [F & I:•Background: Trans**abdominal** sonographic diagnosis has many limitations, including poor visualization with a posterior placenta, patient obesity, or an overdistended bladder.

•Transvaginal sonography provides accurate diagnosis of early pregnancy, ectopic pregnancy, and pelvic masses.

•Objective: to compare the accuracy of a new diagnostic mode, transvaginal sonography, with transabominal sonography in patients with suspected placenta previa.

•The vaginal probe is introduced slowly into the vagina under direct sonographic visualization of the cervix.

•The tip of the probe stops short of the cervix, because a clear picture is produced in the focal zone, inasmuch as the distance between the probe and the cervix is about 3 cm.

°**Vaginal** ultrasound can be used to accurately locate the placenta without causing bleeding.

°**Transabdominal** sonography has several major **disadvantages**:

°°(1) obesity prevents proper imaging by the abdominal route,

°°(2) a full bladder that creates a proper acoustic window for transabdominal sonography may displace the lower uterine segment and produce a false diagnosis of placenta previa,

°°(3) a posterior placenta is less well imaged by the abdominal route and, at times, even the margin of a lateral placenta cannot be well visualized, and

°°(4) the acoustic shadow of the fetal head in a vertex presentation may prevent an accurate localization of a low placenta.

•"Placental migration" is due to the fact that as the lower uterine segment stretches during pregnancy a short distance between the placenta and the inernal os becomes evident.]

Perinatal Medicine

Directions: Each of the questions or incomplete statements below is followed by several suggested answers or completions. Select the BEST answer in each case.

1. The etiology of neural tube defects in diabetics is due to yolk sac response to

    A. electrolyte imbalance
    B. hemoglobin A1c
    C. hyperosmolality
    D. ischemia
    E. ketosis

2. Interpretation of a low maternal serum alpha-fetoprotein in the first trimester

    A. identifies 90% of chromosomal trisomies.
    B. requires a quantiative maternal serum estriol and hPL for interpretation.
    C. must be preceded by a dating ultrasound.
    D. requires a quantiative hCG for interpretation.
    E. uses a low limit cut-off of ≤ 3 MOM.

3. Which of the following is most useful in identifying maternal carbohydrate intolerance postpartum?

    A. 2 hr neonatal plasma glucose
    B. cord plasma C-peptide
    C. cord plasma glucose
    D. fetal and maternal clinical stigmata of carbohydrate intolerance
    E. maternal 3 hr GTT

4. What approximate percentage of patients with rheumatoid arthritis will have a remission during pregnancy?

    A. 25
    B. 50
    C. 75
    D. 90
    E. 95

5. Which of the following antibiotics is preferentially concentrated in the fetus and amniotic fluid?

    A. ampicillin
    B. cefoxitin
    C. ceftizoxime
    D. cephalothin
    E. gentamicin

6. Which of the following tests on maternal serum is useful in distinguishing between open neural tube defects and ventral wall defects?

    A. acetylcholinesterase
    B. carcinoembryonic antigen
    C. pseudocholinesterase
    D. sphingomyelin
    E. α-fetoprotein

7. In considering tocolysis for preterm labor, the enzyme involved in ß-adrenergic receptor **down regulation** is

    A. acetylcholinesterase
    B. adenylate cyclase
    C. cyclic AMP
    D. myosin light-chain kinase phosphatase
    E. phosphodiesterase

8. White matter necrosis seen after intrauterine infection and which is associated with cerebral palsy, is secondary to

    A. disseminated intravascular coagulation
    B. endotoxin
    C. febrile agglutinins
    D. interleukin-1
    E. Jarisch-Herxheimer reaction

9. Which of the following drugs is not primarily metabolized by plasma cholinesterase?

    A. bupivacaine
    B. cocaine
    C. procaine
    D. succinylcholine
    E. tetracaine

10. Compared to singleton pregnancies, the umbilical artery systolic/diastolic values in a normal twin gestation are

    A. $\frac{1}{2}$
    B. 2/3
    C. the same
    D. $1\frac{1}{2}$
    E. double

11. The fetal cerebral structure that can be identified earliest by means of ultrasound is the

    A. cerebellum
    B. choroid plexus
    C. falx cerebri
    D. septum pellucidum
    E. thalamus

12. The earliest time to use umbilical artery velocity studies to diagnose intrauterine growth retardation is (weeks)

    A. 16-18
    B. 20-24
    C. 28-30
    D. 31-33
    E. 34-36

13. Initial diagnostic steps in the management of pregnant women exposed to parvovirus infection should include

    A. amniotic fluid culture
    B. blood culture
    C. serology for specific antibodies
    D. throat culture
    E. ultrasound to determine gestational age

14. Fetal jeopardy in pregnant patients with autoimmune thrombocytopenia purpura can best determined by testing

    A. fetal platelet count by cordocentesis
    B. fetal platelet count by fetal scalp sampling
    C. maternal associated antibody in amniotic fluid
    D. maternal associated antibody in maternal blood
    E. maternal platelet count

15. Total parenteral nutrition given during the first trimester of pregnancy is associated with

    A. fetal anomalies
    B. placental infarction
    C. preterm labor
    D. respiratory quotient greater than 1
    E. small for gestational age infants

16. Which of the following is the most accurate predictor of an adverse neurological outcome in the term neonate?

    A. five minute Apgar score
    B. one minute Apgar score
    C. ten minute Apgar score
    D. ultrasound examination of the newborn head
    E. umbilical cord pH between 7.15-7.20

17. A 22 year old para 0-0-0-0 is diagnosed by ultrasound as having a fetus with gastroschisis at 28 weeks. No other abnormalities are detected. What is the next best plan of management to maximize fetal outcome?

    A. await the onset of labor and deliver by cesarean section
    B. await the onset of labor and deliver vaginally except for obstetrical indications
    C. cesarean section at 28 weeks, without further testing
    D. deliver by cesarean when testing indicates fetal lung maturity
    E. induction of labor at 28 weeks without further testing

18. Ultrasound examination of a twin gestation at 22 weeks, reveals one twin with polyhydramnios, and the other twin with oligohydramnios. The next best step in the further management of the gestation is

    A. amniocentesis of the polyhydramniotic sac and use the fluid to reconstitute the amniotic fluid in the oligohydramniotic sac
    B. amniocentesis of the polyhydramniotic sac
    C. observation
    D. reconstitution of the amniotic fluid in the oligohydramniotic sac
    E. selective feticide of the oligohydramniotic twin

19. During normal pregnancy, what is the shortest cervical length (mm) that is associated with increased risk of preterm labor?

    A. 40
    B. 50
    C. 60
    D. 70
    E. 80

20. Which of the following measurements of respiratory function **increases** as pregnancy progresses?

    A. expiratory reserve volume
    B. functional residual capacity
    C. inspiratory capacity
    D. residual volume
    E. vital capacity

21. What outcome improvement from electively sectioning patients whose fetuses who have open spina bifida can be expected?
Decreased

    A. chance of meningitis
    B. developmental handicap
    C. incidence of RDS
    D. mortality
    E. neurologic handicap

22. The earliest week of embryonic life by which the bronchial tree is completed is

    A. 14
    B. 16
    C. 18
    D. 20
    E. 24

23. A patient who has no other risk factors but an elevated MSAFP value of 2.5 multiples of the median is estimated to be at risk for having a fetus with an open neural tube defect of 1 in 200. After a normal high resolution ultrasound examination, her risk would be correctly estimated as

    A. one in 400
    B. one in 1000
    C. one in 2000
    D. one in 5000
    E. one in 10,000

24. What is the approximate percentage of pregnant alcoholics that will give birth to fetuses with the fetal alcohol syndrome?

    A. 15
    B. 25
    C. 40
    D. 67
    E. 75

25. Infants who survive grade 3 or 4 germinal layer/intraventricular hemorrhage have what frequency (%) of neurological deficits?

    A. < 5
    B. 20
    C. 33
    D. 50-75
    E. 90-95

26. Which part of the brain is primarily affected in microcephaly?

    A. frontal lobe
    B. occipital lobe
    C. parietal lobe
    D. temporal lobe
    E. brain stem

27 Which is the most sensitive test for determining whether a specimen taken during cordocentesis has been contaminated with maternal blood?

    A. ABO and Rh blood typing
    B. hematocrit
    C. human chorionic gonadotropin
    D. Kleihauer-Betke test
    E. α-fetoprotein determination

28. Which of the following is **increased** during a normal pregnancy?

    A. bone resorption of calcium
    B. intestinal absorption of calcium
    C. parathyroid hormone
    D. renal resorption of calcium
    E. serum ionized calcium

29. Which of the following dermatoses of pregnancy is an autoimmune disease?

    A. pruritic urticarial papules and plaques of pregnancy
    B. papular dermatitis of pregnancy
    C. impetigo herpetiformis
    D. prurigo gestationis
    E. herpes gestationis

30. All of the following should be considered in the intrauterine differential diagnosis of fetal cystic hygroma EXCEPT

    A. benign cystic teratoma
    B. meningomyelocele
    C. nuchal edema
    D. subchorionic placenta cyst
    E. ventriculomegaly

31. In which of the following situations would cervical ripening by means intravaginal prostaglandin E2 in an otherwise uncomplicated vertex presentation be **contraindicated**?

    A. Class A diabetes mellitus at term
    B. placental insufficiency at term
    C. postdate pregnancy
    D. premature rupture of membranes at term
    E. previous precipitate delivery

32. All of the following are appropriate in the management of laboring pregnant patients with aortic stenosis EXCEPT

    A. conduction anesthesia
    B. operative assistance for delivery
    C. prophylactic antibiotics
    D. pulmonary artery catheter
    E. volume expansion

Directions: Each set of lettered headings below is followed by a list of numbered words or phrases. For each numbered word or phrase select:

A. if item is associated with (A) only
B. if item is associated with (B) only
C. if item is associated with both (A) and (B)
D. if item is associated with neither (A) nor (B)

    A. cadmium
    B. zinc
    C. both
    D. neither

33. half-life in body measured in decades

34. maternal alkaline phosphatase an indicator of deficiency status

35. concentration in placenta increases with smoking

Directions: For each of the questions or incomplete statements below, ONE or MORE of the answers or completions given is correct. In each case select:

A. if only 1, 2 and 3 are correct
B. if only 1 and 3 are correct
C. if only 2 and 4 are correct
D. if only 4 is correct
E. if all are correct

36. In considering the reliability of chorionic villus biopsy, possible causes of cytogenic discrepancies between trophoblast and fetus include

    1. abnormal single cell lines
    2. chimerism
    3. maternal contamination
    4. meiotic exchanges

37. Sequelae of methamphetamine abuse during pregnancy include

    1. decreased birth weight
    2. decreased head circumference
    3. decreased length
    4. increased incidence of congenital anomalies

38. Endocrine changes associated with early syphilis include

    1. decreased dehyrdroepiandrosterone sulfate in fetus
    2. decreased maternal serum 17 ß-estradiol
    3. increased cholesterol in fetus
    4. decreased maternal progesterone

39. The amount of fat accumulated in the liver in cases of acute fatty liver of pregnancy is correlated with

    1. hematocrit
    2. hemoglobin
    3. platelet count
    4. serum uric acid

40. Clinically useful in the treatment of fetal supraventricular tachycardia

    1. digoxin
    2. quindine
    3. verapamil
    4. transabdominal compression of the fetal cephalic pole

41. Malignant hyperthermia can be triggered in susceptible humans by

    1. amide local anesthetics
    2. catecholamines
    3. depolarizing skeletal muscle relaxants
    4. inhalation anesthetics

42. Clinical effects of low dose (1 to 5 µg/kg/min) dopamine include

    1. dilation of renal blood vessels
    2. increase in glomerular filtration rate
    3. naturiesis
    4. tachycardia

43. Clinically useful in preventing intraventricular hemorrhage in the small preterm infant:

    1. phenobarbital
    2. pancuronium
    3. fresh frozen plasma
    4. exchange transfusion

44. Drugs with a **decreased** clearance during pregnancy include

    1. caffeine
    2. ethylmorphine
    3. hexobarbitone
    4. ritodrine

45. Causes of subnormal insulin requirements during gestation include

    1. increased exercise
    2. placental failure
    3. decreasing renal function
    4. hypothyroidism

46. Clinically useful in managing pregnancies of women who have circulating lupus anticoagulant antibodies

    1. aspirin
    2. umbilical artery flow velocity waveforms
    3. prednisone
    4. cyclosporin

47. Clinically useful in determining fetal pulmonary maturity, amniotic fluid

    1. cholesteryl palmitate
    2. urea nitrogen
    3. phosphatidyl glycerol
    4. acyl transferase

48. Patients are at increased risk for late abortion if they have Group B streptococcus colonization of their

    1. vagina
    2. uterine cervix
    3. urethra
    4. pharynx

49. At 22 weeks a pregnancy is judged to be growth retarded and an ultrasound is ordered. Findings which dictate a karyotype be obtained include

    1. club foot
    2. diaphragmatic hernia
    3. facial defect
    4. ventricular septal defect

50. True statements about neurofibromatosis include

    1. It is inherited as an autosomal dominant.
    2. Non-toxemic hypertension is an invariable feature.
    3. There is an increased incidence of pheochromocytoma.
    4. Chorionic villus sampling can be used to detect affected fetuses.

51. Decreased levels of microvillar enzymes (including alkaline phosphatase, γ–glutamyl transpeptidase) are associated with

    1. chromosomal aneuploidies
    2. fetal structural malformations
    3. normal fetuses
    4. cystic fibrosis

52. The clinical course of patients with diabetic nephropathy who become pregnant is frequently marked by

    1. increased incidence of cesarean section
    2. exacerbation of proteinuria
    3. elevation of blood pressure
    4. development of nephrotic syndrome

53. True statements about chorionic villus sampling include

    1. Use in twin pregnancies has not yet been established.
    2. When mosaicism is observed, subsequent amniocentesis is indicated.
    3. MSAFP (maternal serum alpha-fetoprotein) levels are falsely elevated following CVS, negating their usefulness in second trimester.
    4. Fetal loss is not significantly different from unsampled matched patients.

54. Indicated in the evaluation of the fetus at risk for non-immune hydrops

    1. maternal mean corpuscular hemoglobin
    2. maternal Coombs' test
    3. fetal hemoglobin electrophoresis
    4. fetal karyotype

55. Effects of maternal administration of indomethacin include

    1. closure of the patent ductus in the fetus
    2. decrease in amniotic fluid volume
    3. tocolysis of preterm labor
    4. decrease in fetal levels of ADH

56. Of potential use in limiting cell damage after
hypoxia in the asphyxiated infant

    1. xanthine oxidase inhibitors
    2. free radical scavengers
    3. adenine deaminase inhibitors
    4. 100% oxygen

57. Associated with exencephaly

    1. amniotic band syndrome
    2. anencephaly
    3. encephalocele
    4. omphalocele

58. Oxytocinase

    1. increases the permneability of the
       distal and collecting tubules of the
       kidney.
    2. is produced by the
       syncytiotrophoblast.
    3. levels are decreased in patients who
       are destined to develop
       pregnancy-induced hypertension.
    4. production is induced by oxytocin.

59. Administration of nifedipine to a
hypertensive pregnant patient results in

    1. decreased total peripheral resistance
    2. increase in cardiac output
    3. increased perfusion of uterus
    4. decreased placental blood flow

Perinatal Medicine-References

Directions: Each of the questions or incomplete statements below is followed by several suggested answers or completions. Select the BEST answer in each case.

---

1.   The etiology of neural tube defects in diabetics is due to yolk sac response to

   A.   electrolyte imbalance
   B.   hemoglobin A1c
   C.   hyperosmolality
   *D.   ischemia
   E.   ketosis

---

p.1489   (Pinter E, Reece EA, Ogburn PL JR., Turner S, Hobbins JC, Mahoney MJ, and Naftolin F, "Fatty acid content of yolk sac and embryo in hyperglycemic induced embryopathy and effect on arachidonic acid supplementation" Am J Obstet Gynecol 1988; 159:1484)

1. [F&I:•Background: Diabetes in pregnancy is associated with a high incidence of congenital malformations.

   •Neuroepithelium changes of embryos are accompanied by characteristic signs of injury within the visceral endodermal yolk sac membrane.

   •The typical features of cell damage of the visceral endodermal yolk sac cells included a significant decrease in the size and number of stored lipid droplets.

   °The essential fatty acid arachidonic acid may prevent the embryopathy and alter structural abnormalites of the visceral endodermal yolk sac cells and the neuroepithelial when added to the hyperglycemic medium in which rat embryos were studied.

   °The stored lipid droplets in normal visceral endodermal yolk sacs may constitute a reserve pool of fatty acids.

   •Objective: to analyze the fatty acid composition of major lipid groups of conceptuses cultured in controls, hyperglycemic, and arachidonic acid-supplemented hyperglycemic conditions to determine:

   °1) Whether hyperglycemia induces modification of fatty acid composition within difference lipid groups in the yolk sac and embryo, and

   °2) If so, whether aracidonic acid supplementation could prevent those alterations.

   •Results: Quantitation of fatty acid content in different lipid groups show that the control rat yolk sac always contained higher levels of fatty acids in major lipid groups than does the embryo.

   •Anomalous conceptuses resulting from exposure to excess d-glucose had altered fatty acid levels in major lipid groups.

   °Two of the most remarkable changes were the high embryonic oleic acid content in nonesterified fatty acids and the elevated ratio of oleic acid/stearic acid in embryonic phopholipids of the glucose-treated conceptuses.

   •A variety of conditions including ischemia could activate cell membrane lipases in many tissues resulting in the release of free fatty acids, for example, oleic and arachidonic acids.

°The liberation of these fatty acids because of insufficient blood supply might occur in hyperglycemic-exposed conceptuses, since morphometric analysis showed a significant decrease in the yolk sac and neural tube vascularity.

•The elevated embryonic nonesterified fatty acids and the elevated oleic acid in nonesterified fatty acids, which were preventable with arachidonic acid supplementation, could be markers for essential fatty acid deficiency.

•The inadequate transport of fatty acids to the embryo may be related to the significant decrease in the quantity of rough endoplasmic reticulum in visceral endodermal cells.

°The rough endoplasmic reticulum is the principal site of protein synthesis, including alpha-fetoprotein, which plays a role in the transport of long chain fatty acid.

•Conclusion: Conceptuses grown under hyperglycemic conditions result in structural abnormalities and alterations in the fatty acid content of major lipid groups.

°The addition of relatively high concentrations of an essential fatty acid (arachidonic acid) prevented the malformations of many of the observed abnormalities in fatty acid composition.]

---

2. Interpretation of a low maternal serum alpha-fetoprotein in the first trimester

    A. identifies 90% of chromosomal trisomies.
    B. requires a quantiative maternal serum estriol and hPL for interpretation.
    *C.   must be preceded by a dating ultrasound.
    D. requires a quantiative hCG for interpretation.
    E. uses a low limit cut-off of ≤ 3 MOM.

---

p.1213   (Milunsky A, Wands J, Brambati B, Bonacchi I, and Currie K, "First-trimester maternal serum α-fetoprotein screening for chromosome defects ," Am J Obstet Gynec 1988; 159:1209)

2. [Facts and Issues:•Background: Low maternal serum alpha-fetoprotein values can identify Downs syndrome.

°75-80% of all Down syndrome offspring are delivered unexpectedly by women <35 years of age.

•Objective: to determine the detection efficiency of prospective first trimester maternal serum alpha fetoprotein screening for chromosomal defects in a group of women with an increased risk of having a child with chromosomal defect.

•Results: Eight of 27 of all chromosome defects had maternal serum alpha fetoprotein values ≤0.6 multiples of the median.

•Conclusion: First trimester maternal serum alpha-fetoprotein screening can detect serious field chromosomal defects when preceeded by an ultrasound study to accurately establish fetal age.]

3.   Which of the following is most useful in identifying maternal carbohydrate intolerance postpartum?

    A.   2 hr neonatal plasma glucose
    B.   cord plasma C-peptide
    C.   cord plasma glucose
    D.   fetal and maternal clinical stigmata of carbohydrate intolerance
    *E.   maternal 3 hr GTT

p.1131   (Carpenter MW, Coustan DR, Widness JA, Gruppuso PA, Malone M, and Rotondo LM, "Postpartum testing for antecedent gestational diabetes ," Am J Obstet Gynec 1988; 159:1128)

3. [Facts and Issues:•Background: Gestational diabetes complicates 1.4% to 2.5% of all pregnancies.

•Gestational diabetics are more likely to develop carbohydrate intolerance during future pregnancies and later in life.

•The American College of Obstetricians and Gynecologists does not recommend screening for women younger than 30 years of age.

•Maternal hyperglycemia or glucosuria during the puerperium and neonatal macrosomia, hypoglycemia, polycythemia, and hypocalcemia are nonspecific signs of possible antecedent maternal glucose intolerance during pregnancy.

•Objective: to compare three neonatal variables (cord plasma glucose, cord plasma C-peptide, and 2 hour capillary plasma glucose values) with results of a maternal postpartum, 100 gm, 3-hour oral glucose tolerance test (GTT) to determine which was the most useful in the diagnosis of antecedent gestational diabetes.

•Materials and methods: All participants had a 50 gm, oral, 1-hour screening test at 24 to 28 weeks.

•Control participants (n = 28) had values >130 mg/dl and normal 100 gm, 3-hour, oral GTT results at 35 to 38 weeks.

•These tests were administered after a 3-day preparation with a high-carbohydrate diet.

•Test results were normal if at least three of four values were <95, 180, 155, and 140 mg/dl limits.

•Postpartum GTT values that were evaluated included the individual fasting, 1-hour, 2-hour, and 3-hour concentrations as well as the sum of incremental 1-hour and 2-hour values (incremental 1-hour + 2-hour values = [1-hour - fasting] + [2-hour - fasting] values).

•Diagnosis of gestational diabetes identifies gravid women at risk for perinatal morbidity, including fetal macrosomia, birth trauma, and operative delivery, as well as neonatal hypoglycemia, hypocalcemia, polycythemia, and hyperbilirubinemia.

•There is a detection rate of 53% when historical risk factors alone are used to determine the need for glucose tolerance.

•Variables derived from the postpartum GTT appeared to offer useful information about previous glucose tolerance when performed within the first 48 hours postpartum

    °The incremental 1-hour + 2-hour glucose values of the postpartum GTT function best in this regard.

°At a test threshold of 110 mg/dl, 90.8% of nondiabetic population and 80.0% of those with gestational diabetes would be correctly identified on the basis of these data.

•Conclusion: If antecedent gestational diabetes is suspected at parturition but it is undocumented at 2 hours, 100 gm glucose oral tolerance test may be administered.

°In a normal result, on the basis of incremental 1-hour + 2-hour glucose concentrations (≥110 mg/dl) may justify either further testing in future pregnancies or diagnostic surveillance later in the patient's life.]

4.   What is the approximate percentage of patients with rheumatoid arthritis will have a remission during pregnancy?

    A. 25
    B. 50
    *C.   75
    D. 90
    E. 95

p.896 (McNeill ME, "Multiple pregnancy-induced remissions of psoriatic arthritis: Case report" Am J Obstet Gynecol 1988;159:896)

4. [F & I:•Background: Rheumatoid arthritis is an autoimmune disease.

•Remission of the inflammatory activity of rheumatoid arthritis during pregnancy occurs.

•Transient partial remission of arthritic acitivity occurs in 62% to 75% of patients with rhematoid arthritis who become pregnant.

•High local concentrations of progesterone prolong xenogeneic and allogenic skin grafts and to have profound antiinflammatory effects.

•Pregnancy induced weakening of maternal immunity may relate to changes in estrogen-progesterone ratios.

°Exacerbation of arthritic pain before menstruation suggests a systemic sensitivity to changes in progesterone levels in the late luteal phase of the cycle.

•Immunosuppression during pregnancy results from the action of serum factors on local hormonal immuno-regulation of maternal lymphocytes.

°Among lymphoid cells, immunoregulatory T cells are reported to be the most sensitive to sex hormone action.]

5.   Which of the following antibiotics is preferentially concentrated in the fetus and amniotic fluid?

    A. ampicillin
    B. cefoxitin
    *C.   ceftizoxime
    D. cephalothin
    E. gentamicin

p.573   (Fortunato SJ, Bawdon RE, Welt SI and Swam KF, "Steady-state cord and amniotic fluid ceftizoxime levels continuously surpass maternal levels " Am J Obstet Gynecol 1988;159:570)

5. [F & I:•Objective: to define the optimal antibiotic for intrauterine therapy.

•The ideal drug should

°have an infrequent dosing schedule,

°be minimally protein bound,

°possess minimal toxicity, and

°be active against a broad range of aerobic, anaerobic, and gram-negative pathogens commonly encountered in obstetric infections.

•**Ceftizoxime** would seem an ideal candidate; it is < 30% protein bound, has the lowest molecular weight of all the third-generation cephalosporins, demonstrates along half-life (1.9 hours), possesses excellent broad-spectrum antimicrobial activity, and does not incorporate the N-methyl-thiotetrazole side chain implicated with bleeding disorders, as present in other third-generation cephalosporins.

•Objective: to determine maternal, cord, and amniotic fluid ceftizoxime concentrations in patients undergoing prolonged therapy with ceftizoxime in whom steady-state pharmacodynamics had been achieved.

•Results: A broad-spectrum nontoxic antimicrobial agent can achieve and maintain therapeutic concentrations in the fetus and the amniotic fluid for the duration of its recommended dosing schedule.

•Ceftizoxime levels surpass inhibitory concentrations for the major portion of its dosage schedule when administred in doses of 2 gm every 8 hours.

•No other antimicrobial suitable for single-agent therapy of pelvic infections concentrates in the fetus and amniotic fluid.

•There are consistently higher maternal drug concentrations of cephalothin, cephaloridine, cefuroxime, ceftaxime, moxalactam, clindamycin, mezlocillin, ampicillin, cefoxitin, gentamicin, and cefazolin when compared with the cord and amniotic fluid.]

---

6. Which of the following tests on maternal serum is useful in distinguishing between open neural tube defects and ventral wall defects?

    A. acetylcholinesterase
    B. carcinoembryonic antigen
    *C.   pseudocholinesterase
    D. sphingomyelin
    E. α-fetoprotein

---

p.469   (Drugan A, Syner FN, Belsky R, Koppitch FC, Evans MI, "Amniotic fluid acetylcholinesterase: Implications of an inconclusive result," Am J Obstet Gynec 1988; 159:469)

6. [F & I:•Background: Analysis of amniotic fluid α-fetoprotein levels is essential in making the prenatal diagnosis of neural tube defects.

•Acetylcholinesterase gel electrophoresis is a useful adjunct in patients with elevated α-fetoprotein levels in amniotic fluid and maternal serum: 95.5% of infants with neural tube defects had a positive acteylcholinesterase test result.

°About 50% of cases of omphalocele, fetal demise, cystic hygromas, and hydrops were also associated with positive results.

•The ratio of acetylcholinesterase to pseudocholinesterase activity can distinguish between open neural tube defects and ventral wall defects.

°The ratio is about 10-fold higher in open neural tube defects than in ventral wall defects.

•A false positive rate of acetylcholinesterase gel electrophoresis is <1%.

•Maternal serum acetylcholinesterase-like activity can also be differentiated from true acetylcholinesterase; maternal serum contains only **pseudocholinesterase** and will not be inhibited by the specific inhibitor.

•Classically, acetylcholinesterase is considered a bimodal test-either definitely positive or definitely negative.

•Objectives: to define the gradation of acetylcholinesterase and to categorize the implications of faint "inconclusive" bands which appear in the second position on gel electrophoresis.

•The fetus is the likely source of amniotic fluid acetycholinesterase.

•The amniotic fluid α-fetoprotein level decreases by about 90% from levels in early pregnancy to term; acetylcholinesterase activity is reduced by only 50%.

•Earlier in gestation an inconclusive acetylcholinesterase test result is a more common but a less ominous sign, although it may be associated with fetal malformation.

•**Later in pregnancy, and especially after 20 weeks' gestation, a very high percentage of inconclusive acetylcholinesterase test results in amniotic fluid are associated with a malformed fetus.**

•Abnormal results should prompt a thorough level II ultrasonographic evaluation of the fetus.

»If a karyotype was not determined from the original amniotic fluid sample, a second amniocentesis or umbilical blood sample for karyotyping as well as for repeating the α-fetoprotein measurement and acetylcholinesterase test should be considered essential.

•Of 1099 pregnancies associated with elevated amniotic fluid α-fetoprotein levels noted the association of a positive acetylcholinesterase test result with 99.5% of neural tube, 75% of exomphalos, and 50% of other serious malformations.

•False-positive "inconclusive" results can be explained by contamination with fetal blood or fetal calf serum.

°A vanishing second twin, which occurs in about 20% of twin pregnancies, a twin can account for only a small part of cases.

°Unrecognized previous trauma to the products of conception, can also give a false positive.]

7. In considering tocolysis for preterm labor, the enzyme involved in ß-adrenergic receptor **down regulation** is

    A. acetylcholinesterase
    B. adenylate cyclase
    *C.   cyclic AMP
    D. myosin light-chain kinase phosphatase
    E. phosphodiesterase

p.323   (Gonik B, Benedetti T, Creasy RK, Lee A, "Intramuscular versus intravenous ritodrine hydrochloride for preterm labor management," Am J Obstet Gynec 1988; 159:323)

7. [F & I:•Objective: to examine the efficacy and safety of intravenous versus intramuscular ritodrine hydrochloride for tocolysis in the treatment of preterm labor.

•Patients and methods:

•Criteria for preterm labor include: significant uterine activity (four or more contractions within 20 minutes) and either a documented cervical change by serial examinations or a cervix $\geq$2 cm dilated or at least 80% effaced.

•Patients randomized to the intramuscular treatment group received an initial intramuscular dose of ritodrine hydrochloride 10 mg.

•Injections were uniformly administered in either the gluteal or vastus lateralis muscle group, depending on the subjects institution.

°Subsequent intramuscular injections or 5 to 10 mg were repeated at intervals of 2 to 4 hours.

°The dosage and frequency of injections were individually adjusted by each investigator according to uterine and maternal heart rate responses.

°**The goal was to obtain uterine quiescence, which was defined as fewer than two contractions within 20 minutes.**

•Patients randomized to the intravenous treatment group were administered ritodrine at an initial dose of 100 µg/min.

°This was gradually increased until a maximum dose of 350 µg/min was achieved.

•**Criteria for successful tocolysis included at least 12 continous hours of uterine quiescence with parenteral therapy and a delay in delivery of >24 hours from the initiation of therapy.**

•Treatment failure was determined by the need to discontinue ritodrine therapy because of labor progression or undesirable side effects.

°The need to add an additional tocolytic agent such as magnesium sulfate during the study period was also considered a failure of therapy.

•All patients were maintained on a fluid restriction protocol of $\leq$2500 ml within 24 hours during parenteral therapy.

•Results: Intramuscular administration of ritodrine hydrochloride and ritodrine delivered by the intravenous route were **equally efficacious** for the management of preterm labor.

°Overall success tocolysis (67%) is comparable to that of others in which similar intravenous and intramuscular management schedules have been used.

•Benefits of intramuscular ritodrine therapy:

°Easier administration

°Availability may encourage earlier attempts at tocolysis before transfer to a tertiary care center.

•Overall **less** total drug is needed to adequately inhibit premature uterine activity with the intramuscular route.

•Potential limitations to this route of drug delivery:

°The intramuscular ritodrine is less well titrated to individual responses.

°Local **pain** as a result of repeated injections may limit the patient's acceptance to therapy.

•Prolonged and constant infusion of ritodrine may be less advantageous than intermittent dosing.

°ß-adrenergic receptor down-regulation or tachyphylaxis, occurs with constant administration of ritodrine.

°The mechanism by which this tissue desensitization occurs may involve cyclic adenosine monphosphate-mediated responses.]

---

8. White matter necrosis seen after intrauterine infection and which is associated with cerebral palsy, is secondary to

    A. disseminated intravascular coagulation
    *B.   endotoxin
    C. febrile agglutinins
    D. interleukin-1
    E. Jarisch-Herxheimer reaction

---

p.362   (Bejar R, Wozniak P, Allard M, Benirschke K, Vaucher Y, Coen R, Berry C, Schragg P, Villegas I, Resnik R, "Antenatal origin of neurologic damage in newborn infants. I. preterm infants," Am J Obstet Gynec 1988; 159:357)

8. [F & I:•Background: Periventricular leukomalacia or multifocal necrosis of the cerebral white matter is a frequent ischemic lesion in the inmature brain.

°It is associated with a variety of neurologic deficits in survivors, including cerebral palsy.

°In the acute stage, there are multiple foci of coagulative necrosis associated with congestion and petechial hemorrhages.

°The chronic stage starts 2 or more weeks later, when the necrotic zones degenerate into multiple cystic lesions.

°The cysts are then replaced by glial scars within 3 months.

°Cerebral atrophy develops later in patients with diffuse white matter necrosis.

•White matter necrosis may be identified in living infants with echoencephalography.

°Echolucencies in the white matter representing the cysts are the landmark of the ultrasonic diagnosis of white matter necrosis.

°The presence of multiple cystic lesions differentiate white matter necrosis from intraparenchamyl extension of intraventricular and subependymal hemorrhages which ultrasonically appears hyperechoic zones and the pariventricular white matter.

•Objective: to describe the echoencephalographic anatomic and epidemiologic features of antenatal white matter necrosis in preterm infants.

•Material and methods: Echoencepahlogic technique: Echoencephalograms were performed with a sector scanner with 5 and 7.5 MH transducers.

•The cerebral anatomy was visualized in three planes (coronal, axial, and sagittal) through the fontanelles and cranial sutures.

°The telencephalic white matter was images extensively by modifying the coronal and sagittal planes.

•Diagnosis of white matter necrosis and intraventricular/subependymal hemorrhages:

°**White matter necrosis** was diagnosed when echolucent areas (cysts) were observed in the white matter adjacent to the lateral ventricles.

°The criterion for diagnosis of antenatal white matter necrosis was the presence of echolucencies in the white matter by day 3 after birth.

°This is a conservative diagnosis because cystic lesions in the white matter appear two or more weeks after the acute stage.

°Postnatally acquired white matter necrosis was diagnosed in those instances with echolucencies appearing after day 3.

°**Intraventricular/subependymal hemorrhages** were diagnosed when echogenic material was present i the germinal matrix at the level of the caudate nuclei or in the cerebral ventricular system.

°Intraparenchymal extension of the intraventricular hemorrhage was diagnosed when intraventricular clots continued with echogenic zones in the paraventricular white matter.

°Antenatal white matter necrosis accounted for more than half the total number of infants with white matter necrosis and half of the survivors with white matter necrosis emphasized the extent to which antenatal white matter necrosis may contribute to neurological morbidity in preterm infants.

•The most important finding in this study was the association of antenatal white matter necrosis with fetal bacterial contamination or infection and vascular connections in the placenta of monochorionic twins.

°**There are multiple reports relating white matter necrosis of cerebral palsy with prenatal infection.**

•Chorioamnionitis, prolonged rupture of the membranes and congenital malformations were major predictors of cerebral palsy.

•**Endotoxin** may be the mediator of infection in generating white matter pathologic states.

•Placental vascular connections are very frequent in monochorionic twins.

°Any event that disturbs the balance circulation between the twins may effect these infants.

°Cardiovascular compromise in disseminated intravascular thrombosis associated with multiple ischemic lesions in the brain and other organs occur in monochorionic twins.]

9.   Which of the following drugs is not primarily metabolized by plasma cholinesterase?

     *A.   bupivacaine
     B.   cocaine
     C.   procaine
     D.   succinylcholine
     E.   tetracaine

p.310   (Kambam JR, Perry SM, Entman S, Smith BE, "Effect of magnesium on plasma cholinesterase activity," Am J Obstet Gynec   1988; 159:309)

9. [F & I:•Background: Magnesium potentiates the action of succinylcholine, a depolarizing muscle relaxant, in toxemia of pregnancy.

•Though magnesium has no significant effect on the characteristics of paralysis caused by succinylcholine in nonpregnant patients, the mechanism for the prolongation of the duration of action of succinylcholine in the presence of magnesium in toxemia of pregnancy has not been elucidated.

•Preeclampsia is associated with a significant reduction in plasma cholinesterase activity when this activity is compared with that of both healthy pregnant and nonpregnant women.

°Certain drugs like quinidine are known to cause a further decrease in plasma cholinesterase activity in pregnant women.

•Objective: to study the effect of magnesium sulfate on plasma cholinesterase activity in pregnant patients with preeclampsia.

•Plasma cholinesterase is a glycoprotein responsible for the metabolism of succinylcholine a depolarizing muscle relaxant and all the ester types of local anesthetics including 2-chlorprocaine, procaine, tetracaine, and cocaine.

•The reasons for a decrease in plasma cholinsterase activity level in both healthy pregnant patients and pregnant patients with preeclampsia are not clear.

°Several mechanisms including hypoproteinemia have been suggested.

•Magnesium is a co-factor of all enzymes involved in phosphate transfer.

•In higher than therapeutic concentrations, magnesium alone can cause profound motor paralysis without a significant sensory loss.

•In pregnant patients with preeclampsia and eclampsia, magnesium seems to **prolong** the duration of succinylcholine action whereas in nonpregnant patients, there is no demonstrable prolongation of succinylcholine action.

°Magnesium also prolongs the duration of action of non-depolarizing or curare like muscle relaxants.

°The mechanism for the magnesium induced prolongation of non-depolarizing muscle relaxant action may be from the inhibition of acetylcholine release from the nerve ending at the neuromuscular junction.

•Preeclampsia is associated with a significant reduction in plasma cholinesterase activity compared with that of either nonpregnant patients or healthy pregnant patients.

•Results: **Magnesium has no effect on plasma cholinesterase activity.**

•Conclusion: The prolongation of duration of succinylcholine action in pregnant patients with preeclampsia and eclampsia receiving magnesium sulfate is probably due to the low plasma cholinesterase activity rather than to magnesium administration.]

---

10. Compared to singleton pregnancies, the umbilical artery systolic/diastolic values in a normal twin gestation are

    A. $\frac{1}{2}$
    B. 2/3
    *C.   the same
    D. $1\frac{1}{2}$
    E. double

---

p.205   (Gerson A, Johnson A, Wallace D, Bottalico J, Weiner S, and Bolognese R. "Umbilical arterial systolic/diastolic values in normal twin gestation" Obstet Gynecol 1988;72:205)

10. [F & I:•Background: Doppler ultrasound can be used in singleton pregnancies to evaluate umbilical venous flow, umbilical arterial waveforms, uterine artery waveforms, and velocity of flow and waveforms of the fetal aorta.

°These measurements can be used to predict fetal anemia, intrauterine growth retardation (IUGR), and complications of pregnancy in hypertensive women.

•**In twin pregnancies in which both fetuses were appropriate for gestational age, the systolic/diastolic ration was within the normal range for singletons.**

•Doppler ultrasound measurements of the umbilical artery and umbilical vein were useful in predicting which twin gestations were destined to become discordant later in pregnancy.

°Doppler measurements were used to evaluate the cause of the discordance.

•None of the previous twin Doppler studies has reported gestational age-specific normal values for the umbilical arterial systolic/diastolic ratio.

°In single pregnancies the systolic//diastolic ratio decreases with advancing gestational age.

•Objective: to define normal values of umbilical artery systolic/diastolic ratio during the second and third trimesters in twin gestations that are appropriate for gestational age.

•Conclusion: Umbilical arterial waveforms in twin gestations are the same as the wave forms found in singleton gestations.]

---

11. The fetal cerebral structure that can be identified earliest by means of ultrasound is the

>   A. cerebellum
>   *B.   choroid plexus
>   C. falx cerebri
>   D. septum pellucidum
>   E. thalamus

p.187   (Chitkara U, Cogswell C, Norton K, Mehalek K, and Berkowitz R. "Choroid plexus cysts in the fetus: A benign anatomic variant or pathologic entity?" Report of 41 cases and review of the literature: Obstet Gynecol 1988;72:185)

11 [F & I:•Background: Cysts of the choroid plexus in the ventricular system of the human brain are fairly common, usually asymptomatic and frequently seen at autopsy in all age groups.

•Symptomatic cysts, although rare, have also been described in infants, young children, and adults.

•Choroid plexus cysts in the fetal brain are generally benign and most resolve spontaneously.

•Objectives:

°to determine the incidence of fetal choroid plexus cysts,

°to follow the natural course during intrauterine life and

°to determine whether there is an increased association of chromosomal and/or structural abnormalities in these fetuses.

•The **choroid plexus is the major source of cerebral spinal fluid** and is present in the lateral ventricle, the third ventricle and the fourth ventricle with an extension out of the lateral foramina of Luschka into the cerebellopontile angles.

°During embryonic development, the choroid plexus appears between 6-7 weeks gestation, first in the root of the fourth ventricle, then in the lateral ventricles and lastly in the third ventricle.

°Subsequent growth is rapid and by nine weeks the choroid plexus fills 75% of the lateral ventricle.

°This is followed by a progressive reduction in its size relative to the ventricular volume and further differentiations so that the choroid plexus has assumed its adult appearance by the 20th gestational week.

•**Sonographically, choroid plexus within the lateral ventricles is the first cerebral structure that can be visualized in the fetus.**

•During the late first and early second trimester, the lateral ventricles occupy most of the intracranial cavity, and are filled almost entirely by the echogenic choroid plexus.

°The highly reflective nature of this structure makes it a prominent landmark in the fetal brain that can visualized with ease in the axial coronal and sagittal planes of the fetal head throughout gestation.

•Cysts of the choroid plexus are common and have been found in over 50% of serial autopsy studies occurring with about the same frequency in all age groups.

°They are generally less than 1 cm in diameter and are usually asymptomatic.

°These cysts represent neuro-epithelial folds that subsequently fill with cerebrospinal fluid and cellular debris.

°Cases with obstructive symptoms are always associated with large cysts measuring 2-8 cm in size.

•Sonographically, the cysts appear as echolucent structures within the structures the choroid, and have sharply circumscribed margins.

•Although the benign and transient nature of these cysts in utero has generally been emphasized, at least eight autosomal trisomies have been reported in fetuses with choroid plexus cyst.

°Five of these were trisomy 18, one was trisomy 21, and two were not specified.

•In the 41 cases studied here, only one abnormal karyotype (trisomy 18) was found.

°This fetus was found to have large bilateral choroid plexus cysts at 18 weeks that were still present at 22 weeks gestation; the only other anatomic abnormality suspected was esophageal atresia.

•In 4 of the 8 cases with an associated trisomy, the cysts were large, bilateral and persistent beyond 22 weeks gestation.

•Conclusion: Fetal choroid plexus cysts are fairly commonly observed during a second trimester sonogram.

°They are usually small, 1 cm or less in size, maybe either unilateral or bilateral, and in most cases have either completely disappeared or significantly decreased in size by 22-24 weeks gestation.

°Once resolved, the cysts do not recur in a normal sonogram in late second trimester predicts a normal examination in late pregnancy and in the neonate.

•Because some cases have been associated with anatomic and chromosomal anomalies, particularly **trisomy 18** it is important to conduct a careful sonographic search for other anomalies in all cases.

•Chromosomal studies should be considered and are strongly recommended whenever associated anatomic anomalies are detected or when the cysts are large, bilateral and persistent after 20-22 weeks gestation.]

---

12. The earliest time to use umbilical artery velocity studies to diagnose intrauterine growth retardation is (weeks)

    A. 16-18
    *B.   20-24
    C. 28-30
    D. 31-33
    E. 34-36

---

p.1439 (Gaziano E, Knox GE, Wager GP, Bendel RP, Boyce DJ and Olson J. "The predictability of the small-for-gestational-age infant by real-time ultrasound-derived measurements combined with pulsed Doppler umbilical artery velocimetry," Am J Obstet Gynecol 1987;158:1431)

12 [F & I:•Background: Umbilical artery Doppler velocity waveforms reflect intrauterine growth retardation (IUGR).

•Systolic/diastolic ratio in velocimetry measurements reflect increased peripheral resistance in the umbilical circulation.

•Objectives: to assess the impact of umbilical artery pulsed Doppler studies on the accuracy of IUGR prediction and to compare this technique with real-time ultrasound measurements.

•Lowered diastolic velocities and occasional reversal of flow result in **high** systolic/diastolic ratios, which are characteristic of increased placental resistance.

•A severe decrease in diastolic flow indicates markedly elevated placental vascular resistance, and low or absent diastolic flow may suggest impending fetal death.

•As pregnancy progresses there is a small and gradual fall in umbilical artery resistance reflected as a decrease in the umbilical artery ratio.

•Results: Traditional ultrasound measurements (e.g., estimated fetal weight) when grouped by percentile for gestational age, accurately predict IUGR.

•There is a relatively high predictor status for the systolic/diastolic ratio with respect to birth weight (SGA) variables;

•importance of abdominal circumference as a determinant for weight was reconfirmed.

•Infants with specific inherent genetic defects may be SGA because of factors not related to increased resistance to flow.

•**Once IUGR is predicted, the differential diagnosis between symmetric and asymmetric growth retardation appears mandatory.**

°Rapid karyotype, determination of fetal IgM levels, and differential cranial/umbilical vascular wave patterns, may be essential.]

---

13. Initial diagnostic steps in the management of pregnant women exposed to parvovirus infection should include

    A. amniotic fluid culture
    B. blood culture
    *C.   serology for specific antibodies
    D. throat culture
    E. ultrasound to determine gestational age

---

p.737   (Rodis JF, Hovick TJ Jr., Quinn DL, Rosengren SS, and Tattersall P, "Human parovirus infection in pregnancy" Obstet Gynecol 1988;72:733)

13. [F & I:•Background: Human B19 parovirus is a DNA virus that causes affects humans.

•It causes **erythema infectiosum**, or fifth disease, a common childhood illness with a characteristic rash (slapped-face appearance) and fever.

•In adults, the infection is more variable, with preponderance of arthralgias and arthritis-like symptoms; the rash may not be present.

•Adults may have no clinical evidence of disease even though serologic studies (immunoglobulin M [IgM] and IgG antibodies) would indicate recent infection.

•Parovirus infection during pregnancy may result in **fetal hydrops** and death, whereas other exposed fetuses appear to be unaffected.

•Previous exposure and infection by the parovirus (IgG positive, IgM negative) confers immunity and is not associated with adverse perinatal outcome.

•Objective: to describe managment of four pregnant women exposed and affected by parvovirus and to review the literature.

•If maternal serology indicated recent infection, ie, IgM positive, a level II ultrasound was performed.

•Fetal tissues were examined histologically and the presence of B19 DNA in tissue was detected by a nucleic acid hybridization assay.

•In all cases of fetal hydrops, maternal serology was obtained for cytomegalovirus, toxoplasmosis, syphilis, and rubella.

•Results: Five women who were exposed to children with fifth disease tested, had IgG antibodies but no IgM antibodies suggesting previous exposure.

•All five had full-term deliveries of normal appearing children.

•Four of the women tested had IgM antibodies present indicating recent infection, three of these four had fetuses with hydrops, all of whom died in utero.

•In reviewing the literature of 37 patients who had IgM antibodies, 14 had adverse outcomes including three spontaneous abortions; one anencephalic fetus and one fetus with multiple occular abnormalities.

•Eleven fetuses had hydrops.

•The parvoviruses are small, single-stranded DNA viruses whose limited genetic capacity makes them unusually dependent upon the host cell for their won replication program.

•The immunologic response to inoculation with human B19 parvovirus has been described using adult volunteers.

°Viremia develops approximately 7 days after inoculation and persists for up to 14 days.

°A rash develops approximately 16 days after inoculation, or 8 days after disappearance of viremia.

°Immunoglobulin M antibodies are present in 90% of patients 4-7 days after the onset of symptoms.

•The B19 parvovirus has a well-known predilection for the hematopoietic system.

•Indeed, parvovirus infection is a cause of aplastic crisis in patients with sickle cell anemia.

•The hydrops seen in affected fetuses results from a severe anemia.

•The human parvovirus inhibits multiplication of human erythroid progenitor cells in vitro.

•Outbreaks of fifth disease have seasonal variations of peaks in winter and spring.

•Pediatricians have little trouble clinically diagnosing during outbreaks, based on the characteristic "slapped-face" appearance in febrile children.

•Infections in adults may be quite variable, ranging from asymptomatic infection to a mild flu-like illness or to a more classic erythematous and febrile illness.

•The only significant complication in hematologically normal nonpregnant adults appears to be joint involvement.

•Parvoviruses can cause transplacental infection because

°1) at least some of them are able to proliferate and form inclusions in the walls of small blood vessels; and

°2) they are able to induce a viremia for appreciable duration.

•Parvoviruses are known to cause cerebellar hypoplasia and ataxia in cats as well as anomalies in infected hamsters including anencephaly, micocephaly, face clefts, ectopic hearts and others.

•**Pregnant women should be instructed to avoid contact with children during outbreaks of fifth disease.**

•The first diagnostic step for pregnant women exposed to the parvovirus should include serology for IgG and IgM parvovirus-specific antibodies.

•For the group at high fetal risk (IgM positive) a level II ultrasound should be performed to seek evidence of fetal hydrops and possible congenital anomalies.]

---

14. Fetal jeopardy in pregnant patients with autoimmune thrombocytopenia purpura can best determined by testing

    *A.   fetal platelet count by cordocentesis
    B. fetal platelet count by fetal scalp sampling
    C. maternal associated antibody in amniotic fluid
    D. maternal associated antibody in maternal blood
    E. maternal platelet count

---

p.346 (Moise KJ, Carpenter RJ, Cotton DB, Wasserstrum N, Kirshon B and Cano L, "Percutaneous umbilical cord blood sampling in the evaluation of fetal platelet counts in pregnant patients with autoimmune thrombocytopenia purpura " Obstet Gynecol 1988;71:346)

14. [F & I:•Background: Autoimmune thrombocytopenia purpura complicating pregnancy is associated with fetal thrombocytopenia in 37-70% of cases.

•**Intracranial bleeding** with subsequent psychomotor retardation and neonatal death has occurred in cases of severely depressed fetal platelet counts.

•Attempts to predict the fetal platelet status by testing the maternal hematologic environment have generally been unsuccessful.

•The scalp blood platelet count has been the most widely accepted method for identifying the thrombocytopenic fetus.

°Scalp blood sampling can be performed only in advanced labor, when fetal intracranial hemorrhage may have laready occurred.

•Objective: to report the experience with the use of **percutaneous umbilical blood sampling** in evaluating the fetal platelet status in pregnancies complicated by autoimmune thrombocytopenia purpura.

•Material and Methods: Twenty-one pregnant women with either a previous diagnosis of autoimmune thrombocytopenia purpura or unexplained thrombocytopenia during labor.

•Maternal thrombocytopenia was defined arbitrarily as a platelt count of less than 100,000/μL.

•The diagnostic evaluation in those patients **without** a history of autoimmune thrombocytopenia purpua included

    °antinuclear antibody determination and

    °a coagulation profile consisting of prothrombin time, partial thromboplastin time, and fibrinogen level.

•When the patient presented in labor with newly diagnosed thrombocytopenia, a normal blood pressure and lack of significant proteinuria was used to confirm the **absence of pregnancy-induced hypertension.**

•Peripheral smears were reviewed in milder cases of thrombocytopenia, and the presence of **megathrombocytes** was considered an indication of increased bone marrow production consistent with autoimmune thrombocytopenia purpura.

•When possible, patients were scheduled for elective percutaneous umbilical blood sampling at 38 completed weeks of gestation after documenting normal maternal bleeding time.

    °The procedure was performed in the labor and delivery suite with the usual preoperative preparations in case an emergency cesarean became necessary because of complications.

    °Narcotics and benzodiazepines were administered to the mother before the procedure in an effort to slow fetal movement.

    °Umbilical blood sampling was then done under direct ultrasound guidance.

    °The acquisition of fetal blood was confirmed if the mean corpuscular volume of the fetal red cells was larger than the maternal mean corpuscular volume of a blood sample drawn at the time of the procedure.

    °**Fetal thrombocytopenia was defined as a platelet count of less than 150,000/μL, and severe thrombocytropenia , necessitating delivery by cesarean section, as a fetal platelet count of less than 50,000/μL.**

    °When the platelet count was greater than 50,000/μL, induction of labor was undertaken if the cervical Bishop score was favorable and the patient satisfied dating criteria for 38 or more completed weeks' of gestation.

•Results: Maternal platelet counts drawn at the time for cordocentesis were compared with fetal platelet counts; the degree of maternal thrombocytopenia was **not** predictive of the fetal platelet status.

•There were three cases of of fetal distress related to cordocentesis.

    °Two of the patients were delivered by emergency cesarean performed for persistent fetal bradycardia.

•Nineteen of the 22 fetuses were born by vaginal delivery.

    °Three fetuses were born by abdominal delivery, one for cephalopelvic disproportion and two for fetal distress.

°None of the women experienced bleeding complications as a result of cordocentesis.

•**Because there is no association between the maternal platelet status and the fetal platelet count, direct sampling of the fetal hematologic environment is necessary to identify the thrombocytopenic fetus.**

•There was a significant correlation between fetal platelet counts obtained by cordocentesis and neonatal platelet counts when the interval between the two determinations was less than five days.

•Percutaneous umbilical blood sampling may be superior to scalp blood sampling because it can be performed electively at term before the onset of labor or engagement of the fetal head.

°This would potentially reduce the risk of intracranial bleeding in the severely affected fetus.

°Scalp blood sampling has recently been associated with erroneously low fetal platelet counts.

•Maternal autoimmune thrombocytopenia purpura is rarely associated with severe fetal thrombocytopenia.

•Complications of fetal scalp sampling are rare, although scalp abscesses, blade breakage with retention in the fetal scalp, and fetal death from hemorrhage have been reported.

•Amniotic fluid volume is decreased in late gestation, and the large size of the fetus in relation to the uterine cavity makes visualization of the umbilical cord insertion difficult, especially in cases of posterior placentation.

•Bradycardia associated with cordocentesis is usually transient, lasting less than one or two minutes.]

---

15. Total parenteral nutrition given during the first trimester of pregnancy is associated with

     A. fetal anomalies
     B. placental infarction
     C. preterm labor
     *D.   respiratory quotient greater than 1
     E. small for gestational age infants

---

p.107   (Levine MG and Esser D,"Total parenteral nutrition for the treatment of severe hyperemesis gravidarum: Maternal nutritional effects and fetal outcome" Obstet Gynecol 1988;71:102)

15. [F & I:•Background: Hyperemesis gravidarum can cause severe maternal nutritional deprivation.

•Both enteral and parenteral hyperalimentation are useful.

•Severe maternal nutritional deprivation occurs in several other conditions, including pregnancy complicated by jejunoileal bypass, diabetes, and Crohn's disease.

•Objective: to examine the nutrition state of pregnancy complicated by hyperemesis gravidarum and the effects of total parenteral nutrition on maternal nutrition and fetal outcome when given during the first trimester of pregnancy.

•Severe hyperemesis gravidarum: intractable vomiting requiring hospitalization, with dehydration, electrolyte imbalance, ketonuria, weight loss of greater than 5% of body weight, or other more severe signs, such a neurologic disturbances and liver or renal abnormalities.

°It can resolve spontaneously, but severe complications may occur, including hepatorenal syndrome, Wernicke's encephalopathy, and even death.

•Material and Methods: 9 hospitalized pregnant women with persistent nausea and vomiting, documented weight loss of greater than 5% of body weight, dehydration, ketonuria, and serum electrolyte abnormalities were studied.

•Hyperemesis patients were started on total parenteral nutrition via a silastic Hickman catheter placed in the subclavian vein, using standard technique.

•All hyperemesis patients showed decreased immunologic response, indicating a compromised immunologic and nutritional state.

°None of the patients tested was found to have thyroid abnormalities.

•All patients were started on a total parenteral nutrition solution .

•Patients were monitored with daily electrolytes and glucose determinations.

°All patients required the addition of varying amounts of insulin to the total parenteral nutrition solutions because of hyperglycemia, which commonly occurs because of the increased glucose loads being given.

°The patients were started on a continuous infusion of total parenteral nutrition, and then switched before discharge to nocturnal total parenteral nutrition at a rate of 2 L per night.

•When the patient was able to maintain a nutritional status from oral intake, total parenteral nutrition was decreased.

•Results: Mean respiratory quotient values for the pretreatment hyperemesis group were lower than the control mean respiratory quotient values, indicating a catabolic state; however, the differences were not statistically significant .

•The primary difference between the two control groups versus the pretreatment hyperemesis group was in substrate utilization.

°Pretreatment hyperemesis patients showed preferential utilization of fat, with protein-sparing that was statistically significant when compared with control values.

•Total parenteral nutrition provides a nonprotein calorie source, generally glucose or lipid emulsions; utilizable nitrogen; electrolytes, including magnesium and phosphorus; trace elements; water; and fat-soluble vitamins.

°Glycogen stores can supply only a small amount of the caloric requirement during starvation, whereas adipose tissue, triglycerides, and protein serve as the principle potential energy sources.

°Starvation or severely decreased caloric intake stimulates gluconeogenesis to convert amino acids to glucose using alternate pathways.

°The ketosis that occurs with metabolism of fatty acids can have an adverse effect on the fetus, so prolonged caloric deprivation should be avoided.

•Energy in the form of kilocalories can be measured indirectly by measuring the amount of oxygen consumed and the amount of carbon dioxide produced with respiration, and converting these calories using the standard methods of indirect calorimetry.

°**The respiratory quotient is the ratio of the oxygen consumed and the amount of carbon dioxide produced, measured during an interval of time culminating in a steady respiratory state.**

°For carbohydrate metabolism, the respiratory quotient equals 1.00.

°For the oxidation of fat, oxygen is required for the oxidation of carbon, so the respiratory quotient is less than 1.00.

°Conversely, lipogenesis will yield a respiratory quotient greater than 1.00.

•Nutritional status and pregnancy outcome are not endangered even if there is virtually no extra food intake during pregnancy, chronic or prolonged maternal malnutrition is associated with increased fetal risks.

°Infant birth weight is influenced by maternal prepregnant weight and weight gain during pregnancy.

°Underweight mothers with inadequate weight gain during pregnancy have an increased risk of low birth weight infants and perinatal morbidity and mortality.

•The fetus depends on a constant infusion of glucose for the production of energy and growth, and maternal glucose is the prime source.

°If maternal nutrition is compromised, the fetus may be growth-retarded because of decreased maternal glucose and reduced hepatic glycogen and adipose tissue.

°Decreased caloric intake and nutritional deprivation during hyperplastic growth phases slowed the rate of cell division; if the nutritional deprivation was prolonged, a permanent reduction could be seen in the cell numbers of specific organs, including the brain.

•Fat emulsions have been considered risky because of the possibility of fatty infiltration of the placenta.

°Uterine irritability has also been noted with increased uterine contractions and the possibility of inducing preterm labor.

•Infusion of linoleic acid can lead to increased synthesis of arachidonic acid, which is a precurser of prostaglandins and may be responsible for increased uterine activity.

°In the present study there was no correlation between premature labor or increased uterine irritability and lipid infusion.

•Minimal elevations in fasting blood glucose levels may be important in fetal macrosomia, whether or not maternal gestational diabetes is present.

°Maternal hyperglycemia can cause major complications and fetal anomalies.

°With the addition of insulin to the total parenteral nutrition plus strict glucose monitoring, glucose levels can be maintained in a normal range, thus controlling the amount of glucose delivered to the fetus.

•Conclusion: Total parenteral nutrition given during the first trimester of pregnancy is a safe and effective method of nutritional support.]

16. Which of the following is the most accurate predictor of an adverse neurological outcome in the term neonate?

      A. five minute Apgar score
      B. one minute Apgar score
      *C.   ten minute Apgar score
      D. ultrasound examination of the newborn head
      E. umbilical cord pH between 7.15-7.20

p.121   (Marrin M and Pes BA, "Birth asphyxia: Does the Apgar score have diagnostic value?" Obstet Gynecol 1988;71:120)

16. [F & I:•Objective: to review the accuracy of the one-minute Apgar score as a diagnostic test or marker for the presence of asphyxia.

    •A diagnostic marker is a test that discriminates a particular disease, among the spectrum of all other diseases and states of health.

    •Asphyxia is defined as a condition that occurs when the organ of gas exchange fails.

      °The failure gas exchange, by lung or placenta, is defined by the blood gases; that is, a rise in Pa CO_2 and a fall in PaO_2, ultimately leading to a decrease in pH.

    •These changes result from insufficient gas exchange, and serve as the gold standard for diagnosing asphyxia.

      °Asphyxia was defined by the umbilical cord arterial blood pH, with a value < 7.10 indicating severe asphyxia and < 7.20 indicating at least some asphyxia.

    •Only 27% of infants with a pH < 7.10 had a one-minute Apgar score <7 (ie, **the Apgar score failed to identify severe acidosis In 73% of the cases**).

    •21% with Apgar scores < 7 at one minute had severe acidosis, and only 19% of infants with a five-minute score < 7 had severe acidosis.

    •The sensitivity of a one-minute Apgar score < 4 for an umbilical arterial pH <7.15 was 10.7%, whereas the specificity was 98.7%, indicating that the **score was a poor detector of acidosis** (ie, asphyxia) but was very good at ruling it out.

      °Of all infants with Apgar scores < 4, only 37% had a cord arterial pH < 7.15.

    •Of the infants who had a pH below 7.00, 75% had a one-minute Apgar score less than 7, and 42% had a five-minute score less than 7.

      °Therefore, in infants who were clinically severely asphyxiated, 25% had a "normal" one-minute score and 58% were normal at five minutes.

    •In comparing the accuracy of various Apgar scores for the prediction of adverse neurological outcome with that of the appearance of encephalopathy in the immediate newborn period, **the most accurate Apgar score was a value less than 5 at ten minutes**, with a sensitivity of 43% and a specificity of 95%.

      °The presence of at least moderate clinical encephalopathy was much more accurate, with a sensitivity of 96% and a specificity of 78%.

•Gestational age has been shown to influence the one-minute Apgar score in healthy infants.

°This is due to the decreased motor tone, reduced respiratory effort, and decreased reflex irritability of healthy preterm infants.

•The fetus can suffer a transient period of acidosis with recovery by delivery, so that the infant had a good one-minute Apgar score.

•The diagnosis of asphyxia may be better made by determining the difference between maternal and fetal pH.

•The fetal biophysical profile, particularly a nonreactive nonstress test with absent fetal breathing, has excellent positive and negative predictive values for umbilical cord arterial pH less than 7.20.

•Less than half of newborns with low Apgar scores are asphyxiated by blood gas criteria.

•The one-minute Apgar score appears to be quite good at identifying those who do **not** have asphyxia.

•**The American Academy of Pediatrics suggests that three criteria be met for the diagnosis of perinatal asphyxia: Apgar score of 0-3 at ten minutes, early neonatal seizures, and prolonged hypotonia in the infant.**

•Metabolic acidosis in cord blood helps to confirm suspected hypoxia, and multiple organ dysfunction in the early neonatal period supports the diagnosis of asphyxia.]

---

17. A 22 year old para 0-0-0-0 is diagnosed by ultrasound as having a fetus with gastroschisis at 28 weeks. No other abnormalities are detected. What is the next best plan of management to maximize fetal outcome?

    A. await the onset of labor and deliver by cesarean section
    B. await the onset of labor and deliver vaginally except for obstetrical indications
    C. cesarean section at 28 weeks, without further testing
    *D.   deliver by cesarean when testing indicates fetal lung maturity
    E. induction of labor at 28 weeks without further testing

---

p.912   (Fitzsimmons J, Nyberg DA, Cyr DR and Hatch E, "Perinatal management of gastroschisis" Obstet Gynecol 1988;71:910)

17. [F & I: •Background: Omphalocele arises from a developmental arrest at the stage during which the intestines are normally herniated into the cord.

°The intestines fail to return to the abdominal cavity at ten to 12 weeks' gestation.

°**Omphalocele is frequently associated with other defects, including chromosome abnormalities.**

•In contrast, with **gastroschisis**, there is a normal umbilical ring, but the intestines herniate through a defect in the abdominal wall.

°This defect may result from a **vascular** accident.

•Gastroschisis is less often associated with nongastrointestinal abnormalities than is omphalocele, and infants surviving surgery develop normally.

•Objective: to analyze the outcome of cases of gastroschisis diagnosed antenatally and followed and delivered at a single institution.

•Material and Methods: 16 patients who had a sonographic diagnosis of gastroschisis.

•Usually (but not found in this study) there is a higher prevalence of extracorporeal liver and intrauterine growth retardation among neonates with gastroschisis.

°Extracorporeal liver is probably extraordinarily rare in cases of true gastroschisis; rather, its presence almost certainly indicates omphalocele.

•The timing and route of delivery influence bowel viability and neonatal survival.

•Fibrosis or "peel" on the bowel serosa, present only after 30 weeks' gestation, is related to changes in the osmolarity, sodium, creatinine, and urea in amniotic fluid.

°The abdominal wall defect becomes relatively smaller with advancing gestational age, compressing mesenteric vessels and compromising blood flow to the bowel.

°This could result in preoperative bowel necrosis and affect postoperative bowel viability.

°Delivery before compression of the mesentery may improve the status of the bowel before surgery.

°Abdominal delivery may further enhance such an effect by allowing precise timing of delivery and avoiding further compression of the fetal abdomen and bowel.]

---

18. Ultrasound examination of a twin gestation at 22 weeks, reveals one twin with polyhydramnios, and the other twin with oligohydramnios. The next best step in the further management of the gestation is

    A. amniocentesis of the polyhydramniotic sac and use the fluid to reconstitute the amniotic fluid in the oligohydramniotic sac
    B. amniocentesis of the polyhydramniotic sac
    *C.   observation
    D. reconstitution of the amniotic fluid in the oligohydramniotic sac
    E. selective feticide of the oligohydramniotic twin

---

p.884   (Chescheir NC and Seeds JW, "Polyhydramnios and oligohydramnios in twin gestations" Obstet Gynecol 1988;71:882)

18. [F & I:•Background: Amniotic fluid volume is controlled by a dynamic interaction between the maternal, fetal, and placental compartments.

°In multiple gestations, the fetuses may share not only a common environment, but also a common circulation.

•Objective: to describe seven cases of twins with polyhydramnios and oligohydramnios.

•A "stuck twin" is a growth retarded fetus with oligohydramnios in a twin gestation.

•Perinatal deaths were related to the gestational age at which the fluid disturbances were recognized.

°When the diagnosis was made before 26 weeks' gestation, none of the fetuses survived.

•6/7 cases were associated with monochorionic placentas.

°The underlying pathophysiology may have been **twin-twin** transfusion syndrome.

°This syndrome involves a third circulation through which a small volume of the donor twin's blood is transfused directly into the recipient.

°Over time the donor becomes anemic and growth-retarded, and may develop oligohydramnios, while the recipient becomes plethoric and hypervolemic, and may develop polyhydramnios and even nonimmune hydrops fetalis.

•Twin-twin transfusion syndrome was diagnosed antenatally in each of the 7 pregnancies.

•**No single therapy was clearly associated with an improved outcome, either in the current series or other reports.**

•Therapeutic amniocentisis is associated with premature rupture of membranes and preterm delivery.

•Selective feticide was successful in one pregnancy.

°In this series, although technically successful feticide was associated with continued polyhydramnios, premature rupture of the membranes, and neonatal death.

°The iatrogenic fetal hydrothorax appears to be a safer method of selective feticide than injection of any toxic substance into a possibly shared circulation.

•No intervention has either been uniformly applied or proved uniformly successful.

•If the pregnancy is advanced beyond 26 weeks' gestation, conservative therapy with bed rest and antenatal surveillance offers some probability of successful outcome.]

---

19. During normal pregnancy, what is the shortest cervical length (mm) that is associated with increased risk of preterm labor?

    *A.   40
    B. 50
    C. 60
    D. 70
    E. 80

---

p.943   (Ayers JWT, DeGrood RM, Compton, AA Barclay M andAnsbacher R, "Sonographic evaluation of cervical length in pregnancy: Diagnosis and management of preterm cervical effacement in patients at risk for premature delivery" Obstet Gynecol 1988;71:939)

19. [F & I: •Background: Preterm delivery occurs at a rate of 8% of all live births.

•Two thirds of preterm births are directly attributable to preterm labor and/or premature rupture of the membranes.

•Historic assessments of antecedent preterm delivery or even multifactorial risk scoring systems **fail** to provide predictive correlates for subsequent pregnancy outcome in high-risk populations.

•Premature delivery may be correlated with the development of early effacement and "maturation" of the cervix and lower uterine segment.

•Objectives:.

°1) to delineate the cervical length change in normal term pregnancy, and

---

°2) to apply this normative cervical length to the active antepartum management of women with a previous preterm delivery.

•Material and Methods: 150 healthy gravid patients with uncomplicated singleton gestations were included in the "normal pregnancy" group.

•Cervical sonography was performed serially at four to six-week intervals.

•Cervical length was measured along the clearly discernible, highly echogenic line of cervical glands from external os to the flexion of the uterine corpus and cervix.

•Mean cervical length averaged over 50 mm until 34 weeks' gestation.

°A cervical length value under **40 mm** is less than 2 standard deviations (SD) from the mean of the normal population.

•Eighty-eight multiparous women with a previous second-trimester delivery constituted the study group for the evaluation of cervical length.

•Hysterosalpingograms were performed on 82 of the 88 women before the study pregnancy.

°Patients were grouped according to the following:

°°1) significant müllerian anomalies,

°°2) DES exposure, or

°°3) normal hysterosalpingogram.

•Clinical risk symptoms for preterm delivery were assessed at each prenatal visit. These included:

°Clinical signs.

°°Vaginal **bleeding** after 14 weeks, normal cervix, normal pap smear.

°°Painful and/or persistent **uterine contractions** perceived at rest.

°Sonographic signs.

°°Cervical length **<40 mm.**

°Cervical **shortening** by >50% of initial length.

•For any of the clinical risk factors the patient was placed on **bed rest and intercourse was prohibited.**

•When bed rest alone was not associated with significant decreases in uterine activity, weekly injections of **17-hydroxyprogesterone caporate** (250 mg) were begun, and continued to 35 weeks' gestation.

•Progressive increases in uterine activity or the presence of clinical preterm labor were treated with hospitalization and intravenous **tocolytic agents** administered via a standardized protocol.

•When one or both sonographic cervical length risk factors were noted, without other risk factors, the patient underwent **cervical cerclage.**

°The cerclage sutures were removed in all patients electively at 36-37 weeks, or earlier if intractable preterm labor ensued.

•Results: 8 of the original 150 women in the control group delivered before 35 weeks' gestation.

°5 of these with no antecedent risk factors demonstrated cervical length shortening of greater than 50% before delivery.

°3/8 exhibited no cervical length shortening before preterm delivery.

•Serial evaluation of high-risk patients revealed that 70 of 88 patients met the sonographic criteria for preterm cervical effacement, underwent cervical cerclage.

°The median gestational age at cerclage was 20 weeks, and the range was nine to 30 weeks.

°The mean cervical length of cerclage patients was 31 mm.

°After the double purse-string procedure, the mean cervical length was increased to 54 mm.

•Independent of etiology, preterm labor and delivery are often preceded by gradual premature cervical effacement and which may be detected by sector scan sonographic evaluation of cervical length.

•Significant findings included:

°1) a consistent mean cervical length of 52 ± 12 mm through 33 weeks' gestation, and

°2) progressive effacement and cervical length shortening beginning at 33 weeks.

•Using a cervical length of 40 mm as the minimum standard of normal pregnancy, sonographic measurement of cervical length has a high predicative value (96%), sensitivity (93%), and specificity (50%) for subsequent term delivery.

•Of the women with an **abnormal uterine cavity, 90%** demonstrated significant preterm cervical effacement, and underwent cerclage.

•High risk patients with a normal hysterosalpingogram, show sonographic cervical length shortening less frequently.

•**Unexpected finding:** the high incidence of clinical risk symptoms-uterine contractions and vaginal bleeding-seen in women with **both** normal and abnormal hysterosalpingogram findings.

°Vaginal bleeding occurred more often in women with sonographic evidence of cervical effacement than in those where cervical length remained in the normal range.

°**Vaginal bleeding in the second trimester is a potentially ominous sign for significant anatomical cervical effacement.**

•Whether premature cervical length shortening is an effect of premature labor or symptom of cervical incompetence could not be determined from this study.]

20. Which of the following measurements of respiratory function **increases** as pregnancy progresses?

       A. expiratory reserve volume
       B. functional residual capacity
       *C.   inspiratory capacity
       D. residual volume
       E. vital capacity

p.177 (South-Paul JE, Rajagopal KR, Tenholder MF,"The effect of participation in a regular exercise program upon aerobic capacity during pregnancy " Obstet Gynecol 1988;71: 175)

20. [F & I:•Objectives: to determine if

°pregnancy causes a decrease in physical fitness as measured by maximal oxygen consumption between the second and third trimesters

°the maintenance of a regular exercise program during the second half of pregnancy has a positive effect on fitness.

•Materials and Methods: Women between the ages of 19-35, both primigravidas and multigravidas, entered the study at the beginning of the second trimester of pregnancy.

•The subjects were screened to exclude endocrine, cardiac, neurologic, hypertensive, or pulmonary diseases.

•Smokers and identified substance abusers were excluded.

•Patients with polyhydramnios, anemia (hemoglobin less than 10 g/dL), previous delivery of an abnormal infant, or weight greater than 50% above ideal body weight were also excluded.

•Each subject, in a postabsorptive state, completed a graded exercise test between 1 and 3 PM in a pulmonary function laboratory.

°Each subject performed the exercise in a sitting position on a Collins cycle ergometer.

•Subjects in the control group were asked to maintain their usual daily activities.

•The exercise group was enrolled in a ten-step exercise program conducted three times per week for one hour in a supervised physical therapy department.

°The exercise program included a warm-up phase, which consisted of a one-eighth-mile walk; pelvic strengthening exercises; strengthening of the spinal extensors, hamstrings, and calf muscles, and push-ups in the plantar grade position.

°This was followed by aerobic activity performed on the Fitron cycle ergometer.

°A heart rate of 60% of the measured maximal heart rate during the initial exercise test (20 weeks' gestation) was used as the guideline for determining the initial level of training exercise.

°Subsequently, the duration of training exercise was progressively increased by two minutes each session, up to a level of 80% of the measured maximal heart rate.

°The aerobic segment was followed by a cool-down period during which subjects walked for one-eighth of a mile.

•Seven women remained in the nonexercising group and ten in the exercise group.

•Results: At maximal exercise, the change in respiratory frequency from 20 to 30 weeks' gestation was the same for the exercise and the control groups (approximately 30 breaths per minute).

•The changes from 20-30 weeks in respiratory quotient, heart rate, multiples of resting metabolic oxygen requirements, and oxygen consumption per kilogram at maximal exercise **were comparable** between the two groups.

•The **absolute oxygen consumption at maximal exercise increased** by a mean of 225 mL in the **exercise** group.

•The control group increased their oxygen consumption by a mean of 99 mL.

•The tidal volumes at maximal exercise also varied between the two groups, with a mean increase of 43 mL from 20-30 weeks in the control group versus a mean increase of 177 mL in the exercise group.

•Minute ventilation at maximal exercise increased proportionately to the increase in oxygen consumption in both groups.

•As pregnancy progresses the enlarging uterus displaces the diaphragm, so that the effective vertical diameter of the chest is decreased by approximately 4 cm.

°There is, as a result, a reduction in expiratory reserve volume and residual volume.

°**Inspiratory capacity is increased**, with a relatively stable vital capacity.

°The decreased functional residual capacity, due mainly to the decrease in expiratory reserve volume, results in a lower ventilatory reserve.

•Pregnancy is associated with an increase in maternal blood volume, heart rate and stroke volume.

°Cardiac output in increased, which facilitates increased oxygen consumption.

°These changes occur primarily in the second trimester.

°Oxygen consumption also increases with exercise and throughout the last trimester of pregnancy.

°The maximal oxygen consumption near term has been reported at 16-32% above that in the nonpregnant state.

°The concurrent, progressive weight gain contributes to the increased oxygen consumption expected near term.

°These normal cardiopulmonary adaptations to pregnancy minimize any significant impact of the decreased ventilatory reserve on oxygen consumption.

•During the first two trimesters of pregnancy, increasing **progesterone** levels are known to drive ventilation, with a resultant decrease in pCO_2.

°Despite some anatomic limitation to ventilation as pregnancy progresses, additional alveoli can be recruited when the pregnant woman is erect, especially during exercise.

°These changes are not sufficient to overcome the progesterone effect.

°The resulting hypocapnia is associated with "dyspnea" and hyperventilation throughout pregnancy.

°This dyspnea is reported to occur in 60-70% of pregnant women.

•Results: Changes in tidal volume and maximal oxygen uptake in the exercise group, as compared with controls were found.

°Normal nonpregnant individuals **decrease their physiologic dead space** with exercise, and unless pregnant women have lung disease, they should respond in the same manner.

°With training, tidal volumes increase while frequency remains relatively unchanged at comparable work levels.

°The tidal volume increase in the exercising group was **four** times that seen in the control group.

•Oxygen consumption per kilogram per minute was also **increased** at maximum levels exercise; 9% in the exercising group as opposed to 2% in the control group.

•The control group demonstrated higher minute ventilation at lower oxygen consumptions, and appeared **less efficient** (ie, they had greater work of breathing) than their exercising counterparts.

•The exercising group was able to achieve higher oxygen consumptions without disproportionate increases in minute ventilation at equivalent work.

•Conclusion: Pregnancy does not reduce maximal oxygen consumption between the second and third trimesters of pregnancy, a period during which detraining could have been substantial.

•**Fitness, as measured by increased maximal oxygen consumption per kilogram, may be improved by participation in a supervised exercise program.**

°Support evidence for improved efficiency includes increases in tidal volume at a stable respiratory frequency, increases in oxygen consumption/kg/minute, and stable ventilatory equivalent for oxygen in the exercising group.]

---

21. What outcome improvement from electively sectioning patients whose fetuses who have open spina bifida can be expected? **Decreased**

    *A.   chance of meningitis
    B. developmental handicap
    C. incidence of RDS
    D. mortality
    E. neurologic handicap

---

p.533 (Bensen JT, Dillard RG, Burton BK, "Open spina bifida: Does cesarean section delivery improve prognosis? " Obstet Gynecol 1988;71:532)

21. [F & I: Objective: to test the hypotheses that cesarean section delivery improves the prognosis for infants with open spina bifida.

•Materials and Methods: 72 infants with open spina bifida, of whom 40 were born vaginally and 32 by cesarean section.

•The **indications** for cesarean section were as follows:

°breech presentation (nine),

°previously diagnosed open spina bifida and/or hydrocephalus (seven),

---

°failure to progress in labor (five),

°repeat cesarean section (five),

°vaginal bleeding (two),

°cephalopelvic disproportion (two),

°fetal distress (one), and

°maternal intestinal obstruction (one).

°Thirteen (40%) of the cesarean patients had labor before delivery.

•The distribution and size of lesions were similar in the vaginal and cesarean groups, as was the development of hydrocephalus.

°Of the infants born vaginally, the presentation was vertex in 31 and breech in 9.

•Results: There was **no significant difference in mortality** between infants in the vaginal delivery and the cesarean groups.

•Five of the forty infants delivered vaginally, and three of the thirty-two infants born by cesarean section died before initial nursery discharge.

•Only four of 72 infants in the study population developed neonatal meningitis.

°Three of these were delivered vaginally and one by cesarean.

•At one year of age, height, weight and head circumference were **similar** in the vaginal and cesarean section groups.

•The **neurologic and developmental findings** were **similar** in the two groups.

•Breech delivery, a common occurrence in infants with spina bifida, may lead to mechanical trauma to the already handicapped muscles and nerves of the lower extremities.

•Conclusion: The study was unable to demonstrate any improvement in outcome up to one year of age in infants with open spina bifida who were delivered by cesarean section.

•Theoretically it is less likely that cesarean section would be beneficial in preserving neurologic function.

•The spinal cord damage and resulting handicaps are presumably **long-standing** in infants with spina bifida, as evidenced by the frequently seen positional deformities of the lower extremities, which result from the **decreased movement.**

°Early in gestation, the fetal spinal cord is **trapped** at the site of the spinal lesion, usually in the lumbosacral area at a time when the cord is normally migrating upward to reach its usual termination point at about the level of the first lumbar segment.

°Further damage to the neural tissue at delivery could conceivably affect reflex function, but would be unlikely to increase handicap.

•Nineteen patients who were sectioned **before** the onset of labor were compared with those who delivered vaginally and there was no difference noted.

•The **benefit** of cesarean section might be **decreased bacterial contamination** of the open lesion leading to a decreased incidence of neonatal meningitis.

°Central nervous system infections are clearly linked to an increase in mortality and a decrease in intellectual potential in infants with spina bifida.

°A larger series might be needed to detect any difference.]

---

22. The earliest week of embryonic life by which the bronchial tree is completed is

    A. 14
    *B.   16
    C. 18
    D. 20
    E. 24

---

p.800   (Blott M, Nicolaides KH, and Greenough A, "Pleuroamniotic shunting for decompression of fetal pleural effusions " Obstet Gynecol 1988;71:798)

22. [F & I:•Background: Congenital diaphragmatic hernia and pleural effusions, which cause prolonged intrathoracic compression of the fetal lung are associated with pulmonary hypoplasia and neonatal death.

•Material and Methods: 11 women with singleton pregnancies, at 22-35 weeks gestation, were studied because of unexplained fetal pleural effusions diagnosed by ultrasonography performed because of maternal **polyhydramnios.**

•Results: Pleural effusions were successfully drained in all cases.

•Results: 8 newborns survived and 3 died.

°Of the survivors, one had congenital diaphragmatic hernia which was successfully corrected, and another had trisomy 21 and an atrial septal defect.

°None of the infants had any respiratory problems in the neonatal period.

•Of the three infants who died in the neonatal period

°one died on the tenth day from pseudomonas **septicemia;**

°the second infant had **congenital diaphragmatic hernia** and had severe respiratory difficulties form birth and died on day two.

°The third was delivered because of **premature labor** requiring high pressure ventilation and developed bilateral pneumothoraces.

•The bronchial tree is normally fully developed by the **16th week** of intrauterine life, whereas alveoli start to form at 24 weeks' gestation and continue to develop after birth.

•Pleural effusions that develop in the late second trimester of pregnancy are unlikely to have interfered with the development of the bronchial tree, but could lead to alveolar maldevelopment and hypoplasia, which can be prevented by chronic drainage.]

---

23. A patient who has no other risk factors but an elevated MSAFP value of 2.5 multiples of the median is estimated to be at risk for having a fetus with an open neural tube defect of 1 in 200. After a normal high resolution ultrasound examination, her risk would be correctly estimated as

> A. one in 400
> B. one in 1000
> *C.   one in 2000
> D. one in 5000
> E. one in 10,000

p.205   (Richards DS, Weeds JW, Katz VL, Lingley LH, Albright SG, Cefalo RC, "Elevated maternal serum alpha-fetoprotein with normal ultrasound: Is amniocentesis always appropriate? A review of 26,069 screened patients. " Obstet Gynecol 1988;71: 203)

23. [F & I:•Background: Many malformations associated with elevated MSAFP values can be detected sonographically, and ultrasound may clarify situations in which MSAFP values appear elevated because of incorrect clinical gestational age, multiple gestation, or fetal death.

•When sonography is nondiagnostic, an amniocentesis to assess amniotic fluid alpha-fetoprotein (AFP) and acetylcholinesterase levels is performed to detect or exclude the presence of an open neural tube defect.

•Objective: to report the experience of a large screening program in which risk is reassessed when specialized ultrasound examination is adequate and normal.

•Material and Methods: Maternal serum alpha-fetoprotein values less than 2.25 multiples of the median indicate no significantly increased risk of an open neural tube defect, and no further testing is recommended.

°Specific cutoff levels are modified by race and by historic risk factors, such as diabetes or a positive family history of a neural tube defect.

•Samples of MSAFP between 2.25-3.0 multiples of the median are repeated.

°Counseling and further testing are offered for a second elevation.

•If the initial MSAFP value is 3.0 multiples of the median or greater, sonographic evaluation is made available before a repeat serum test.

•Before initial counseling, the patient's probability of carrying a fetus with a neural tube defect is calculated based on clinical risk factors and the magnitude of the MSAFP elevation.

•Procedure-related risk of pregnancy loss from amniocentesis is 0.5-1.0%.

•After counseling, a detailed ultrasound examination, which includes a general anatomic survey and measurements for gestational dating is performed.

°Placenta, fetal abdominal wall, urinary tract, and amniotic fluid volume are evaluated.

°Examination of the central nervous system includes longitudinal (coronal and oblique) and serial transverse views of the spine, and evaluation of the skull and intracranial anatomy, with particular attention to the posterior fossa.

•If the ultrasound images are considered clear enough, and no explanation is found for the elevated MSAFP, then the original risk estimate, which was based on the MSAFP and clinical history before ultrasound, is **reduced by 90%**.

•The primary goal of MSAFP screening is to identify otherwise low risk pregnancies that are increased risk for open neural tube defects.

°Maternal serum alpha-fetoprotein screening for neural tube defects has a sensitivity of 80-85%, with a specificity of 96-98% depending on the protocols and cutoffs used.

°The positive predictor value of abnormal MSAFP tests is only 2-4%.

°Even when women are excluded for incorrect dates, multiple gestation, and fetal death, only 5% with an abnormal MSAFP had an infant with a neural tube defect.

•Optimal views of relevant anatomy are required.

°Transverse views, to looks for integrity of the skin and normal relationships of the ossification centers at each spinal segment, are necessary in addition to longitudinal views.

°Cranial signs, including ventricular dilation, decreased biparietal diameter, scalloping of the parietal bones, and crowding of the cerebellar hemispheres, are present in a high percentage of cases with neural tube defects, and these secondary signs should be sought to optimize the sensitivity of the ultrasound examination.

•If the ultrasound examination is normal, patients are given **revised** risk estimates for neural tube defects.

•This revision is based on an estimated detection sensitivity of 100% for anencephaly and 80% for open spine defects.

°Because each of these constitutes one half of the total number, these numbers are combined to give a 90% sensitivity for open neural tube defects.

°When the estimated probability was reduced by 90%, many patients whose MSAFP values were mildly elevated had a risk estimate less than that in the general unscreened population.

°Two-thirds of the patients declined amniocentesis after considering the revised risk estimates.

°Of the 22 patients in this series with neural tube defects, 20 were detected by ultrasound.

°For the 2 patients not detected the MSAFP elevations were **high** enough (3.6 and 7.7 multiples of the median) that the adjusted risk estimates after normal ultrasound were still above general population.

•Conclusion: A policy of altering risk estimates based on ultrasound before proceeding to amniocentesis is appropriate only if the following criteria are met:

°1) An accurate risk estimate must be known, based on the degree of elevation of MSAFP and on family history.

°2) Patients with abnormal values should receive thorough counseling from trained counselors knowledgeable about neural tube defects and their detection.

°3) Ultrasound should be performed with high resolution equipment by examiners who are experienced at detecting neural tube defects.

°4) If suboptimal views are obtained of the fetal spine or intracranial anatomy, alteration of risk estimates is inappropriate.

°5) After the ultrasound examination, nondirective counseling should be provided, detailing the probability and consequences of an unrecognized fetal anomaly compared with the advantages and procedure-related risks of amniocentesis.]

24. What is the approximate percentage of pregnant alcoholics that will give birth to fetuses with the fetal alcohol syndrome?

    A. 15
    B. 25
    *C.   40
    D. 67
    E. 75

p.61 (Ylikorkala O, Hlamesmäki E, Viinikka L.Urinary prostacyclin and thromboxane metabolites in drinking pregnant women and in their infants: Relation to the fetal alcohol effects: Obstet Gynecol 71:61,1988)

24. [F & I: •Background: Approximately 40% of pregnant alcoholics, and one of every 600-700 unselected parturients, give birth to infants with fetal alcohol syndrome.

•Objective: to study prostacyclin and thromboxane A_2 production in drinking pregnant women and in their newborn infants.

•Material & Methods: 22 drinkers gave birth to infants with fetal alcohol effects.

°This diagnosis was based on the presence of at least two of the following criteria:

°°intrauterine growth retardation (IUGR) (less than the tenth percentile; 18 of 22),

°°facial characteristics (20 of 22), and

°°neurologic aberrations (16 of 22).

•The effect of ethanol on the urinary excretion of prostacyclin and thromboxane A_2 metabolites is unknown

•In healthy **nonpregnant** volunteers, an acute dose of ethanol **inhibited** thromboxane A_2 synthesis in platelets.

•Results: Increased excretion of prostacyclin and thromboxane A_2 in drinking women must be compared cautiously with the above data because the study patients were pregnant and abused alcohol chronically.

°The site of prostanoid stimulation in these drinkers remains unknown, but probably originated from the kidneys.

•Ethanol can stimulate prostacyclin and thromboxane A_2 synthesis from exogenously added arachidonic acid in in vitro preparation and in human fetal tissues.

°If maternal alcohol abuse leads to renal arachidonic acid production by cellular damage or stimulation of renal phospholipases, the excretion of prostacyclin and thromboxane A_2 metabolites would be increased.

°Increased urinary excretion of prostacyclin and thromboxane A_2 metabolites could be secondary to ethanol intake or secondary nutritional changes.

°Smoking among drinkers can be a confounding factor, but no relation between smoking and prostanoid excretion was noted.

°Smoking may cause reduced synthesis of prostacyclin and other metabolites of arachidonic acid.

•Fetal and maternal ethanol concentrations equilibrate readily because ethanol freely crosses the placenta.

°Maternal drinking was accompanied by changes in **neonatal** prostacyclin and thromboxane A_2 similar to those in the mothers.

°Only infants with fetal alcohol effects had increased prostacyclin output.

°°The ratio between prostacyclin and thromboxane A_2 metabolite excretion was lower only in infants with fetal alcohol effects.

•Conclusion: Fetal alcohol effects may be associated with changes in fetal (neonatal) prostacyclin/thromboxane A_2 balance.

°Ethanol **inhibits** prostacyclin and thromboxane A_2 synthesis from endogenous arachidonic acid in human fetal tissues in vitro, but it stimulates those syntheses starting from exogenous arachidonic acid.

°Maternal drinking results in increased release of fetal arachidonic acid, which is converted to prostacyclin and thromboxane A_2 .

•Aspirin could be useful in preventing fetal alcohol effects, and preeclampsia.

°Subcutaneous aspirin (150 mg/kg), a prostaglandin synthesis inhibitor, significantly reduced the incidence of alcohol-induced fetal damage in mice,

°indomethacin, another prostaglandin synthesis inhibitor, blocked the ethanol-induced rise in embryonic brain prostaglandins and protected against brain hypoplasia in hens.]

---

25. Infants who survive grade 3 or 4 germinal layer/intraventricular hemorrhage have what frequency (%) of neurological deficits?

    A. < 5
    B. 20
    C. 33
    *D.   50-75
    E. 90-95

---

p.1386 (Anderson GD, Bada HS, Sibai BM, Harvey C, Korones SB, Magill HL, Wong SP, and Tullis K, "The relationship between labor and route of delivery in the preterm infant," Am J Obstet Gynecol 1987;158:1382)

25. [F & I:•Background: Germinal layer/intraventricular hemorrhage is a well-recognized cause of serious morbidity and mortality in the premature infant.

°Reported incidence ranges from 40% to 90% among those infants with birth weight ≤1500 gm or gestation ages ≤34 weeks.

•It is important to distinguish early onset from late onset hemorrhage because the influence, if any, of obstetric factors becomes remote the later the onset of the hemorrhage from delivery.

•Objective: to evaluate the effects of the active phase of labor and mode of delivery on the frequency of germinal layer/intraventricular hemorrhage in the preterm infant, particularly early onset hemorrhages.

•Material and Methods: Eighty nine infants with ultrasound estimated fetal weights of ≤1750 gm were studied.

°Twenty eights (31.5%) had germinal layer/intraventricular hemorrhages in one hour after birth, and an additional 50 infants (70%) had germinal layer intraventricular beyond one hour after birth.

•Findings of hemorrhages in the ultrasound scan were graded from 1 to 4, wherein

°grade 1 referred to hemorrhages confined to the germinal layer,

°grade 2 referred to intraventricular hemorrhage,

°grade 3 referred to intraventricular hemorrhage with ventricular dilatation, and

°grade 4 included associated parenchymal hemorrhage or extension.

•Infants who weighed ≤1500 gm underwent ultrasound head scans at delivery and a 1, 6, and 24 hours of age and then daily for the first 7 days of life.

°Infants who weighed 1501 to 1750 gm underwent ultrasound scans at delivery and at 1, 6 and 24 hours and 7 days of age.

•The 89 infants delivered of 86 women were initially divided into three groups.

°53 infants delivered vaginally.

°10 infants whose mothers had cesarean section after entering the active phase of labor.

°26 infants whose mothers had cesarean section before entering the active phase of labor.

•Results: the main **indications** for cesarean section in the infants of women with **no** active phase of labor was **hypertensive disorder of pregnancy,**

°with **unfavorable cervix** in 9 infants,

°**abruptio placentae or placenta previa** in 7 infants,

°**abnormal presentation** in 4 infants, and

°**fetal distress** in 3 infants.

•The primary indication for cesarean section in the 10 women who entered the **active phase of labor** was

°**abnormal presentation** in 8 infants, and

°**fetal distress** in 2 infants.

°Only 2 of the women in this group had cervical dilatation >6 cm.

•6 infants in breech presentation were delivered **vaginally**; 2 of the 6 had germinal layer/intraventricular hemorrhage.

•Of the 36 infants delivered by **cesarean section**, 15 were in **breech** presentation and 6 of 15 had germinal layer/intraventricular hemorrhage.

•Ten women had the diagnosis of placenta previa or abruptio placentae (three infants were delivered vaginally and seven by cesarean section).

°Five of these infants had germinal layer/intraventricular hemorrhage (three in the cesarean group and two in the vaginal group).

•Most of the infants of women who had cesarean section before the active phase of labor developed a germinal layer/intraventricular hemorrhage >1 hour after delivery; in the other two groups, however, most of the infants who developed germinal layer/intraventricular hemorrhage did so within the first hour after delivery.

•The frequency of germinal layer/intraventricular hemorrhage in the first hour of life was significantly **lower** in the infants delivered by cesarean section before the active phase of labor as compared with the other two groups.

•**None** of the 8 infants delivered by cesarean section before the active phase of labor with grades 1 or 2 hemorrhage had progression of their hemorrhage to grades 3 or 4.

•There was no difference in the umbilical cord blood gas values between the infants who did or did not develop germinal layer/intraventricular hemorrhage.

•Infants who did not develop germinal layer/intraventricular hemorrhage were **further in gestation** and were heavier when compared with the infants that developed germinal layer/intraventricular hemorrhage ≤1 hour after delivery, or those who developed germinal layer/intraventricular hemorrhage ≥1 hour after delivery.

•The majority of infants predisposed to develop germinal layer/intraventricular hemorrhage who delivered **vaginally**, will develop the hemorrhage during labor, delivery or in the first hour of life.

•The majority of infants delivered by **cesarean section** after entering the active phase of labor who are predisposed to germinal layer/intraventricular hemorrhage will do so within ≤1 hour after delivery.

•The infant of the women delivered by cesarean section before the active phase of labor is not protected from developing germinal layer/intraventricular hemorrhage; only the time at which the infant will develop hemorrhage is shifted to later in neonatal life.

•**Infants who survive with grades 3 or 4 hemorrhage have approximately a 50% to 75% frequency of neurologic deficits compared with the 15% frequency of neurologic deficits in the infants who survive with grades 1 to 2 hemorrhage.**

»Thus, the overall frequency of germinal layer/intraventricular hemorrhage may not be as important as the percent of germinal layer/intraventricular hemorrhages that **progress** to either grade 3 or 4.

»One may speculate that abdominal delivery before the active phase of labor may prevent the most serious form of germinal layer/intraventricular hemorrhage rather than the overall frequency of hemorrhage.

•41%of infants whose mothers were in labor had germinal layer/intraventricular hemorrhage within 1 hour after delivery, compared with 8% who had delivered who had delivered by cesarean section.

•The missing link in the pathogenesis of germinal layer/intraventricular hemorrhage may well occur between the onset of the second stage of labor and the time of cord clamping or first breath.

°Among the causes suggested for this hemorrhage are hypoxic-ischemic insult, thrombosis of deep cerebral vessels, increased venous or subependymal capillary pressure, and cerebral hyperperfusion during episodes of hypoxemia.

°Autoregulation of cerebral blood flow is impaired in distressed neonates and therefore possibly also in distressed fetuses.

°Compression of the fetal head during labor and delivery might alter intracranial capillary and venous pressures.

26. Which part of the brain is primarily affected in microcephaly?

    *A.   frontal lobe
    B. occipital lobe
    C. parietal lobe
    D. temporal lobe
    E. brain stem

p.1062 (Goldstein I, Reece EA, Pilu G, O'Connor TZ, Lockwood CJ, and Hobbins JC, "Sonographic assessment of the fetal frontal lobe: A potential tool for prenatal diagnosis of microcephaly," Am J Obstet Gynec 1988; 15:1057)

26. [F & I:•Background: True **microcephaly** can be diagnosed by serial measurements of fetal head growth.

•Many of the present measurements for diagnosing microcephaly require reduced measurements <3 SD below the mean.

•The antenatal diagnosis of microcephaly was only 56% accurate in one study.

•Microcephaly occurs from 1/6250 to 1/8500 births.

•Associated anomalies are frequent and include agyria, absence of the corpus callosum, or ventricular enlargement secondary to atrophy of the cortex.

°Strong correlation also exists between microcephaly and **mental retardation**.

•Microcephaly is most often associated with the decrease size of the frontal fossa and a flattening of the frontal bone with the other lobes of the fetal brain remaining unchanged.

•Objective: to determine normal dimensions of the anterior cranial fossa and the frontal lobe of the fetal brain to provide normative data against which fetuses suspected to have microcephaly or any other lesion affecting the anterior fossa could be evaluated.

•Typical features of the microcephalic fetus include a cone-shaped head, a large face, large ears, and narrowing, receding, and flattening of the forehead, sometimes referred to as "pinhead" or "birdhead".

•The method used involved the traditionally occipital frontal diameter in addition to two other measurements: frontal lobe and the thalamic frontal lobe measurements.

•measures below the the tenth percentile are considered diagnostic of microcephaly.]

27   Which is the most sensitive test for determining whether a specimen taken during cordocentesis has
been contaminated with maternal blood?

>   A.   ABO and Rh blood typing
>   B.   hematocrit
>   *C.   human chorionic gonadotropin
>   D.   Kleihauer-Betke test
>   E.   α-fetoprotein determination

p.1187   (Forrestier F, Cox WL, Daffos F, Rainaut M, "The assessment of fetal blood samples," Am J
Obstet Gynec   1988; 15:1184)

27. [F & I:•Background: In the presence of **maternal infection**, contamination of fetal blood samples
with maternal blood will cause a false positive diagnosis of fetal infection.

•The presence of maternal blood cells in a specimen for investigation of fetal karyotype makes the
specimen useless, but amniotic fluid or sodium citrate have negligible effects.

•Investigation of **disorders of hemostasis (platelets or coagulation factors)** is most
severely affected by amniotic fluid contamination because **amniotic fluid activates some
coagulation factors** and can cause platelet aggregation.

•Three major differences distinguish maternal from fetal blood in considering distribution curves of
hematological indexes:

°1.   There is only 1 peak of leukocytes in the fetus (corresponding to lymphocytes and nucleated
erythrocytes);

°2.   The average erythrocyte volume is much higher in the fetus; and

°3.   Red cell distribution width is broader in the fetus.

•The Kleihauer test relies on detecting differences in hemoglobins present in adult and fetal red cells and
in theory should be able to detect a maternal blood contamination of as little as 0.5%.

°Accurate results are not possible because of the gradual appearance of hemoglobin A in fetal
erythrocytes.

°After staining, erythrocytes containing only hemoglobin A appear as empty "cell ghosts"; those
containing mainly or exclusively hemoglobin F stain darkly and those with both hemoglobin A
and F have an intermediate level of staining.

•Blood smears stained for differential count will clearly show amniotic fluid squames.

•Erythrocyte antigen expression is different in the fetus compared with the adult; **I** antigen is present
only on adult erythrocytes, **i** antigen is present only on fetal erythrocytes.

°Monoclonal antibody agglutination (anti-i and anti-I) is simple to perform and will detect a
maternal blood contamination of 5%.

•**ß-hCG** is of maternal origin, has a steep gradient across the placenta, and is found in only **minute**
quantities in fetal blood, although higher levels are found in amniotic fluid.

°It is most sensitive in determining if the sample is contaminated and allows detection of as little
of 0.2% maternal blood or 1% amniotic fluid contamination.

•**Coagulation factors V or VIII** will detect both amniotic fluid and sodium citrate contamination but must be interpreted with caution.

°Less than 1% contamination with amniotic fluid activates coagulation and falsely increases the activities of V and VIII when tested against adult reference plasma.

°These values need to be compared with vitamin K-dependent factors, such as IX or II, which are not activated by amniotic fluid.

•Concentration of α-**fetoprotein** is markedly higher in fetal serum, and the test is **not** useful to detect contamination of fetal blood specimens.

•In a fetus who has received a transfusion of adult blood products, either whole blood, platelets, or pure factor concentrates, the assessment of subsequent samples needs to be performed carefully.

°If the transfused product has **maternal** platelets, then the ß-hCG levels are subject to error.

°If whole adult blood has been given, then the hematologic indexes will be altered, but the ß-hCG level should not have changed.

°In a fetus with **ß-thalassemia**, the hematologic indexes will show a relative microcytosis, which may cause confusing results in a mother with **iron deficiency.**

•Conclusion: **Maternal blood** is detected with ß-hCG, hematologic indexes, and erythrocyte antigens.

•**Amniotic fluid** is detected with ß-hCG , coagulation factors, hematologic indexes (dilution), and blood smear.

•**Sodium citrate** is detected with coagulation factors and hematologic indexes (dilution).]

---

28. Which of the following is **increased** during a normal pregnancy?

    A. bone resorption of calcium
    *B.   intestinal absorption of calcium
    C. parathyroid hormone
    D. renal resorption of calcium
    E. serum ionized calcium

---

p.899   (Belizan JM, Villar J and Repke J, "The relationship between calcium intake and pregnancy-induced hypertension: Up-to-date evidence " Am J Obstet Gynecol 1987;158:898)

28. [F & I:•Background: At term, fetal calcium accumulation totals approximately 30 gm.

°It increases sharply from week 30 of gestation, and **80% of total fetal calcium is deposited during the third trimester.**

°The transport of ionized calcium from the mother to the fetus increases from about 50 mg/24 hours at 20 weeks of gestation to a maximum of about 350 mg/24 hours at 35 weeks.

•Renal calcium excretion **increases** during pregnancy.

•Calcium excretion and creatinine clearance are significantly correlated suggesting that the increase in calciuria during pregnancy is due to the increase in the glomerular filtration rate.

•Pregnancy may be a physiologic state of "obligatory" high urinary calcium output and the levels of maternal intake >2.0 gm/day are necessary to provide for fetal requirements.

•**Maternal bone calcium tends to be preserved during pregnancy.**

•Intestinal absorption can increase from 27% before pregnancy to as high as 50% during gestation.

•**Total** maternal **calcium** levels **decrease** progressively during pregnancy, because of both a decrease in albumin levels and a small reduction in ionized calcium.

•**Parathyroid hormone** levels **increase** compensatorily.

°There is an inverse relationship between total calcium during pregnancy and parathyroid hormone levels with the group with >2 gm calcium intake per day having the lowest parathyroid levels at term.

•The only compensatory mechanism fully developed during gestation is an **enhanced intestinal absorption**, while renal and bone reabsorption is diminished.

°This process increases parathyroid hormone secretion and results in a **"physiologic hyperparathyroidism"** during pregnancy.

•Selected subgroups of subjects can benefit more dramatically than others from calcium supplementation.

°Those with initial low total serum calcium levels, greater body weights, lower initial serum parathyroid hormone levels, or lower initial plasma renin activity constitute these groups.

°An interaction of parathyroid hormone and serum calcium with plasma renin activity may be present in this selective effect.

•Healthy women of childbearing age who were receiving a daily supplementation of 1.0 gm of elemental calcium had a significant reduction in diastolic blood pressure in comparison with a control group receiving placebo.

•Steps in the genesis of pregnancy-induced hypertension may be as follows:

°(1) In populations with a **lower** calcium intake than required during pregnancy there is an **increase** in serum parathyroid hormone levels.

°(2) An **increase** in parathyroid levels would involve an **increase** in free intracellular (cytosolic) calcium .

°°Parathyroid hormone increases the intracellular cytosol concentration of calcium in several types of cells, such as kidney, liver, and HeLa cells.

°°Two mechanisms can mediate the action of calcium on vascular smooth muscle cells.

°°An increase in cellular membrane permeability to calcium and an activation of adenyl cyclase and an increase of cyclic adenosine monophosphate, with a consequent liberation of calcium from the mitochondria to the cytosol.

°(3) The concentration of intracellular free (cytosolic) calcium in vascular smooth muscle cells determines the degree of tension in and is the trigger for muscular **contraction**.

°(4) The **vasoconstrictive** effect results with a rise in blood pressure resulting from an increase in the vascular smooth muscle tension.

•Individuals with hyperparathyroidism have higher blood pressure.

°An increase in ionized calcium concentration in platelets is observed in women with pregnancy induced hypertension.

•Calcium has a role in renin secretion.

•A **decrease in renin** production is manifested by an **increase in calcium concentration**, and inversely a decrease in calcium concentration produces a rise in renin liberation.

»Conclusion: It is premature to recommend calcium supplementation to all pregnant women with the prevention of pregnancy-induced hypertension as the only objective since there are no reports that document an inverse relationship between calcium intake and blood pressure.]

---

29. Which of the following dermatoses of pregnancy is an autoimmune disease?

    A. pruritic urticarial papules and plaques of pregnancy
    B. papular dermatitis of pregnancy
    C. impetigo herpetiformis
    D. prurigo gestationis
    *E.   herpes gestationis

---

p.417   (Alcalay J, Ingber, Kafri B, and Segal J, "Hormonal evaluation and autoimmune background in pruritic urticarial papules and plaques of pregnancy," Am J Obstet Gynecol 1988;158:417.)

29. [F & I:•Background: Gravidas can have the same kind of skin diseases as nonpregnant patients.

°A small group of dermatoses unique to pregnancy include herpes gestationis, impetigo herpetiformis, prurigo gestationis, papular dermatitis of pregnancy, and pruritic urticarial papules and plaques of pregnancy.

•Since its original description in 1979, pruritic urticarial papules and plaques of pregnancy has been recognized as a distinct clinical entity.

•Results: No severe maternal complications or cases of prematurity, postmaturity, or spontaneous abortion have been documented.

°No hormonal alterations in patients with pruritic urticarial papules and plaques of pregnancy were found when compared with normal pregnant women.

•No major known autoimmune background is responsible for the eruption of pruritic urticarial papules and plaques of pregnancy.]

---

30. All of the following should be considered in the intrauterine differential diagnosis of fetal cystic hygroma EXCEPT

    A. benign cystic teratoma
    B. meningomyelocele
    C. nuchal edema
    D. subchorionic placenta cyst
    *E.   ventriculomegaly

---

p.223   (Pijpers L, Reuss A, Stewart PA, Wladimiroff JW, and Sachs ES. "Fetal cystic hygroma: Prenatal diagnosis and management" Obstet Gynecol 1988;72:223)

---

30 [F & I:•Objective: to present the diagnosis, management, and genetic consequences of cystic hygromas.

•Cystic hygroma, a congenital malformation of the lymphatic system, arises as a consequence of a lag in the normal formation of a communication between the developing jugular lymph sacs and the internal jugular vein at 40 days' gestation.

•Cystic hygromas are endothelium-lined, single or multiloculated fluid-filled cavities found mainly the the posterior cervical region, but also occasionally in the anterior neck, axilla, chest wall, or groin.

•The differential diagnosis of cystic hygroma should include meningomyelocele, benign cystic teratoma, nuchal edema, encephalocele, and subchorial placental cyst.

•The ultrasonic diagnosis should be based upon at least two bilaterally symmetrical, echofree areas in the postnuchal region usually divided by septa, a completely formed cranial vault, and a constant location of the masses with respect to the occiput even during fetal motion.

°A thorough ultrasound examination of the entire fetus should be carried out to exclude other congenital malformations.

•Abnormal karyotypes such as trisomy 13, 18, and 21 are known to be associated with hygroma colli.

°**Chromosome analysis is therefore required for parental genetic counseling.**

•In the case of monosomy or trisomy, the recurrence risk will be very low.

°Chorionic villus sampling or amniocentesis can be offered in subsequent pregnancies.

°When normal karyotypes are found, nonchromosomal syndromes, which have a recurrence risk up to 25% should be considered.

•**The ultimate prognosis of cystic hygroma is poor.**]

---

31. In which of the following situations would cervical ripening by means intravaginal prostaglandin E2 in an otherwise uncomplicated vertex presentation be **contraindicated**?

    A. Class A diabetes mellitus at term
    *B.   placental insufficiency at term
    C. postdate pregnancy
    D. premature rupture of membranes at term
    E. previous precipitate delivery

---

p.57   (Williams JK, Lewis JL, Cohen GR, and O'Brien WF, "The sequential use of estradiol and prostaglandin E2 topical gels for cervical ripening in high-risk term pregnancies requiring induction of labor" Am J Obstet Gynecol 1988;158: 55)

31. [F & I:•Objective: : to examine the safety and efficacy of 200 mg estradiol valerate topical cervical gel used sequentially with 2 mg PGE2 vaginal gel as a ripening agent compared with a placebo followed by the PGE2 gel.

•Measures included the change in Bishop score, length of induction, presence of uterine contractions, and maximum dose of oxytocin.

•Materials and Methods: The estradiol gel was prepared by mixing 200 mg of estradiol valerate with 5 ml of hydroxyethyl cellulose gel.

•The PGE2 gel was prepared by mixing a 20 mg PGE2 vaginal suppository with K-Y Jelly to a volume of 20 ml and supplied as 2 ml unit (2 mg).

•Estradiol valerate may alter bonding in collagen fibers, resulting in increased cervical compliance.

•Both estradiol and dehydroepiandrosterone sulfate, given intravenously, can cause cervical ripening.

•Results: Estradiol vaginal gel was **not** efficacious in cervical ripening, either as a single agent over a 6 hour period or as an additive to improve the efficacy of PGE2 gel.

•A total of 85% of patients receiving the PGE2 gel experienced some contractions, with 20% of patients going into active labor without oxytocin, despite the low PGE2 dosage (2 mg.)

•The high rate of uterine activity caused by the prostaglandins is a continued drawback in their use as an ideal "ripening" agent, especially in the case of potential uteroplacental insufficiency.

°They also fail to demonstrate a ripening effect separate from that caused by uterine activity.]

---

32. All of the following are appropriate in the management of laboring pregnant patients with aortic stenosis EXCEPT

      A. conduction anesthesia
      B. operative assistance for delivery
      C. prophylactic antibiotics
      D. pulmonary artery catheter
      *E.   volume expansion

---

p.117   (Easterling TR, Chadwick HS, Otto CM and Benedetti TJ, "Aortic stenosis in pregnancy" Obstet Gynecol 1988;71:113)

32. [F & I:•Background: Significant aortic stenosis is uncommon in women of childbearing age.

•Objective: to report the experience with 5 cases of aortic stenosis in pregnancy.

•Management of pregnancy complicated by aortic stenosis requires accurate assessment.

°Unlike in mitral stenosis, clinical symptoms appear very late in the course of the disease.

°Once patients complain of angina, shortness of breath, or syncope, their risk of sudden death may be out of proportion to the severity of their clinical symptoms.

•Intracardiac pressure gradients can be accurately measured noninvasively by Doppler echocardiography.

•Calculation of aortic valve area provides an index of the stenosis that is independent of changes in transaortic volume flow.

•**Reduced activity was the mainstay of antepartum care.**

•Delivery was delayed until fetal pulmonary maturity was confirmed.

°Labor was induced in some patients.

°Cesarean section was performed only for obstetric indications.

•The first stage of labor was managed according to usual obstetric standards.

°As expected, the patients were very susceptible to supine hypotension.

•The second stage was managed with minimal pushing and operative assistance when adequate station was achieved.

•The third stage was managed aggressively to avoid potential hemorrhage.

•Prophylactic antibiotics were administered to all patients.

•The pulmonary artery catheter was used in four of five patients.

•Unlike the afterload imposed by hypertension, the systemic circulation and especially the coronary circulation are subjected to reduced rather than elevated pressures.

•Coronary blood flow is impaired by systemic afterload reduction, increased ventricular diastolic pressure, and tachycardia which reduces diastolic perfusion time.

°All may result in angina.

•Preload must be maintained for the left ventricle to generate an adequate cardiac output across the stenotic aortic valve.

°Given a noncompliant ventricle, small changes in fluid loading result in large changes in filling pressures.

•Critical aortic stenosis creates a narrow window of appropriate fluid loading.

°Small decreases in preload due to hemorrhage or regional anesthesia may result in decreased cardiac output and clinical hypotension.

°Small increases in vascular volume may produce dramatic increases in filling pressures, resulting in pulmonary edema.

•The goal of hemodynamic management should be to maintain filling pressures within the narrow therapeutic window and to avoid tachycardia.

•Immediately postpartum, filling pressures frequently rose, requiring a diuretic.

•Effective analgesia can prevent the tachycardia associated with labor pain.

•Regional anesthesia can be used if adequate time is given to carefully titrate the block and initiate compensatory actions to correct hemodynamic changes induced by the anesthetic.

•Patients with congenital aortic stenosis should be informed of a 14-26% risk of carrying a fetus with congenital heart disease.

°Fetal echocardiography may be useful.]

Directions: Each set of lettered headings below is followed by a list of numbered words or phrases. For each numbered word or phrase select:

A. if item is associated with (A) only
B. if item is associated with (B) only
C. if item is associated with both (A) and (B)
D. if item is associated with neither (A) nor (B)

A. cadmium
B. zinc
C. both
D. neither

33. half-life in body measured in decades   Ans: A

34. maternal alkaline phosphatase an indicator of deficiency status   Ans: B

35. concentration in placenta increases with smoking   Ans: A

---

p.69   (Kuhnert BR, Kuhnert PM, Zarlingo TJ, "Associations between placental cadmium and zinc and age and parity in pregnant women who smoke," Obstet Gynecol 71:67,1988)

33-35. [F & I: •Background: Infants delivered by older smokers are at higher risk of impaired fetal growth than those delivered by younger smokers.

°zinc is needed for fetal growth

°cadmium toxicity could decrease zinc in the placenta of older patients who smoke.

°This altered relationship may interfere with the passage of zinc to the fetus.

•There is a relationship between the ratio of placental zinc to placental cadmium (Zn/Cd), birth weight, and retention of both cadmium and zinc in the placenta of smokers.

•The nutritional status of trace elements such as zinc and chromium may become less favorable with increasing parity.

•Cadmium has a very long half-life in the body and accumulates in tissues with age.

°The accumulation in smokers is five to six times that in nonsmokers.

•Objectives:

°to examine the relationship between placental cadmium and placental zinc in smokers and nonsmokers and

°to test the hypothesis that older, multiparous smokers have altered ratios of placental zinc to placental cadmium.

•Placental cadmium and placental zinc increase with smoking.

°Cadmium induces the formation of the binding protein metallothionein, which can bind both cadmium and zinc.

°This results in less zinc available to the infants of smokers.

•Results: The ratio of placental zinc to placental cadmium **decreased** with increasing age, and was always **lower** in smokers than in nonsmokers.

°zinc transfer is altered by the cadmium and less zinc crosses the placenta and reaches the infant.

•There is an increase in placental cadmium with increasing parity in smokers.

°The explanation for a relationship between parity and placental cadmium in smokers is that the half-life of disappearance of cadmium from the body is measured in **decades.**

•The decrease in two indices of zinc status (placental zinc and plasma alkaline phosphatase) with age and parity suggests that body stores of zinc may be lower in older women who have had more children.

•**No** relationship was found between plasma zinc and age or parity.

•The placental Zn/Cd ratio is significantly related to birth weight in smokers: the lower the ratio, the lower the birth weight.]

Directions: For each of the questions or incomplete statements below, ONE or MORE of the answers or completions given is correct. In each case select:

A.   if only 1, 2 and 3 are correct
B.   if only 1 and 3 are correct
C.   if only 2 and 4 are correct
D.   if only 4 is correct
E.   if all are correct

---

36. In considering the reliability of chorionic villus biopsy, possible causes of cytogenic discrepancies between trophoblast and fetus include

1.   abnormal single cell lines
2.   chimerism
3.   maternal contamination
4.   meiotic exchanges

---

p.642   Ans: B   (Butler WJ, Schwartz CE, Sauer SM, Wilson JT, and McDonough PG, "Discordance in deoxyribonucleic acid analysis of fetus and trophoblast." Am J Obstet Gynecol 1988;158:642)

36. [F & I:•Background: First trimester chorionic villi sampling offers several advantages over other methods of prenatal diagnosis, but there is concern about the accuracy of testing trophoblast to determine fetal status.

°There are cytogenic discrepancies between fetus and trophoblast.

°There are abnormal single-cell lines and mosaicism not reflected in karyotypes of multiple fetal tissues.

°Diagnostic errors may result from assay mistakes, maternal contamination, or differential gene expression or mutation.

•Trophoblast molecular genetic constitution may not reflect fetal status.

•Chorionic villus sampling requires that the fetal karyotype, metabolic phenotype, or genotype be inferred from extraembryonic tissue. This is unlike amniocentesis, where fetal cells are obtained from amniotic fluid for analysis.

•Cytogenic discrepancies between the fetus and placenta usually reside in the placenta because only a few cells of the inner cell mass directly contribute to embryonic development.

°Most cytogenic abnormalities involve the presence of a **trisomic or polyploidic** cell line, usually as a mosaic with accompanying normal cell line.

°Cell lines with chromosome breaks, fragments, and rearrangements have been reported in 1% to 2% of cytotrophoblast cells under direct analysis.

•Unequal recombination can occur at meiosis or mitosis.

°Most exchanges occur between sister chromatids during **mitosis**.

°Meiotic exchanges could not account for allelic variations between fetus and trophoblast, but certainly result in different cell populations exhibiting a variation in individual fragment lengths and band patterns.

•There may be **mitotic crossing-over** in human cells.

°There are regions of high-recombination activity, and certain genetic diseases, such as Bloom's syndrome, may result from recombination which favors oncogene rearrangement and neoplasia.

°The cytotrophoblast is a relatively immature, mitotically active cell type and is suspected of having an increased tendency for such recombination.

•**Sister chromatid exchange**, as a mechanism to account for the high rate of unequal recombination in the hypervariable minisatellite regions, has been identified in direct preparations of chorionic villi by incubation with 5-bromodeoxyuridine.

•Results: Variations in the DNA "fingerprints" of four paired fetus-trophoblast specimens supports the hypothesis of active mitotic DNA rearrangement in trophoblast.]

---

37. Sequelae of methamphetamine abuse during pregnancy include

1. decreased birth weight
2. decreased head circumference
3. decreased length
4. increased incidence of congenital anomalies

---

p.542   Ans: A   (Little BB, Snell LM and Gilstrap LC III, "Methamphetamine abuse during pregnancy: Outcome and fetal effects " Obstet Gynecol 1988;72:541)

37. [F & I:•Objective: to evalute pregnancy and fetal outcome in a group of methamphetamine abusers.

•Results: Maternal methamphetamine abuse was associated with a significantly decreased birth weight, length and head circumference.

•Significantly more amphetamine abusers use tobacco but no separate effect of cigarette smoking on birth weight, length or head circumference was found.

•Mean gestational length and Apgar scores were not significantly different between the methamphetamine exposed in comparison groups.

•Cocaine, methamphetamine, and cocaine plus methamphetamine are associated with an increased rate of both prematurity and intrauterine growth retardation,and altered neonatal behavioral patterns.

•Conclusion: There was not statistical power to support a statement that methamphetamine abuse during pregnancy presents a risk.

•Impurities such as lead oxide and cyanide have been found to contaminate methamphetamines sold illegally, and may be determintal to pregnancy as well.

•Conclusion: Fetal growth was significantly delayed in infants whose mothers abused methamphetamines throughout pregnancy, including the first trimester.

•The frequency of congenital anomalies was **not** significantly increased in the drug-exposed group.

•Although there was a slight excess of major congenital anomalies in infants exposed in utero to methamphetamines, the statistical power of the study was not sufficient to determine wheter this was associated with maternal drug abuse.]

---

38. Endocrine changes associated with early syphilis include

1. decreased dehyrdroepiandrosterone sulfate in fetus
2. decreased maternal serum 17 ß-estradiol
3. increased cholesterol in fetus
4. decreased maternal progesterone

---

p.1330 Ans: A (Parker CR, and Wendel GD, "The effects of syphilis on endocrine function of the fetoplacental unit" Am J Obstet Gynecol 1988;159:1327)

38. [F&I:•Background: Estrogen formation in the human placenta is regulated by the availability of precursor, i.e., dehydroepiandrosterone sulfate, produced by the fetal adrenal glands.

•The accelerated rate of deh:yroepiandrosterone sulfate formation during the last 10 to 12 weeks of gestation appears to be facilitated by an enhanced rate of assimilation of low-density lipoprotein-cholesterol by the fetal adrenal glands.

°Failure of normal adrenal development, such as in cases of fetal anencephaly, is associated with subnormal levels of dehydroepiandrosterone sulfate and hypercholesterolemia in fetal blood and relative hypoestrogenism in the maternal compartment.

•Objective: to determine whether syphilis, a stress associated pregnancy complication, would have similar effects on the fetoplacental unit.

•Serum levels of progesterone in women with syphilis during pregnancy arc normal or somewhat increased, therefore, the capacity of placental steroid biosynthesis probably is not compromised by maternal syphilis infection.

°A relative deficiency of 17ß-estradiol and estriol occurs in the sera of women infected with syphilis.

°The reduction of estriol levels among women whose fetuses had congenital syphilis is due to decreased dehydroepiandrosterone sulfate secretion by fetal adrenal glands.

•Because fetal serum levels of estriol were subnormal in both affected and nonaffected neonates, despite the fact that dehydroepiandrosterone sulfate levels were normal in the noninfected infants of women with syphilis, placental aromatase activity or hepatic 16-hydroxylase activity may be deficient.

•Infected and noninfected infants of women with syphilis were found to have excessive serum levels of cortisol.

•Fetal serum cholesterol levels appear to be inversely related to the steroidogenic activity of the fetal adrenal gland especially the fetal zone of the adrenal gland.

•Low serum dehydroepiandrosterone sulfate level and hypercholesterolemia caused by excessive low density lipoprotein-cholesterol occurs in neonates chronically "stressed" in utero because of severe maternal hypertension and in infants having maldevelopment of the fetal adrenal glands because of anencephaly.

•Hypercholesterolemia that occurs in newborn infants with congenital syphilis is due to reduced uptake and utilization of low-density lipoprotein by the fetal adreanl glands in utero.

•Infants having congenital syphilis have moderate fibrosis of the adrenal glands and it is unclear whether the defect in adrenal steroidogenesis is due to a local infectious process or to a systemic stress response to syphilis.]

---

39. The amount of fat accumulated in the liver in cases of acute fatty liver of pregnancy is correlated with

    1.   hematocrit
    2.   hemoglobin
    3.   platelet count
    4.   serum uric acid

---

p.1046   Ans: E   (Minakami H, Oka N, Sato T, Tamada T, Yasuda Y, and Hirota N, "Preeclampsia: A microvesicular fat disease of the liver? ," Am J Obstet Gynec   1988; 159:1043)

39. [Facts and Issues:•Background: Acute fatty liver of pregnancy is an uncommon but potentially fatal disorder that may complicate the third trimester.

•Acute fatty liver of pregnancy is considered an independent clinical entity whose definitve diagnosis requires histologic examination of the liver.

•A microscopic feature of acute fatty liver of pregnancy is microvesicular fat vacuolation of the hepatocytes.

•The syndrome of hemolysis, elevated liver enzymes, and low platelet count in the third trimester is a form of preeclampsia, even though it may lack the traditional signs of this disorder.

•Objective: to confirm the hypothesis that three clinical conditions, acute fatty liver of pregnancy, the syndrome of hemolysis elevated liver enzymes and low platelet count, and preeclampsia with liver dysfunction are part of the same spectrum.

•Results: It is not possible to differentiate histologically between acute fatty liver of pregnancy, the syndrome of hemolysis, elevated liver enzymes, and low platelet count, and preeclampsia.

»Conclusion: Preeclampsia, hemolysis, elevated liver enzymes and low platelet count syndrome and acute fatty liver of pregnancy are one in the same disorder.

°On the basis of the extent of fat accumulation on the liver, acute fatty liver of pregnancy may be considered one of the most severe forms of preeclampsia.

°The amount of fat in the liver is correlated with serum concentrations of uric acid, a reliable laboratory indicator for preeclampsia and also with the platelet count which is reported to decrease in preeclampsia.

°These findings suggests the preeclamptic patient may show microvesicular fat disease.

•Failure of plasma expansion may be associated with the development of preeclampsia which is a hyperviscosity syndrome.

°The total blood flow may be decreased in preeclampsia.

•Hemoconcentration leading to hypoperfusion of the liver might further enhance the fatty change of the liver in severely affected patients.]

---

40. Clinically useful in the treatment of fetal supraventricular tachycardia

  1. digoxin
  2. quindine
  3. verapamil
  4. transabdominal compression of the fetal cephalic pole

---

p.861   Ans: E   (Fernandez C, De Rosa GE, Guevara E, Velazquez H, Pueyrredon HR, Casavilla F, and Suarez LD, "Reversion by vagal reflex of a fetal paroxysmal atrial tachycardia detected by echocardiography" Am J Obstet Gynecol 1988;159:860)

40. [F & I:•Fetal paroxysmal supraventricular tachycardia may cause cardiac failure, nonimmune hydrops, and prenatal sudden death.

•Digoxin, quinidine, procainamide, verapamil, and ß-blockers, can be used in pregnancy during fetal rhythm disturbances, with dissimilar results.

•Vagal maneuvers are effective for reverting tachyarrhythmias in fetuses during delivery.

°vagal reflex is induced by transabdominal compression of the fetal cephalic pole.

•Transabdominal compression of the fetal cephalic pole should be considered as initial or concomitant treatment of fetal tachyarrhythmias after week 32 of pregnancy at which time a sufficient maturity of the autonomic nervous system is generally observed.]

---

41. Malignant hyperthermia can be triggered in susceptible humans by

  1. amide local anesthetics
  2. catecholamines
  3. depolarizing skeletal muscle relaxants
  4. inhalation anesthetics

---

p.831   Ans: E   (Shime J, Gare D. Andrews J, and Britt B, "Dantrolene in pregnancy: Lack of adverse effects on the fetus and newborn infant" Am J Obstet Gynecol 1988;159:831)

41. [F & I:•Background: Malignant hyperthermia is an autosomal dominant myopathy of humans.

•Malignant hyperthermia reaction is a paroxysmal hypercatabolic reaction of skeletal and heart muscle.

•Reactions may be triggered in susceptible humans by depolarizing skeletal muscle relaxants, inhalation anesthetics, amide local anesthetics, and catecholamines.

•There have been no deaths related to malignant hyperthermia during any regional anesthetic.

°In addition to anesthetics, environmental stress, muscle injury, and heavy exercise have been implicated in a general sympathetic stress phenomenon that may trigger a malignant hyperthermia crises.

•Intravenous administration of dantrolene sodium is a recognized treatment of malignant hyperthermia crisis.

•Objective: to evaluate the effects on the fetus and newborn of oral dantrolene used prophylactically in pregnant women.

•Results: Dantrolene sodium is a hydantoin derivative first synthesized in 1967, whose initial use was to treat muscle spasm.

°Dantrolene prevents the efflux of calcium ions and acts on skeletal muscle, smooth muscle, and cardiac muscle.

•35% of an oral dose is absorbed by the intestine.

°Hydroxlation takes place in the liver, and the major metabolite is partially active.

•The half-life of dantrolene is 6 to 8 hours.

•Hepatotoxicity occurs in approximately 1% of patients.

•Side effects of dantrolene include muscle weakness, drowsiness, dizziness, nervousness, nausea, comiting, feelin of inebriation, flurred speech, ataxia, and blurred vision.

•Dantrolene probably crosses into breast milk.

•Because of the limitations of oral dantrolene for malignant hyperthermia prophylaxis, an alternative approach has been considered.

•Preoperative intravenous dantrolene has been administered before anesthetic induction.

•The gastrointestinal side effects were avoided; however, other side effects such as phlebitis are reported.

°The half-life of the dantrolene after an intravenous bolus was 12 hours.

°Booster doses of dantrolene could be given intravenously every 8 to 12 hours to maintain a therapeutic blood level throughout labor and delivery.

•At present dantrolene is recognized as a prophylactic and therapeutic agent for malignant hyperthermia reactions

•There were no discernible adverse effects of dantrolene with respect to the fetus or neonate.]

---

42. Clinical effects of low dose (1 to 5 μg/kg/min) dopamine include

    1.   dilation of renal blood vessels
    2.   increase in glomerular filtration rate
    3.   naturiesis
    4.   tachycardia

---

p.605   Ans: A (Kirshon B, Lee W, Mauer MB, and Cotton DB, "Effects of low-dose dopamine therapy in the oliguric patient with preeclampsia " Am J Obstet Gynecol 1988;159:604)

---

42. [F & I:•Background: The oliguric patient with severe preeclampsia can be treated by fluid challenge, vasodilatory therapy, and diuretics.

•Patients with a **low pulmonary capillary wedge pressure, hyperdynamic** ventricular function, and moderate **elevation of systemic vascular resistance** respond to ⟦FLUIDS⟧.

•Patients with a **normal or elevated pulmonary capillary wedge pressure and cardiac output** accompanied by **normal systemic vascular resistance** respond to ⟦(PRELOAD OR AFTERLOAD REDUCTION).⟧

•Therapy for patients with an **elevated wedge pressure, systemic vascular resistance,** and **depressed ventricular function** consisted of ⟦FLUID RESTRICTION AND AGGRESSIVE AFTERLOAD REDUCTION.⟧

•Dopamine, a selective renal vasodilator, is indicated for patients with oliguria who have a normal or elevated pulmonary capillary wedge pressure and normal ventricular function.

°The cause of oliguria in these patients may in part be due to renal artery vasospasm.

°Dopamine may also be beneficial in the rare instance of elevated pulmonary capillary wedge pressure and systemic vascular resistance accompanied by depressed ventricular function.

•Objective: to determine if dopamine is effective in the treatment of oliguria in severe preeclampsia.

•In **low** doses (1 to 5 ug/kg/min) dopamine, an endogenous catecholamine, selectively dilates renal vessels and increases renal blood flow, sodium excretion, and glomerular filtration rate.

°The cortical component of renal blood flow increases during low-dose dopamine infusion.

•In the absence of identifiable prerenal, postrenal, or nephrotoxic causes, acute oliguria associated with pregnancy-induced hypertension may be the result of decreased renal blood flow and a redistribution of the flow away from the cortex.

•At **higher** doses, dopamine exerts a potent inotropic effect.

°In nonpregnant adults, high-dose dopamine causes α-adrenergic effects to predominate and the salutary effects on renal blood flow are lost.

•Results: Low-dose therapy was uniformly accompanied by a significant rise in the patient's urine and cardiac output.

°A concomitant decline in systemic vascular resistance occurred, but blood pressure remained unchanged.

°Dopamine was well tolerated.

°The increased cardiac output should be beneficial to both renal and placental perfusions.

°The improvement in urine output may be accounted for by the increases in cardiac output and renal vasodilatation.

•The absence of fetal distress during dopamine therapy implies that placental perfusion was not compromised.

•Patients with severe preeclampsia may have elevated left ventricular filling pressures on the basis of an elevated systemic vascular resistance and not increased volume.

°The most dramatic responses of urine output and urinary indices to dopamine were seen in the patient with the highest initial pulmonary capillary wedge pressure.

°A pulmonary capillary wedge pressure of at least 8 mm Hg implied euvolemia.

°Dopamine may be most effective in reversing the oliguria of preeclampsia when pulmonary capillary wedge pressures are moderately elevated.

°This is consistent with the concept that patients with severe preeclampsia are often volume contracted, despite having normal pulmonary capillary wedge pressures.

•Dopamine produces its renal effects by increasing renal blood flow and glomerular filtration.

°This is accomplished via stimulation of the kidney's dopaminergic receptors, which usually results in a marked natriuresis.

°°Because sodium is a major component of urinary osmolality, a dopaminergic-induced natriuresis should result in an increased fractional excretion of sodium and osmolar clearance.

•Conclusion: When severe oliguria develops in patients with severe preeclampsia, invasive hemodynamic monitoring may be helpful in defining the cause of the oliguria.

•Low central venous and capillary wedge pressures imply the need for volume repletion.

»Markedly elevated pulmonary capillary wedge and central venous pressures, accompanied by elevated systemic vascular resistance and depressed ventricular function, warrant aggressive afterload reduction and consideration of dopamine therapy.]

---

43. Clinically useful in preventing intraventricular hemorrhage in the small preterm infant:

1. phenobarbital
2. pancuronium
3. fresh frozen plasma
4. exchange transfusion

---

p.777   Ans: A (Morales WJ, Angel JL, O'Brien WF, Knuppel RA, and Marsalisi F, "The use of antenatal vitamin K in the prevention of early neonatal intraventricular hemorrhage " Am J Obstet Gynecol 1988;159:774)

43. [F & I:•Background: Periventricular-intraventricular hemorrhage remains the most devasting neurologic event in the perinatal period and occurs in 35% to 45% of neonates who weigh <1500 gm at birth.

•About 65% of neonatal deaths are associated with intraventricular hemorrhage; 20% of survivors have moderate to severe motor and sensory impairment.

•Objective: to ascertain the efficacy of antenatal vitamin K in the prevention of early neonatal intraventricular hemorrhage.

•Material and methods: Criteria for inclusion was anticipated preterm delivery at or before 32 week's gestation with certain complications being excluded.

•Patients were randomized to

°group I, vitamin K therapy: 10 mg intramuscularly every 5 days until delivery, or

---

°group II, no vitamin K treatment.

•Antenatal **corticosteroids** (betamethasone) and/or phenobarbital were adminstered to the mother as per protocols.

•Grading of intracentricular hemorrhage was based on that proposed by Papille et al.:

°grade I, subependymal hemorrhage;

°grade II, intraventricular hemorrhage without ventricular dilatation;

°grade III, intraventricular hemorrhage with ventricular dilatation; and

°grade IV, intraventricular hemorrhage with parenchymal hemorrhage.

•Grade III and IV lesions were combined and interpreted as severe intraventricular hemorrhage.

•Respiratory distress syndrome (RDS) was graded as follows:

°mild: requiring positive pressure ventilation with a forced inspiratory oxygen value of <40%;

°moderate: mechanical ventilation with a forced inspiratory oxygen value of 40% to 70%; and

°severe: mechanical ventilation with a forced inspiratory oxygen value >70%.

•Intraventricular hemorrhage in the immature brain is the result of **rapid changes** in cerebral vascular perfusion, associated with loss of autoregulation and oftern in association with perinatal hypoxemia and hypercarbia.

°Neonatologists avoid wide fluctuations in arterial blood pressure and rapid volume expansion and with the use of pancuronium and phenobarbital while the neonate is undergoing mechanical ventilatory assistance.

°Despite these improvements in neonatal medicine, the incidence of this serious complication remains ≈ 40% in infants who weigh <1500 gm.

•About 30% of intraventricular hemorrhages occur soon after birth, and most occur within 72 hours of life.

•The earlier the lesion appears, the more progressive the lesion and the worse the prognosis, justify the need for effective antenatal intraventricular hemorrhage prophylaxis.

•Maternally adminstered phenobarbital may be useful in the prevention of intraventricular hemorrhage.

°Its mechanism of action includes transient abolition of rapid mean arterial pressure changes, decreased cerebral flow, decreased catecholamine release and decreased cerebral metabolic rate.

•Coagulation profiles were not different in cord blood between infants who developed intraventricular hemorrhage and those who did not, except for a low level of factor V in the intraventricular hemorrhage group.

°Only factor VII levels were significantly decreased in the presence of grade IV hemorrhage.

•Autopsy-proved intraventricular hemorrhage has been associated with a disseminated intravascular coagulation pattern in infants that died of RDS.

°Early hypocoagulability is determined by platelet count, fibrinogen level and and clotting times have been positively correlated with the developments of grades II to IV lesions during the first 72 hours of a premature infants life.

•Intraventricular hemorrhage and low thrombotest levels are correlated.

•Maternal serum vitamin K1 levels correlate with cord blood levels supporting the theory of transplacental passage of vitamin K.

•At least four hours are required to observe changes in the coagulation profile.

°The benefits of antenatal vitamin K as prophylaxis against intraventricular hemorrhage are limited if delivery occurs <4 hours after maternal adminstration.

•Conclusion: There is a significant improvement in prothrombin time and partial thromboplastin time in infants whose mothers were given 10 mg of vitamin K at least four hours before birth.

°Clinically, this resulted in a marked decrease in the occurrence of intraventricular hemorrhage expecially of the severe grades.]

---

44. Drugs with **a decreased** clearance during pregnancy include

    1. caffeine
    2. ethylmorphine
    3. hexobarbitone
    4. ritodrine

---

p.331   Ans: E   (Caritis SN, Lin LS, Venkataramanan R, Wong LK, "Effect of pregnancy on ritodrine pharmacokinetics," Am J Obstet Gynec   1988; 159:328)

44. [F & I:•Background: The kinetics of ritodrine have been studied primarily in non-pregnant female or male volunteers.

°Ritodrine is conjugated in the liver to the glucuronide and sulfate forms which are excreted by the kidneys.

°Some of the drug is excreted without conjugation, particularly after intravenous administration.

•Because renal blood flow, plasma volume, and protein concentrations vary in the pregnant and nonpregnant states, it is reasonable to expect that the distribution, metabolism or excretion of ritodrine may differ in pregnant and nonpregnant subjects.

•Objective: to determine if ritodrine kinetics differ in the pregnant and nonpregnant states.

•Results: There are significant differences in the pharmacokinetics of ritodrine in pregnant and nonpregnant rhesus monkeys.

•The volume of distribution of ritodrine in pregnancy is considerably **less** than that in the nonpregnant state which suggests that ritodrine binding to extravascular tissue is reduced in pregnancy.

•Because hepatic blood flow was unaltered in pregnancy and renal plasma flow and glomerular filtration are increased in pregnancy, pregnant patients might be expected to eliminate ritodrine **more rapidly** than do nonpregnant patients.

•A **slower clearance** of ritodrine in pregnancy suggests a reduced capacity to conjugate ritodrine in the liver.

°A dose of ritodrine results in higher plasma concentrations because of the smaller volume of distribution in pregnancy.

°The total amount of ritodrine delivered to the liver per unit time is substantially greater in pregnancy because blood flow to the liver is similar in pregnant and nonpregnant states.

•This suggests an inhibition in pregnancy of enzymes required for ritodrine conjugation.

°Similar effects of pregnancy on hepatic metabolic activity are seen with other drugs.

°Progesterone and estradiol are competitive inhibitors of microsomal oxidases for drugs such as ethylmorphine and hexobarbitol.

°Estrogens have a cholestatic effect that may prolong the half-life of certain drugs.

°A well-recognized example of the effect of pregnancy of drug metabolism is caffeine, a drug eliminated primarily by hepatic metabolism.

°**In pregacy, the clearance of caffeine is approximately one fourth that in the nonpregnant state.**

•If ritrodrine clearance is **reduced** in human pregnancy, a given dosage will produce higher ritodrine concentrations in pregnancy than expected from that in men and nonpregnant women.

°Some side effects of ritodrine therapy such as chest pain, shortness of breath, and vomiting may be related to the plasma concentration or the rate of rise of plasma concentration.

°These side effects might be minimized if ritodrine infusion regimen was altered to reflect the pharmacokinetics of the drug in pregnancy.]

---

45. Causes of subnormal insulin requirements during gestation include

    1. increased exercise
    2. placental failure
    3. decreasing renal function
    4. hypothyroidism

---

p.444   Ans: E   (Jovanovic-Peterson L, Peterson CM, "De novo clinical hypothyroidism in pregnancies complicated by type I diabetes, subclinical hypothyroidism, and proteinuria: A new syndrome," Am J Obstet Gynec   1988; 159:442)

45. [F & I:•Background: Laboratory evidence of thyroid abnormalities in patients with type I (insulin dependent) diabetes is as high as 40%.

°This may be the result of the generalized autoimmune response found in most such patients that may progress to either hyperthyroidism or hypothyroidism.

•Pregnancy is associated with an increased prevalence of thyroid abnormalities.

•Objectives:

°to document the prevalence of new onset clinical hypothyroidism during pregnancy complicated by type I diabetes mellitus and

°to elucidate prognostic indicators of incipent decreased thyroid function based on evidence of first trimester subclinical hypothyroidism.

•Results: Abnormalities of thyroid function tests may be present in up to 50% of pregnant women with type I diabetes with a **normal serum T4 level as determined by RIA.**

•Women with diabetes at risk for the development of clinical hypothyroidism during gestation had abnormal thyroid tests (elevated antithyroid antibody levels or elevated TSH levels) during the first trimester and developed urinary proteinuria >4 gm/24 hr during gestation concomitant with a relatively low insulin requirement, low T4 level and elevated TSH level.

°The insulin requirement rose to normal within two weeks of thyroid replacement.

°The degree of proteinuria did not change with thyroid replacement.

°Proteinuria and autoimmune thyroid disease is independant of thyroid globulin in microsomal antibody levels.

•**The normal increase in serum T4 levels during gestation is attributed to estrogen-induced elevations of thyroid binding globulin.**

°The level of free or metabolically active hormone is unchanged.

°The thyroid gland must increase T4 production to maintain adequate levels of free hormone.

°Women who become hypothyroid during gestation may have compromised thyroid reserve inadequate to meet the demands of pregnancy combined with a loss of protein-bound hormone into the urine.

•Patients with new onset clinical hypothyroidism failed to showed the normal incremental increase in insulin requirment at 20 ± 2 weeks gestation.

°The insulin requirement is relatively uniform in pregnancies complicated by diabetes.

°Hypothyroidism is a cause of subnormal insulin requirements during gestation; other causes include decreased food consumption and subsequent weight loss, increased exercise, placental failure and/or decreasing renal function.

°The hypothyroid diabetic pregnant women in this study sustained renal function as reflected by normal values for creatinine clearance despite proteinuria between 4 and 11 gm/24 hr.

•Type I diabetic pregnant women should be monitored by determinations of T4 and TSH levels and thyroid antibody titers.

°Studies should include free T4 and/or free T4 index.

•**The best evidence of true hypothyroidism is the elevated TSH levels.**

•Without a free T4 measurement, it is impossible to conclude that the T4 RIA level is truly low because it might be low due to the loss of thyroid binding globulin, as is seen in nephrotic syndrome.

•The fetus has an independant pituitary-thyroid axis by 20 weeks of gestation and is probably not at risk from maternal hypothyroidism; however women who develop hypothyroidism during gestation warrant further thyroid surveillance post partum.

•Conclusion: There is a group of patients with subclinical thyroid dysfunction in the first trimester of pregnancy which may progress to clinical hypothyroidism probably due to chronic thyroiditis.

•Pregnant women with diabetes who have no evidence of thyroid dysfunction in the first trimester despite developing proteinuria will not develop progressive thyroid dysfunction.

•Pregnant women with diabetes with sub-clinical thyroid disease in the first trimester, who do not have significant proteinuria, will not progress to clinical hypothyroidism during pregnancy.]

---

46. Clinically useful in managing pregnancies of women who have circulating lupus anticoagulant antibodies

    1. aspirin
    2. umbilical artery flow velocity waveforms
    3. prednisone
    4. cyclosporin

---

p.215   Ans: A (Trudinger B, Stewart G, Cook C, Connelly A, and Exner T. "Monitoring lupus anticoagulant-positive pregnancies with umbilical artery flow velocity waveforms" Obstet Gynecol 1988;72:215)

46 [F & I:•Background: A high incidence of pregnancy loss, both early and late, is associated with the presence in maternal blood of the lupus anticoagulant autoantibody.

°Seven fetuses out of 160 reported survived without treatment, and all were growth retarded.

•Successful pregnancy outcome with fetal survival has been achieved by treating the mother with aspirin and prednisone throughout pregnancy.

°A high dose of prednisone is required to suppress antibody activity, and such therapy is not without risk.

°Aspirin has been used because thrombosis dominates the clinical presentation.

°The most common pathologic finding is decidual and placental vascular thrombosis and placental infarction.

•Vascular pathology in the placenta may be monitored using umbilical artery flow velocity waveforms with Doppler ultrasound.

°The waveforms are analyzed by indices that measure downstream resistance, such as the systolic/diastolic (A/B) ratio or pulsatility indices.

°A high resistance indicated by a high S/D ratio has been correlated with vascular pathology.

•Objective: to report umbilical artery flow velocity waveforms in six pregnancies of four women positive for lupus anticoagulant to detect the development of placental vascular pathology.

•The key points in management were detailed antenatal care, with very close fetal surveillance from 24 weeks onward, and a preparedness to deliver the pregnancy at any time after 28 weeks when an increasing umbilical placental vascular resistance was indicated by a rising umbilical artery systolic/diastolic ratio.

•Results: All pregnancies were delivered **electively** in the third trimester and produces and live born infant that survived the neonatal period.

•An interesting feature of 5 of the pregnancies was the birth of an infant with a weight appropriate for gestational age.

°Thrombosis in the placental vessels over a long period may be expected to lead to chronic placental insufficiency and fetal growth retardation.

°The appropriate birth weight and the development of abnormality in the umbilical artery waveform over only a short form suggests an acute process causing rapid deterioration in fetal welfare.

•In the usual situation of placental insufficiency not associated with lupus anticoagulant, the change in the umbilical artery waveform precedes by several weeks any fetal heart rate monitoring evidence of impending fetal death.

•Prednisone and aspirin were not used in the management of these patients, but these patients did not have other clinical features of active systemic lupus erythematosus that might have indicated such therapy.

°The process of thrombosis (possibly attenuated) can occur during therapy.

°Aspirin alone may be sufficient to prevent the acute thrombotic process in the fetal placental circulation.

•Because it is possible to record umbilical artery flow velocity waveforms from 14 to 16 weeks onward, beginning study at that time in the high-risk patients would be better than commencing at 24-28 weeks.

°This would permit detection of patients developing placental vascular pathology before 24 weeks.

°Although early delivery is not a therapy option in this group, it is possible that drug therapy instituted then may be of benefit in maintaining the uteroplacental and umbilical-placental circulation.]

---

47. Clinically useful in determining fetal pulmonary maturity, amniotic fluid

    1.   cholesteryl palmitate
    2.   urea nitrogen
    3.   phosphatidyl glycerol
    4.   acyl transferase

---

p.361   Ans: A (Ludmir J, Alvarez JG, Landon MB, Gabbe SG, Mennuti MT and Touchstone JC, "Amniotic fluid cholesteryl palmitate in pregnancies complicated by diabetes mellitus " Obstet Gynecol 1988;71:360)

47. [F & I:•Background: Amniotic fluid cholesteryl palmitate appears to be as very sensitive and specific predictor for the risk of respiratory distress syndrome (RDS) in normal pregnancies.

°RDS does not occur when the cholesteryl palmitate concentration is 41 µg/mg or higher.

•Objective: to measure amniotic fluid cholesteryl palmitate concentration from pregnancies complicated by diabetes mellitus and compare it with concentrations from a nondiabetic population to determine whether diabetes and glycemic control could affect the concentration of cholesteryl palmitate.

•Results: No difference in total lecithin concentration was noted between groups.

•The appearance of phosphatidyglycerol may be delayed in pregnancies complicated by diabetes.

°Many clinicians rely on the presence of amniotic fluid phosphatidylglycerol before undertaking elective delivery of the diabetic patient.

•The source and possible role of cholesterol esters in amniotic fluid are unknown.

°Cholesteryl palmitate may be a transport intermediate for palmitic acid, which facilitates esterification to yield saturated phosphatidylcholine.

°Cholesteryl palmitate may also be involved in the storage of fatty acids in the lung for later esterification.

•Amniotic fluid cholesteryl palmitate levels are significantly lower in pregnancies complicated by diabetes than in control patients at the same gestational age.

°This difference was even greater for insulin-dependent diabetics, despite good glycemic control as demonstrated by normal third-trimester glycosylated hemoglobin values.

•An increased concentration of nonesterified fatty acids may be present in the fetal lung when pregnancy is complicated by diabetes.

°Nonesterified fatty acids could inhibit new synthesis of palmitic acid and possibly cholestryl palmitate by type II pneumocytes.

°If there is an increase in nonesterified fatty acids in diabetics, and if these fatty acids contribute to fetal macrosomia, then LGA status might be expected to be associated with lower levels of cholesteryl palmitate in amniotic fluid.

°Although lower cholesteryl palmitate levels were obtained in LGA infants of diabetic mothers, the difference was not statistically significant.

•Another possible mechanism for decreased levels of cholesteryl plamitate in pregnancies complicated by diabetes could involve different levels of activity for acyl transferase enzyme, allowing the reaction between cholesterol and phosphatidylcholine.]

---

48. Patients are at increased risk for late abortion if they have Group B streptococcus colonization of their

    1. vagina
    2. uterine cervix
    3. urethra
    4. pharynx

---

p.30   Ans: A (Daugaard HO, Thomsen AC, Henriques U, Østergaard A, "Group B streptococci in the lower urogenital tract and late abortions" Am J Obstet Gynecol 1988;158: 28)

48. [F & I:•Background: There is a correlation between early rupture of the fetal membranes, preterm delivery, and the occurrence of group B streptococci in the lower urogenital tract.

°The group B streptococci in the urine has been associated with a significant increase in the frequency of primary rupture of membranes and preterm delivery.

•Objective: to compare the occurrence of group B streptococci in the urine, cervix, and vagina of women with spontaneous abortion and women with uncomplicated pregnancy and to evaluate the abortion rate in women with group B streptococci in the urine.

•Material and Methods: Women admitted to the hospital with signs of threatened abortion, such as vaginal bleeding, contractions, or escape of amniotic fluid, between 12 and 28 weeks of gestations were included.

°Examinations for group B streptococci was performed on clean-voided midstream urine specimens with a calibrated loop technique and on swabs from the uterine cervix and vagina.

•Amniotic fluids samples were collected by transabdominal puncture and examined for occurrence of group B streptococci.

•A total of 150 women with signs of abortion were included. Abortion occurred in 71 women and recovery occurred in 79.

•Group B streptococci occur in the lower urogenital tract of approximately 20% of pregnant women and seem to predispose to premature rupture of the membranes and preterm deliveries.

•Group B streptococci were isolated significantly more frequently from the lower urogenital tract of women with abortion than from a control group.

°A causal relationship seems reasonable, as group B streptococci were isolated as the only bacterial species from amniotic fluid collected by transabdominal amniocentesis in some of these patients with intact membranes.

°Group B streptococci were cultured from the blood and other viscera of two fetuses with histologic evidence of inflammation who were delivered by these mothers.

•The isolation of group B streptococci from amniotic fluid in patients with intact membranes suggests that the bacteria are capable of crossing the membranes.

•The occurrence of antibody-coated bacteria in amniotic fluid suggests that bacterial have been in contact with immunocompetent tissue, as IgA, IgG, and IgM antibodies.

•The women at risk seem to be those who have group B streptococci in the urine.

°The degree of significance between the colonization rate in the urine of women with signs of abortion and in that of normally pregnant women was high.

°In patients with symptoms delivery occurred significantly more frequently in women with group B streptococci, than in those without.

•Results: Abortion occurred in 85% of women with group B streptococci in the urine, and 42% of women with no group B streptococci in the urine.

°The occurrence of bacteria in the urine indicates a high degree of pathogenicity of the bacteria or a decreased defense of the host, because real urinary tract infection was confirmed in only a few cases by symptoms including associated pyuria.]

49. At 22 weeks a pregnancy is judged to be growth retarded and an ultrasound is ordered. Findings which dictate a karyotype be obtained include

    1.   club foot
    2.   diaphragmatic hernia
    3.   facial defect
    4.   ventricular septal defect

p.408   Ans: A (Benacerraf BR, Miller WA,and Frigoletto FD, "Sonographic detection of fetuses with trisomies 13 and 18: Accuracy and limitations," Am J Obstet Gynecol 1988;158:404)

49. [F & I:•Objective: to examine the accuracy and ability of prenatal sonography to identify fetuses with trisomies 13 and 18 and

•to identify the most common sonographic abnormalities associated with these chromosomal defects.

•**Trisomy 18** has an incidence of 0.3/1000 births and is one of the most common chromosomal defects associated with multiple malformations.

•The most common abnormalities seen in fetuses with trisomy 18

°a fixed, clinched fist with overlapping index finger,

°limb reduction abnormalities,

°rocker-bottom or clubfeet,

°congenital heart disease,

°hernias such as diaphragmatic, umbilical, or inguinal,

°abnormalities of the kidneys,

°poor growth, and

°associated polyhydramnios.

•**Trisomy 13** has an incidence of one in 5000 births.

•Features of trisomy 13 include

°holoprosencephaly and associated facial abnormalities of the midline,

°polydactyly,

°congenital heart disease,

°omphalocele, and

°polycystic kidneys.

•Fetuses with trisomy 13 and 18 have a poor outcome.

°The mean survival for an infant with trisomy 13 is 130 days and 48 days for infants with trisomy 18.

•Because fetuses with trisomy 18 have associated severe intrauterine growth retardation, there is a high rate of cesarean section for fetal distress in pregnancies with trisomy 18.

•The high rate of an associated chromosomal abnormality in a fetus with congenital clubfoot was 22.2%.

•Three fetuses with trisomy 18 had diaphragmatic hernias.

•Trisomies 13 and 18 have a very high rate of congenital heart disease (90% to 99%).

•Ventricular septal defects and other minor defects represent a large proportion of these cardiac anomalies and are known to be less optimally identified sonographically, particularly in the second trimester, and therefore not helpful in suggesting further work-up for the vast majority of cases.

•Conclusion: Abnormalities of the face, particularly when associated with other congenital abnormalities, and anomalies of the hands and feet, as well as diaphragmatic hernia, represent indications for prenatal cytogenetic diagnosis.]

---

50. True statements about neurofibromatosis include

    1. It is inherited as an autosomal dominant.
    2. Non-toxemic hypertension is an invariable feature.
    3. There is an increased incidence of pheochromocytoma.
    4. Chorionic villus sampling can be used to detect affected fetuses.

---

p.388   Ans: A   (Blickstein I, Lancet M, and Shoham Z, "The obstetric perspective of neurofibromatosis," Am J Obstet Gynecol 1988;158:385)

50. [F & I:•Neurofibromatosis is a common hereditary trait in humans.

•The term neurofibromatosis was coined after the German pathologist Friedrich Daniel von Recklinghausen's report in 1882, but the condition was described earlier by Smith in 1849.

•The earliest obstetric description was probably by Brickner, in 1906, who termed the disease "fibroma molluscum gravidarum."

•The classical von Recklinghausen's neurofibromatosis is inherited in an autosomal-dominant way.

    °Both sexes are equally affected.

    °The penetrance is almost 100% but the expressivity is highly variable.

•**Expressivity** is the **extent** to which an inheritable trait is manifested by an **individual** carrying the principle gene or genes that determine it.

•**Penetrance** is the **frequency** in which an inheritable trait manifested by **individual**S carrying the principle gene or genes conditioning it.

•The **mutation rate is very high,** since only 50% to 60% of affected individuals have inherited the disease from one of their parents and the remainder show new mutations.

    °A high mutation rate suggests that neurofibromatosis is a heterogeneous entity and may be caused by several mutations.

•Affected children born to affected mothers had an overall severity **greater** than that of diseased children born to affected fathers or children with new mutations.

•Progression of neurofibromatosis is always **unpredictable** but always unidirectional to higher grades.

•The neural crest is the source of cellular elements affected by the gene defect.

•**Nerve growth factor**, a protein responsible for growth and differentiation of neural crest-derived cells, seems to have a central role in the pathogenesis of neurofibromatosis.

•Pathogenesis of neurofibromatosis: hypothesis #1:

°The primary defect resides in the secretory membrane system of the Golgi complex and the endoplasmic reticulum and causes a defect in cell-cell interactions.

°Mast cells probably participate in this mode of pathogenesis.

•Hypothesis #2 indicates a hypothalamic defect that influence pigmentation, growth, and neural function.

•Nerve growth factor has been detected in normal amniotic fluid.

•Hyperpigmentation doesn't seem to be a consideration in pregnancy.

•Neurofibromas appear about puberty.

°Their size and number increase steadily in both men and women, but growth is especially noticed during gestation.

•During pregnancy massive hemorrhage into the rapidly growing tumor may cause profound anemia.

°The growth of pelvic tumors during pregnancy can cause dystocia.

°Macrocephaly seems to develop after birth.

°At least 2% of patients with neurofibromatosis have a distortion of the spine.

°When affecting the lower spine, kyphoscoliosis can cause fetal malposition and lead to dystocia because of pelvic contraction.

°Cardiopulmonary function may be compromised by the deformed thoracic cage.

•During pregnancy, central nervous system tumors grow and can produce acute morbidity requiring neurosurgery because of the life-threatening symptoms.

•The incidence of **pheochromocytoma** in patients with neurofibromatosis is 1% to 5%.

°During gestation, symptoms of a chromaffin tumor can be confused with those of essential hypertension and preeclampsia.

°Pregnancy in a patients with pheochromocytoma is frequently catastrophic, with mortality figures of 40% to 50%.

°Profound postpartum shock, often after a slight trauma, suggests the diagnosis.

°°Fluctuating hypertension, especially in the first two trimesters of gestation, concomitant with neurofibromatosis, suggests pheochromocytoma.

•Neurofibromatosis affects the smaller arteries and arterioles in a distinct manner, and these changes may lead, in extreme cases, to rupture with massive hemorrhage.

•Management: Before conception each patient should undergo evaluation and grading.

•Patients with grade III to IV should be advised not to conceive and the need for tubal sterilization should be discussed.

°Patients with a minimal or mild form (*formes frustes*) of the disease should be further evaluated.

•Assays for pheochromocytoma, and brain and spine radiologic examination should be done.

•During pregnancy patients with neurofibromatosis should be carefully evaluated by the high-risk pregnancy unit.

°There is no available antenatal diagnosis of affected fetuses.

•Contraception: **Hormonal contraception** in patients with neurofibromatosis may have **adverse** affects because sex steroids affect the disease.

°Barrier methods and intrauterine contraceptive devices are alternatives to the use of steroids, provided that no pelvic tumor is present that may reduce the safety and efficacy of the devices.

°Tubal sterilization appears to be the safest choice and is definitely indicated in the moderate and severe (grade III to IV) forms of neurofibromatosis.]

---

51. Decreased levels of microvillar enzymes (including alkaline phosphatase, γ–glutamyl transpeptidase) are associated with

    1. chromosomal aneuploidies
    2. fetal structural malformations
    3. normal fetuses
    4. cystic fibrosis

---

p.947   Ans: E   (Gilbert F, Tsao KL, Mendoza A, Mulivor R, Gluckson MM and Denning CR, "Prenatal diagnostic options in cystic fibrosis " Am J Obstet Gynecol 1987;158:947)

51. [F & I:•Background: **Cystic fibrosis** is the most common autosomal recessive disorder in the white population.

•Prenatal diagnosis in cystic fibrosis is the result of two events.

°First ,the discovery that pregnancies resulting in cystic fibrosis-affected homozygotes are often characterized by **reduced** levels of certain microvillar enzymes (including alkaline phosphatase, γ– glutamyl transpeptidase, and leucine aminopeptidase) in amniotic fluid in the second trimester.

°°This reflects a **partial intestinal obstruction** that develops in most cystic fibrosis-homozygous fetuses in the second trimester, blocking the outflow of intestinal contents, including sloughed mucosal cells (containing microvillar enzymes), into amniotic fluid.

°Second, the report of tight linkage between the gene for cystic fibrosis and deoxyribonucleic acid (DNA) sequences mapped to the long arm of chromosome 7 (7q).

•Objective: to determine limitations of amniotic fluid enzyme analysis and/or DNA family studies.

•In microvillar enzyme analysis in amniotic fluid both false positive and false negatives occur.

°**False positives** (i.e. predicted to be affected prenatally and then found to be unaffected after birth) have been found with chromosomal aneuploidies, fetal structural malformations, and in a normal fetus.

°Reduced enzyme activities in the amniotic fluid in each instance could be the result of intestinal obstruction, which can be pathologic (e.g., caused by intestinal malrotation, extrinsic obstruction by a tumor, or vascular malformation, etc.) or may reflect a transient, physiologic variation (e.g., the result of inspissated or thickened meconium).

°**False negatives** (i.e. predicted unaffected prenatally and then proved affected after birth) may result from misdating of the pregnancy (the levels of microvillar enzyme activities in the amniotic fluid generally decrease between weeks 16 and 21 in gestation), and possibly from clinical variation in the disease.

•The combined frequency of false positives and false negatives in different series ranges from 2% to 10%, which gave microvillar enzyme analysis of the amniotic fluid for cystic fibrosis a predictive accuracy as high as 98%.

•Problems with cystic fibrosis-linked recombinant DNA probes are:

°(1) Not every family is appropriate for testing.

°(2) Not every family is informative.

°(3) The interpretation of results can be complicated by recombination in meiosis.

•During the formation of sperm and egg, the chromosome number is halved (from 46 to 23 in humans).

°Early in the chromosome reduction divisions (meiosis), the two members of a chromosome pair join and frequently exchange segments or sequences between themselves.

°This exchange is called **recombination**, and the likelihood of recombination between two genes on a chromosome is directly proportional to the distance separating them on the chromosome (i.e. the farther apart the genes, the greater the chance of recombination).

°Three generally available markers linked to cystic fibrosis are **close** to one another and the cystic fibrosis gene; the recombination frequencies of each in a large number of families studied are between 0% and 5%.

•Conclusion: Counseling of families with a cystic fibrosis-affected person is as follows:

°For families in which a living child with cystic fibrosis and both parents are available, DNA screening with the available chromosome 7q-specific probes is recommended.

°If they are **fully informative** (both parents heterozygous for at least one 7q-specific marker), they have two prenatal diagnostic options; a first-trimester test (chorionic villus biopsy) or second-trimester amniocentesis.

°If a couple is only **partially informative** (only one parent heterozygous), they can have an amniocentesis in the second trimester with both the amniotic fluid microvillar enzyme studies and restriction fragment length polymorphism analysis of fetal amniocytes.

°For families in which DNA analysis is **inappropriate or uninformative,** the only available option is amniocentesis with microvillar enzyme analysis of the amniotic fluid.

°°This option is offered to couples with an a priori one in four risk for cystic fibrosis (previous child with cystic fibrosis) and to those with a family history of cystic fibrosis and a reduced risk (e.g., given a white population frequency of 1/1600 with a "carrier" frequency of 1/20, the risk for a pregnancy in a couple in which one partner is a known carrier is 1/80; for a couple in which one partner's sibling is affected, the risk of an affected fetus is 1/120, etc.)

°**In pregnancies with a risk less than one in four, it is important that the couple understand that the risk of a false positive or a false negative (2% to 10%, depending on the series) is greater than the actual numerical risk.**

•Presently, prenatal testing for cystic fibrosis cannot be offered to the general public because the only available test, amniotic fluid microvillar enzyme analysis, has a false positive risk that is considerably higher (2% to 5%) than the a priori population risk for cystic fibrosis (1/1600).]

---

52. The clinical course of patients with diabetic nephropathy who become pregnant is frequently marked by

    1.   increased incidence of cesarean section
    2.   exacerbation of proteinuria
    3.   elevation of blood pressure
    4.   development of nephrotic syndrome

---

p.64   Ans: E   (Reece AE, Coustan DR, Hayslett JP, Holford T, Coulehan J, O'Conner TZ, and Hobbins JC. "Diabetic nephropathy: Pregnancy performance and fetomaternal outcome," Am J Obstet Gynec   1988; 159:56)

52 [F & I:•Background: Diabetic nephropathy is a complication of diabetes mellitus and occurs in 30% to 40% of patients with insulin-dependent (type I) and approximately 50% of subjects with noninsulin-dependent diabetes (type II).

•In type I disease, renal insufficiency eventually occurs in all patients who exhibit macroproteinuria, whereas in type II disease a deterioration is found in only 5% to 10%.

•There are five stages in the course of type I diabetic nephropathy.

°1. Early hypertrophy-hyperfunction.

°2. Glomerular lesions without clinical disease.

°3. Incipient nephropathy characterized by microproteinuria.

°4. Overt nephropathy characterized by macroproteinuria.

°5. End-stage diabetic renal disease.

•Pregnancies complicated by overt clinical nephropathy are at increased risk for fetomaternal morbidity and perinatal mortality.

•Objectives: to examine the effects of diabetic nephropathy on maternal blood chemistry and renovascular function during pregnancy,

°to assess maternal and neonatal outcomes, and

°to evaluate maternal and infant status at long-term follow-up.

•Material and Methods: Patients were classified as having **diabetic nephropathy** if the urinary protein level was ≥300 mg/24 hr before the third trimester.

•Patients were classified as having **renal insufficiency** if the creatinine level was >1.2 mg./dl or creatinine clearance was <90 ml/min in the absence of urinary tract infection and other causes of primary or secondary renal disease.

•The severity of the proteinuria was categorized as mild (300 to 499 mg/24 hr), moderate (500 to 3000 mg/24 hr), and severe or nephrotic syndrome (>3 gm/24 hr).

•A major goal in maternal management was normalization of blood glucose levels (average plasma values <120 mg/dl).

•Patients were usually not treated with antihypertensive medications unless the diastolic blood pressure exceeded 105 mm Hg, because fetal and maternal outcomes are reported to be satisfactory even in mild to moderate hypertension (diastolic pressure >90 and <110 mm Hg).

•Preferred medications to control hypertension included α-**methyldopa or hydralazine.**

•Patients taking diuretics for hypertension before pregnancy maintained the same therapy (hydrochlorothiazide or furosemide) throughout pregnancy.

•Because the diagnosis of preeclampsia is difficult to confirm in patients with nephropathy, criteria for diagnosis included worsening of hypertension (>15% increase in systolic or diastolic blood pressure) or deterioration of renal function associated with multisystemic involvement, resulting in abnormal liver function tests and coagulation studies, particularly elevation in the fibrin split products and thrombocytopenia.

•Pregnancies were allowed to continue to term and were delivered vaginally if possible, after the establishment of fetal pulmonic maturity.

•Anemia (hemoglobin <10 gm/dl) in 13 pregnancies (42%), preeclampsia in 11 (35%), and congestive heart failure in 2 (6%), were also found.

•In utero fetal deaths occurred in two patients (6%), with the remaining 29 pregnancies culminating in the birth of a living child at a mean gestational age of 36 ± 2.7 weeks.

°Stillbirths occurred at 28 and 24 weeks in two patients with poor blood glucose control.

•Two neonates had birth defects (ventricular septal defect and a large patent ductus arteriosus), and in both of these pregnancies the maternal first trimester glucose control had been unsuccessful.

•Antepartum fetal heart rate testing results were abnormal in seven pregnancies (23%) and were the most common indication for a primary cesarean section.

°Other indications included malposition in two (6%), worsening maternal disease in three (10%).

•Among the seven pregnancies delivered because of abnormal antepartum fetal heart rate testing respiratory distress syndrome occurred in 5 (84%).

•At the initial antepartum visit 39% had renal insufficiency, 26% exhibited heavy proteinuria (>3.0 gm/24 hr), and 26% had a diastolic blood pressure ≥90 mm Hg.

•During the course of pregnancy the incidence of renal insufficiency increased to 45% and included four subjects with a serum creatinine value ≥2.0 mg/dl and an increase in heavy proteinuria to 71%.

•Diastolic hypertension (≥90 mm Hg) was observed at some time during pregnancy in 18 patients (58%).

•Proliferative retinopathy was present in 68% of cases.

•The decline in glomerular filtration rate and increase in proteinuria during pregnancy in these patients remains unexplained.

•The severity of proteinuria regressed postpartum to levels comparable to first trimester or preconception values.

°This pregnancy-related transient increase in protein excretion in patients with preexisting proteinuria parallels those of normal pregnancy, and may be from an increase in the amount of filtered protein, a decrease in tubular reabsorption of filtered protein, or both.

•The natural course of diabetic nephropathy in this series was not adversely affected by pregnancy.

•Complications of fetal growth and development were considerable and included stillbirths (6.5%), primary cesarean section (48.5%), major congenital abnormalities (nearly 10%).

°Preterm deliveries occurred in 32% of pregnancies and 16% of infants were small for gestational age.

•In addition, neonatal complications of respiratory disease, hypoglycemia, and hyperbilirubinemia were high.

°These rates occurred despite reasonably good control of blood glucose levels in second and third trimesters.

•The low infant birth weight in the present series most strongly correlated with gestational age and serum creatinine level.]

---

53. True statements about chorionic villus sampling include

    1.   Use in twin pregnancies has not yet been established.
    2.   When mosaicism is observed, subsequent amniocentesis is indicated.
    3.   MSAFP (maternal serum alpha-fetoprotein) levels are falsely elevated following CVS, negating their usefulness in second trimester.
    4.   Fetal loss is not significantly different from unsampled matched patients.

---

p.211   Ans: C (Green JE, Dorfmann A, Jones SL, Bender S, Patton L, Schulman JD, "Chorionic villus sampling: Experience with an initial 940 cases. " Obstet Gynecol 1988;71: 208)

53. [F & I:•Background: Chorionic villus sampling offers several advantages over amniocentesis.

°It is performed at nine to 11 weeks of gestation, compared with 14.5-16 weeks for amniocentesis.

°Earlier diagnosis provides the possibility for earlier pregnancy termination, which appears to reduce the social and psychological burdens of second-trimester abortion as well as the fivefold increased risk of maternal mortality associated with abortion during the 16-24th week gestation.

°Whereas karyotyping using amniocentesis requiring 1.5-4 weeks to complete, chorionic villus sampling offers cytogenetic analysis results within several days.

°Genetic disorders can be diagnosed immediately by analysis of sample tissue obviating extended processing.

•Complication rates in chorionic villi sampling are similar to those of amniocentesis, chorionic villi sampling may become the preferred prenatal diagnostic method.

•Objective: To report an initial 1000 chorionic villus sampling procedure experience.

•Materials and Methods: Chorionic villus sampling was not performed if the patient had an acute vaginal infection, positive cervical culture for *Neisseria gonorrhoeae,* or active herpes until treated.

•Sampling was generally performed during the ninth through 11 week of gestation, although a few samples were obtained in the eighth or 12th weeks

•Villus tissue was obtained under ultrasound guidance by passing a Portex catheter transcervically to the chorion frondosum.

•All patients had follow-up sonograms one to two weeks after sampling, and most had follow up sonography again at 16 weeks of gestation

•The indication for chorionic villus sampling in approximately 90% of patients was **maternal age** close to or > 35 at delivery.

•At initial ultrasound evaluation, 108 patients (10.3%) were determined to have abnormal gestational sacs, and chorionic villus sampling was not performed.

°All these cases resulted in spontaneous abortion.

•Several patients with a twin pregnancy or abnormal vaginal bleeding did not have chorionic villus sampling performed.

•Over 80% of patients required only one catheter insertion.

•Chorionic villi could not be obtained in six cases.

°In five cases, this failure was due to the presence of obvious cervical fibroids on sonography.

•Chorionic villus sampling was performed in nine sets of twins, and fetal loss occurred in one of these sets.

•Most patients bled for one to several days after the procedure.

•One case of marked oligohydramnios was discovered in the second trimester, and was associated with bilateral cystic renal disease.

•Complications: Two patients developed symptoms of possible intrauterine infection within two weeks after chorionic villus sampling.

°In one, there was a fetal loss.

°There were 3 other fetal deaths within one week of chorionic villus sampling with no maternal symptoms and no sonographic abnormalities.

°There were two pregnancies in which chorionic villus sampling was followed by persistent maternal vaginal staining for several weeks in the presence of a subchorionic hematoma, followed by fetal death.

°One of these pregnancies was twins.

•Results: Thirty-nine cytogenetic abnormalities, representing 4.2% of the patients sampled were discovered.

°Mosaicism on direct preparations accounted for one-third of these aberrations.

°**Amniocentesis was always recommended when mosaicism was detected** by chorionic villus sampling, amniocentesis detected no cytogenetic abnormalities in the 12 mosaic cases for which this was performed.

•Amniocentesis was ultimately performed on 34 gravidas representing 3.6 of those who intended to have fetal diagnosis by chorionic villus sampling.

°In 6 patients amniocentesis was required because chorionic villus tissue could not be obtained, and in 12 patients because mosaicism was detected.

•Ten percent of patients chorionic villus sampling were found to carry abnormal gestational sacs by ultrasound.

•Concern has been raised that villus sampling might falsely elevate MSAFP levels, resulting in an inappropriately increased number of amniocentesis for MSAFP determination.

°**MSAFP levels from patients who underwent chorionic villus sampling were not significantly different from those in controls at 15-18 weeks' gestation.**

•Patients who who have chorionic villus sampling should be informed in advance that there is about a 2-3% chance that subsequent amniocentesis might also be indicated.

Conclusion: Chorionic villus sampling in singleton pregnancies is a relatively safe procedure with risks similar to those with amniocentesis.

•Twin pregnancies can be analyzed by chorionic villus sampling when both sacs are clearly delineated and easily accessible.]

---

54. Indicated in the evaluation of the fetus at risk for non-immune hydrops

    1.   maternal mean corpuscular hemoglobin
    2.   maternal Coombs' test
    3.   fetal hemoglobin electrophoresis
    4.   fetal karyotype

---

p.189   Ans: E   (Hsieh FJ, Chang JM, Huang HC, Lu CC, Ko TS, Chen HY, "Umbilical vein blood flow measurement in nonimmune hydrops fetalis " Obstet Gynecol 1988;71: 188)

54. [F & I:•Background: Some nonimmune hydrops fetalis, such as fetal supraventricular tachycardia, responds to in utero treatment.

°Nonimmune hydrops fetalis, e.g., that associated with hemoglobin Bart's, is fatal and causes severe maternal morbidity.

•Hemoglobin Bart's hydrops fetalis is a severe form of α–thalassemia with autosomal recessive inheritance and a 25% recurrence rate in each pregnancy.

°It is the major cause of nonimmune hydrops fetalis in Southeast Asia and Taiwan.

•**Pulsed Doppler duplex sonography** is able to measure the fetal blood flow in utero noninvasively.

•High fetal umbilical vein blood flow occurs in pregnancies complicated by rhesus-isoimmunization.

•Objective: to investigate the hemodynamic characteristics of nonimmune hydrops fetalis by measuring umbilical vein blood flow.

•Materials and Methods: Twenty-two cases of nonimmune hydrops fetalis had umbilical vein blood flow measured.

•Tests to find the underlying cause of nonimmune hydrops fetalis included:

°1) maternal mean corpuscular volume and **Coombs' test,**

°2) fetal cord blood sampling (taken by percutaneous ultrasound guided fetal blood sampling or obtained at delivery) for hemoglobin electrophoresis and karyotyping, and

°3) autopsy for pathology examination.

°tests to rule out perinatal infection.

•Results: Among the 22 cases of nonimmune hydrops fetalis, 15 proved to be hemoglobin Bart's hydrops fetalis.

°The remaining 7 cases included one case of fetal lung sequestration, one case of fetal congenital heart disease (ventricular septal defect plus atrial septal defect), one case of fetal trisomy 16, and four cases of unknown etiology.

•The mean umbilical **vein** blood velocity in fetuses with hemoglobin Bart's hydrops fetalis was consistently higher than that of non-Bart's group.

•Explanations are as follows:

°1) The fetus attempts to compensate for insufficient tissue oxygenation by increasing its umbilical circulation; or

°2) There is an alteration of blood viscosity due to the decreased red cell mass caused by fetal hemolytic anemia.

•In hemoglobin Bart's hydrops fetalis, there is total absence of α-globin chain synthesis.

°The affected fetus is grossly hydropic, with marked hemolytic anemia and hepatosplenomegaly.

•Because hemoglobin Bart's has a very **high** oxygen affinity, the bulk of hemoglobin in these fetuses **cannot deliver oxygen** effectively to the tissues.

°The cause of hydropic change and death is **severe hypoxia.**

°The mechanism of increased blood velocity in hemoglobin Bart's fetalis may be similar to that in Rh-isoimmunization, ie, compensatory increase of umbilical circulation and lower blood viscosity resulting from fetal hemolytic anemia.

•The **umbilical vein diameter was increased** in the group with hemoglobin Bart's hydrops.

°Some active vasodilatation in the umbilical vessel contributed to the umbilical vein dilation observed in Rh-isoimmunization.]

---

55. Effects of maternal administration of indomethacin include

   1.   closure of the patent ductus in the fetus
   2.   decrease in amniotic fluid volume
   3.   tocolysis of preterm labor
   4.   decrease in fetal levels of ADH

---

p.53   Ans: A   (Kirshon B, Moise Jr KJ, Wasserstrum N, Ou C-N, and Huhta JN,"Influence of short-term indomethacin therapy on fetal urine output" Obstet Gynecol 1988;71:51)

55. [F & I:•Background: Indomethacin in preterm labor has been used to inhibit prostaglandin (PG) synthesis.

   °Indomethacin can close a patent ductus arteriosus in premature infants; but has been associated with transient renal dysfunction.

•Objective: to evaluate the effect of maternal indomethacin on fetal urine output when used to treat preterm labor.

•Material and Methods: 8 patients ranging from 27-32 weeks' gestation with premature labor and normal amniotic fluid volume.

•Fetal bladder volume was obtained sonographically.

•Three classes of prostaglandins-PGE, PGF, and PGI-have been isolated from renal medullary extracts of man and several animal species.

•The preponderance of evidence suggests that class E PGs antagonize the peripheral action of ADH by blocking its stimulation of cyclic adenosine monophosphate.

•Prostaglandins may also directly influence ADH release by a central effect.

•Inhibitors of PG synthesis may potentiate the effects of ADH.

   °The increase in ADH levels after PG synthesis inhibition is a cause of decreased urine output.

•Results: Urine production declines markedly during maternal indomethacin therapy.

   °The decline in fetal urine output was observed as early as five hours after initiation of indomethacin therapy.

•There was no correlation between maternal serum indomethacin levels and fetal urine output.]

---

56. Of potential use in limiting cell damage after hypoxia in the asphyxiated infant

   1.   xanthine oxidase inhibitors
   2.   free radical scavengers
   3.   adenine deaminase inhibitors
   4.   100% oxygen

---

p.765   (Pietz J, Guttenberg N, and Gluck L, "Hypoxanthine: A marker for asphyxia" Obstet Gynecol 1988;72:762)

---

56. [F & I:•Background: Perinatal asphyia is a major cause of neonatal mortality and morbidity,but is poorly defined.

•A specific biochemical indication of the degree of asphyxia is needed.

•Concentrations of lactate and base deficit in blood are elevated in conditions other than hypoxia, and oxygen levels in blood are to transient to provide reliable information about prolonged asphyxia.

•The blood concentration of hypoxanthine may be a measure of hypoxia.

•Hypoxanthine is a metabolic product of the energy-rich phosphorylated nucleotide adenosine triphospate.

•Hypoxia is associated with accelerated catabolism of adenosine monophosphate (AMP) to hypoxanthine, a major way in which cells restore their intra-cellular energy charge.

•The salvage of hypoxanthine to inosine monophosphate is blocked because the formation of phosphoribosylpyrophosphate is dependent on the presence of ATP.

•Furthermore, the catabolism of hypoxanthine to uric acid is inhibited during hypoxia because xanthine oxidase is an oxygen-dependent enzyme.

•These three factors thus combine to cause accumulation oh hypoxanthine during hypoxia.

•Objective: to compare serum hypoxanthine levels in asphyxiated and nonasphyxiated newborns.

•Material and methods: Forty-two newborns.

•Results: The levels of hypoxanthine were significantly higher among asphyxiated newborns than among non-asphyxiated ones.

•Asphyxiated infants have a significantly higher serum hypoxanthine level than non-asphyxiated controls.

•Tissues exposed to high levels of hypoxanthine and oxygen are severely damaged.

•Tissue damage can be limited after hypoxia by inhibiting the conversion of hypoxanthine by xanthine oxidase has been successful.

•The finding that hypoxanthine accumulates during hypoxia coupled with the knowledge that hypoxanthine's conversion to uric acid causes tissue damage after oxygen is resupplied suggests current methods of resusitation should be re-evaluated.]

---

57. Associated with exencephaly

1. amniotic band syndrome
2. anencephaly
3. encephalocele
4. omphalocele

---

p.899   Ans: E   (Henricks SK, Cyr DR, Nyberg DA, Raabe R, and Mack LA, "Exencephaly-Clinical and ultrasonic correlation to anencephaly," Obstet Gynec 1988; 72:898)

57. [Facts and Issues:•Background: Exencephaly is defined as acrania with a large amount of brain tissue present.

°It may be an embryologic precursor of anencephaly, an anomaly incompatible with neonatal life

•Sonographically, exencephaly may resemble other nonfatal cranial malformations such as encephalocele.

•Exencephaly is an uncommon malformation of the fetal cranium.

°It is differentiated pathologically from anencephaly by increased massive residual brain tissue but clinically both conditions are incompatible with life.

•The abnormal central nervous system development seen in anencephaly and exencephaly may be from failure of the neural tubes to close, rupture of the brain stem caused by excessive accumulation of neural tube fluid, and failure of junction of the intrinsic primitive blood vessels.

•All theories conclude that exencephaly is an embryologic precursor to anencephaly.

•The final common pathway for these theories would be the failure of closure of the telencephalic, diencephalic, and mesencephalic regions of the neural plate.

•Pathologically, the exencephalic brain is convered by a highly vascular layer of epithelium.

°Two relatively equivalent cerebral hemispheric remnants are present, with a reddish mass of disorganized tissues, remnants of deep cerebral neural elements, blood vessels, fibrous tissues, and fluid filled spaces.

°This is called the *anencephalic area cerebrovasculosa.*

°Gyri and sulci are shallow, flattened, and disorganized with the rare appearance of normal midline strucutres.

•Central nervous tissue is dysplastic with little or no neuronal differentiation.

°Very little normal cortex is present and the subarachnoid area is obliterated.

•The sonographic appearance of exencephaly is representative of pathologic correlates.

°The most striking sonographic finding is the large amount of disorganized cerebral tissue arising from the base of the cranium.

•Identification of the fetal brain without the surrounding calvarium raise the possibility of exencephaly.

°Differentiation from massive encephalocele may be difficult but careful examination of the skull should allow this distinction.

°Concurrent anomalies consistent with amniotic band syndrome may aid the diagnosis.]

58. Oxytocinase

1. increases the permneability of the distal and collecting tubules of the kidney.
2. is produced by the syncytiotrophoblast.
3. levels are decreased in patients who are destined to develop pregnancy-induced hypertension.
4. production is induced by oxytocin.

p.851　Ans: E　(Wood PL and Durham BH, "Change in plasma cystyl aminopeptidase (oxytocinase) between 30-34 weeks' gestation as a predictor of pregnancy-induced hypertension," Obstet Gynec　1988; 72:850)

58. [Facts and Issues:•Background: Cystyl aminopeptidase (oxytocinase; vasopressinase; aminoacyl-peptide hydralase EC 3.4.11.3) is a placental enzyme that degrades cystine peptides such as oxytocin and vasopressin.

•Synthesis may be induced by oxytocin itself.

°Serum activity levels increase as normal pregnancy progresses and then decrease slowly after delivery.

•Objective: to measure the enzyme levels propectively in normal women with uncomplicated pregnancies throughout the second and third trimester.

•Vasopressin is secreted alongside oxytocin from the posterior pituitary as a result of the effect on the hypothalamus of a change in tissue fluid osmotic pressure.

°It increases the permeability of the distal and collecting tubules of the kidneys, altering the tonicity of the urine.

•Oxytocinase has a broad specificity, and inactivates vasopressin and oxytocin at the same rate.

•Results: There are higher levels of the enzyme in women developing hypertension in pregnancy.

•The rate of gain of body water in women who developed preeclampsia was within the limits for normal pregnancy until thirty weeks.

°The gain beyond thirty weeks was more rapid than in normal pregnant women who had generalized edema.

•There is a significantly lower rise in cystyl aminopeptidase levels from 30 weeks in women who later develop hypertension.

•The differences between normal and hypertension groups between 30-34 weeks may indicate a comparatively decreased breakdown of vasopressin by cystyl aminopeptidasein the hypertensive groups.]

59. Administration of nifedipine to a hypertensive pregnant patient results in

1. decreased total peripheral resistance
2. increase in cardiac output
3. increased perfusion of uterus
4. decreased placental blood flow

p.1444   Ans: A   (Ahokas RA, Sibai BM, Mabie WC, and Anderson GD, "Nifedipine does not adversely affect uteroplacental blood flow in the hypertensive term-pregnant rat" Am J Obstet Gynecol 1988;159:1440)

59. [F&I:•Background: Very high blood pressure directly damages small arteries and arterioles and experimental evidence suggests that this damage occurs within ten minutes after a short term rise ≥150 mm Hg mean blood pressure.

•Severe chronic essential hypertension during pregnancy is associated with the risk of convulsions, fatal cerebral hemorrhage, left ventricular failure, renal inpairment and disseminated intravascular coagulation.

•Nifedipine, a dihydropyridine calcium channel blocker, is a particularly effective antihypertensive agent with extremely low toxicity and teratogenicity.

°It causes vasodilation by interfering with the excitation-contraction coupling of vascular smooth muscle by blocking the entrance of ionized calcium through slow channels in the plasma membrane into the cell.

°It induces a prompt consistent and predictable pressure reduction in patients with severe primary hypertension by diminishing peripheral vascular resistance with a rise in cardiac output and pulse rate.

°Nifedipine effectively suppresses uterine smooth muscle like activity arresting preterm labor.

•Objective: to investigate the short-term effects of nifedipine on maternal hemodynamics and the utero-placental circulation in hypertensive term-pregnant spontaneously hypertensive laboratory animals.

•Result: Nifedipine significantly alters maternal hemodynamics in the hypertensive term pregnant spontaneously hypertensive rat.

°It lowered blood pressure by decreasing total peripheral resistance which was accompanied by a significant increase in cardiac output.

°Heart rate was not significantly affected so the increase in cardiac output must have been caused by increased stroke volume.

°A reduction in total peripheral resistance was from a generalized decrease in the vascular resistance of all regions of the body with the exception of the skin which remained unchanged.

•Nifedipine induces significant increase in perfusion of reproductive organs.

°The increase in blood flow was the result of increased blood flow to the uterine wall (endometrium/myometrium) and the ovaries because of large decreases in the vascular resistances.

•Nifedipine reduced uterine placental resistance which confirms the fact that the uterine placental vasculature is not maximally dilated in the hypertensive pregnant spontaneously hypertensive rat.

°If the uteroplacental vasculature in a normotensive animal is already near maximally dilated, reduction in blood pressure induced by nifedipine would be expected to cause a fall in uterine perfusion.

•Conclusion: Lowering the maternal blood pressure with nifedipine does not appear to place the fetus at under risk of hypoxemia and acidemia caused by reduction in placental perfusion.

°However, the direct effects of nifedipine used long term cannot be ascertained.]

INDEX